Learning
Medical
Terminology

Learning Medical Terminology

A Worktext

Miriam G. Austrin, B.A., R.N.

Consultant in Allied Health Careers and Medical Office Management
Former Coordinator-Director, Medical Assistant Program
St. Louis Community College
St. Louis, Missouri

Harvey R. Austrin, Ph.D.

Diplomate in Clinical Psychology
American Board of Professional Psychology
Emeritus Professor of Psychology
Saint Louis University
St. Louis, Missouri

ninth edition

with 173 *illustrations*

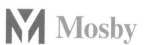 Mosby

An Affiliate of Elsevier

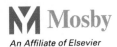
An Affiliate of Elsevier

Publisher: Don Ladig
Executive Editor: Jeanne Rowland
Senior Developmental Editor: Carolyn Kruse
Project Manager: Linda McKinley
Production Editor: Rich Barber
Designer: Liz Young
Manufacturing Manager: Debbie Larocca

ninth edition

Printed in China
Composition, editing, and production by Top Graphics

Mosby, Inc.
11830 Westline Industrial Drive
St. Louis, Missouri 63146

International Standard Book Number 0-323-00279-X

04 05 06 07 08 / 9 8 7 6 5 4 3

In Loving Memory of Our Parents

Benjamin and Bertha Gottschalk

and

Benjamin and Rose Austrin

Preface

Organization

In this ninth edition of *Learning Medical Terminology* we have maintained the basic structure that has been so popular in previous editions. Section I, The Basic Foundation of Medical Terminology, is composed of four chapters that introduce the basics of medical language. These chapters present the word parts used to build medical terms in easily read chart form. This section may be used as the basis for a short course in medical terminology, with the additional sections serving as enrichment resources, or for independent study. The concentration of foundational material within the first four chapters allows for flexibility in how the subsequent chapters are used, according to the instructor's convenience and the student's area of interest.

We have retained the extensive lists of prefixes, suffixes, roots, and combining forms that students and instructors have found particularly helpful. The arrangement of the roots and their combining forms into categories (external and internal anatomy) and groupings (verbs and adjectives, body fluids, substances, chemicals, and colors) is another feature that helps the learner organize information.

Sections II, III, and IV—The Body Shell and Its Supports, The Internal Mechanisms of the Body, and The Adaptive and Defense Mechanisms of the Body—use the systems approach, connecting medical language directly to the anatomy of each body system. Each chapter starts with an interesting fact relating to the system described. New questions have been added to the reviews and exercises throughout the text. Content has been rearranged within selected chapters, and substantial revisions have been made to reflect current knowledge.

Six appendixes provide supplemental information on abbreviations and symbols, Latin and Greek combining forms for English numbers, the metric system and equivalents, hospital records and reports, medical insurance, and medical specialties.

Study Aids

- To assist the student in retaining the chapter contents, over 1550 review and exercise questions (with answers) are incorporated throughout the text.
- To further reinforce and add enjoyment to the learning process, we have included a crossword puzzle and a hidden words puzzle for Chapters 1 through 17.
- There are 16 full-color anatomic plates at the front of the book, in addition to over 150 illustrations within the chapters.
- As in previous editions, we have integrated review sections with subject presentation so that material is presented in manageable units. This feature also allows students to rehearse information before they complete the chapter exercises.

New to This Edition

- In this edition, in response to user suggestions, we have separated the genitourinary system into two chapters, The Urinary System and The Reproductive System, for a more consistent length of chapters.
- Also as requested by users, the answers to Review Questions, Exercises, and Puzzles have been moved to the back of the text, and the pages have been perforated so that they can be removed for programs that use the exercises for homework and tests.

- Related Terms lists (previously called Glossaries) have been revised, with new entries and deletions of obsolete material. These lists, with phonetic pronunciation, contain additional medical terms, designed to capture student interest, help them to enjoy the learning process, and reinforce their understanding of the text. Related Terms are grouped as descriptions of anatomic parts, diseases and disorders, surgical procedures, and laboratory tests, and they reflect current knowledge.
- A new design highlights tables, the Review and Exercises sections, and the Related Terms lists for easy navigation.

Ancillaries

For the student
- An *audiotape* of the material covered in Chapters 1 through 4 helps in learning to pronounce medical terms.

For the instructor
- An *instructor's manual* contains tips on teaching, including setting up courses of different lengths ranging from a 3-month course to a two-semester one. Medical historical background and folklore are included as well, plus a chapter-by-chapter test bank of about 1000 questions.
- A *computerized test bank* contains questions in electronic form to facilitate construction of tests and examinations.

Application

Learning Medical Terminology lends itself to classroom use, with interval checks in Review sections and chapter comprehension in Exercises. However, this text is also designed so that a motivated student can use it as a self-teaching instrument, with little or no supervision. The "Austrin approach"—building a strong foundation in medical terminology—is flexible enough to accommodate both classroom and independent formats.

Whatever method you choose, we hope that your study of medical terminology will be an interesting and rewarding start to your career as a health care professional.

ACKNOWLEDGMENTS

We gratefully acknowledge Diane A. Klein, M.S., B.M.E., M.P.H., a specialist in Public Health and Wellness, and Michael S. Austrin, M.A., a professional in strategic health planning, managed care, and insurance issues, as contributing authors in the areas of medical insurance, managed care, and health maintenance programs.

We are indebted to cartoonist Mike Peters and Tribune Media Services, Inc., for allowing us to use strips from "Mother Goose and Grimm" relating (in their own unique way) to medical terminology. We also give special thanks to Mike Royal, R.Ph., of the Washington University/St. Louis AIDS Medical Trials Unit, and to Kathy Mullen, M.L.S., of the St. Louis College of Pharmacy Library, for their assistance in clarifying fine points in the treatment of AIDS.

Our very special thanks are offered to Jeanne Rowland, Carolyn Kruse, and Tamara Myers for their many helpful suggestions and hand-holding, and our appreciation goes to the entire production team. Last, but by no means least, we would like to recognize the contributions made by the instructors and students who generously provided us with constructive criticism and suggestions.

Miriam G. Austrin
Harvey R. Austrin

Contents

section III

The Internal Mechanisms of the Body

Color Plates

ANTERIOR VIEW OF SKELETON

Axial skeleton is shown in blue. Appendicular system is
bone colored.

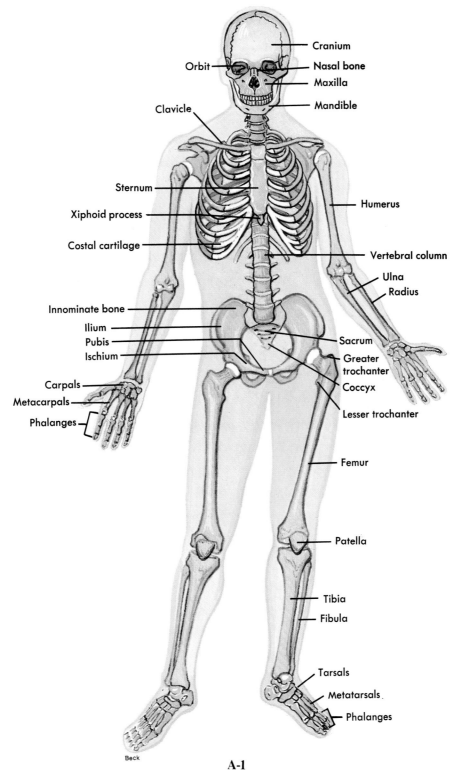

Cranium

Orbit

Nasal bone

Maxilla

Mandible

Clavicle

Sternum

Humerus

Xiphoid process

Costal cartilage

Vertebral column

Ulna

Radius

Innominate bone

Ilium

Pubis

Sacrum

Ischium

Greater
trochanter

Carpals

Coccyx

Metacarpals

Lesser trochanter

Phalanges

Femur

Patella

Tibia

Fibula

Tarsals

Metatarsals

Phalanges

Beck

POSTERIOR VIEW OF SKELETON
Axial skeleton is shown in blue. Appendicular system is
bone colored.

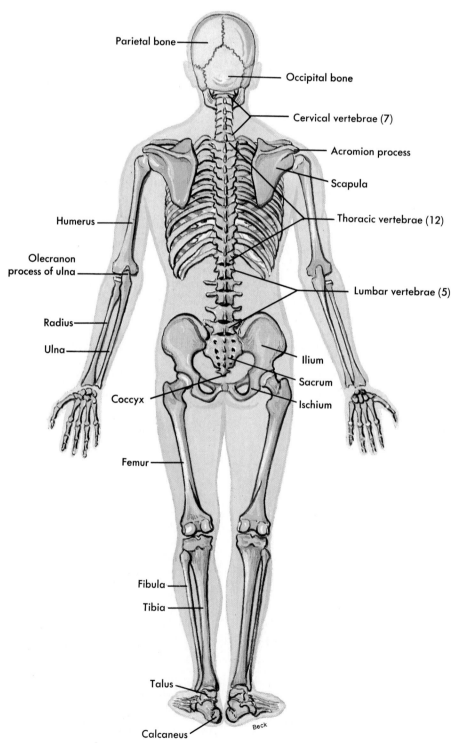

Parietal bone

Occipital bone

Cervical vertebrae (7)

Acromion process

Scapula

Humerus

Thoracic vertebrae (12)

Olecranon
process of ulna

Lumbar vertebrae (5)

Radius

Ulna

Ilium

Sacrum

Coccyx

Ischium

Femur

Fibula

Tibia

Talus

Calcaneus

Beck

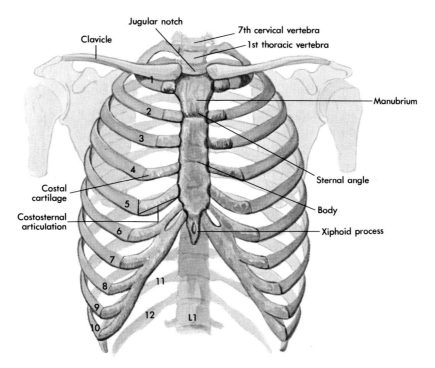

THORAX AND RIBS

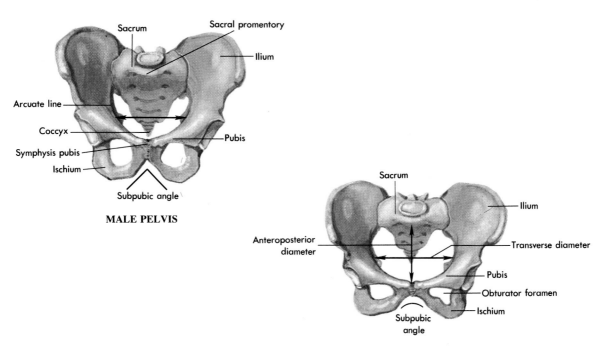

MALE PELVIS

FEMALE PELVIS

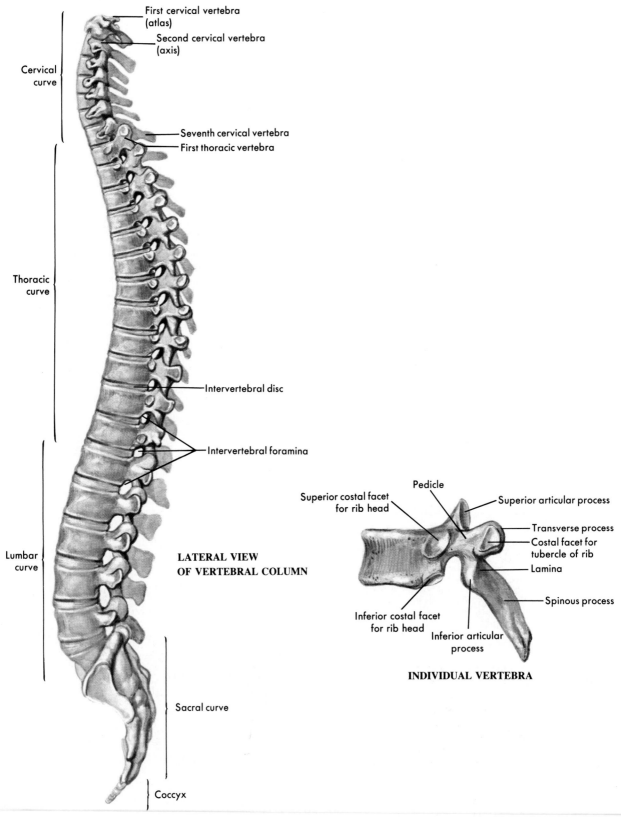

First cervical vertebra (atlas)

Second cervical vertebra (axis)

Cervical curve

Seventh cervical vertebra

First thoracic vertebra

Thoracic curve

Intervertebral disc

Intervertebral foramina

Lumbar curve

**LATERAL VIEW
OF VERTEBRAL COLUMN**

Sacral curve

Coccyx

Pedicle

Superior costal facet for rib head

Superior articular process

Transverse process

Costal facet for tubercle of rib

Lamina

Spinous process

Inferior costal facet for rib head

Inferior articular process

INDIVIDUAL VERTEBRA

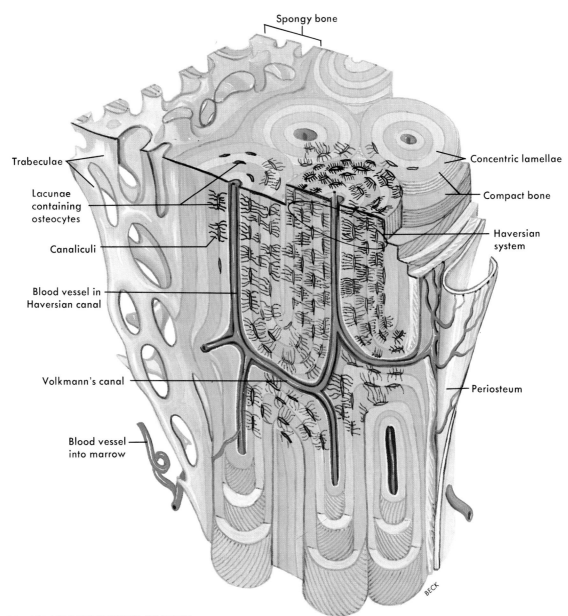

Spongy bone

Trabeculae

Lacunae
containing
osteocytes

Canaliculi

Blood vessel in
Haversian canal

Volkmann's canal

Blood vessel
into marrow

Concentric lamellae

Compact bone

Haversian
system

Periosteum

BECK

MICROSCOPIC STRUCTURE OF BONE
Haversian systems, several of which are shown here,
compose compact bone. Note the structures that make
up one haversian system: concentric lamellae, lacunae,
canaliculi, and a haversian canal. Shown bordering the
compact bone on the left is spongy bone, a name
descriptive of the many open spaces that characterize
it.

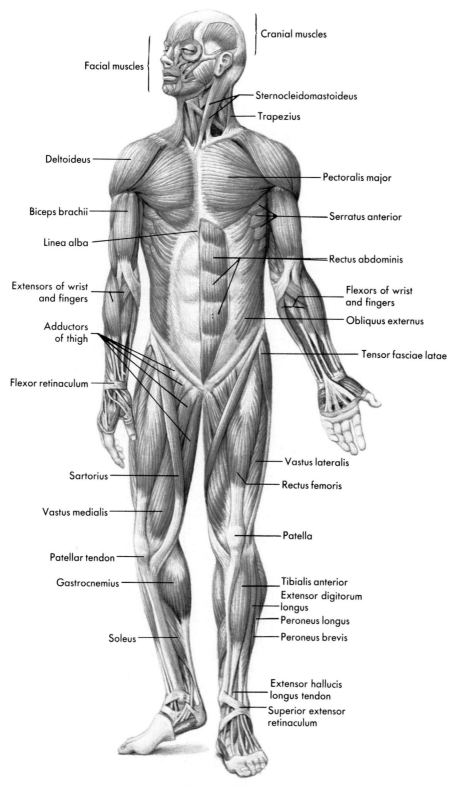

Cranial muscles

Facial muscles

Sternocleidomastoideus

Trapezius

Deltoideus

Pectoralis major

Biceps brachii

Serratus anterior

Linea alba

Rectus abdominis

Extensors of wrist and fingers

Flexors of wrist and fingers

Adductors of thigh

Obliquus externus

Flexor retinaculum

Tensor fasciae latae

Vastus lateralis

Sartorius

Rectus femoris

Vastus medialis

Patella

Patellar tendon

Tibialis anterior

Gastrocnemius

Extensor digitorum longus

Peroneus longus

Peroneus brevis

Soleus

Extensor hallucis longus tendon

Superior extensor retinaculum

ANTERIOR VIEW

A-6

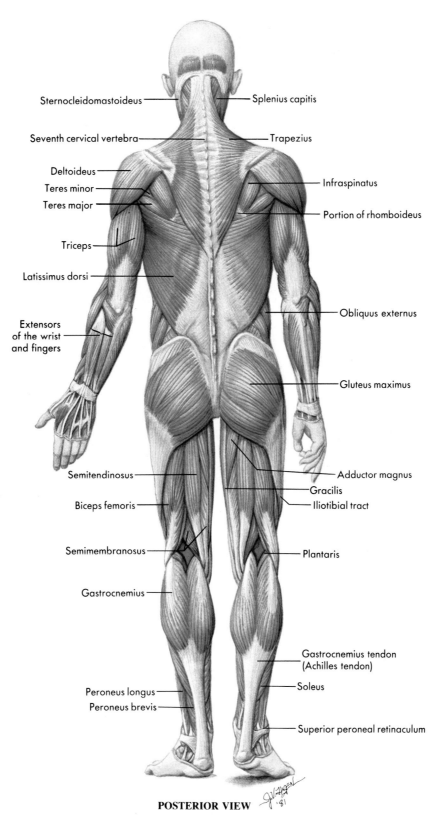

Sternocleidomastoideus

Splenius capitis

Seventh cervical vertebra

Trapezius

Deltoideus

Teres minor

Teres major

Infraspinatus

Portion of rhomboideus

Triceps

Latissimus dorsi

Extensors
of the wrist
and fingers

Obliquus externus

Gluteus maximus

Semitendinosus

Adductor magnus

Gracilis

Iliotibial tract

Biceps femoris

Semimembranosus

Plantaris

Gastrocnemius

Gastrocnemius tendon
(Achilles tendon)

Soleus

Peroneus longus

Peroneus brevis

Superior peroneal retinaculum

POSTERIOR VIEW

A-7

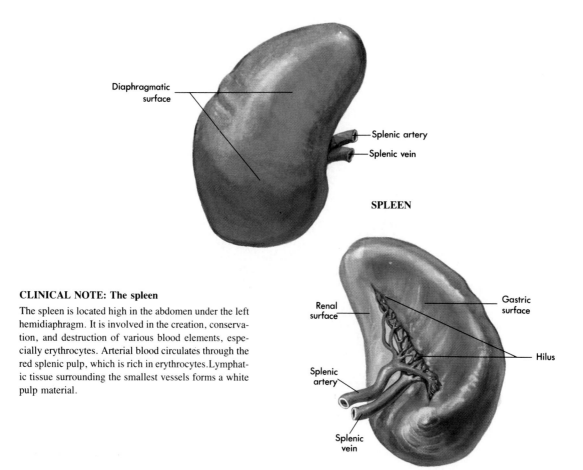

Diaphragmatic surface

Splenic artery

Splenic vein

SPLEEN

Renal surface

Gastric surface

Hilus

Splenic artery

Splenic vein

CLINICAL NOTE: The spleen

The spleen is located high in the abdomen under the left hemidiaphragm. It is involved in the creation, conservation, and destruction of various blood elements, especially erythrocytes. Arterial blood circulates through the red splenic pulp, which is rich in erythrocytes. Lymphatic tissue surrounding the smallest vessels forms a white pulp material.

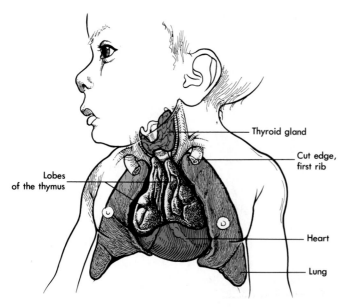

Thyroid gland

Cut edge, first rib

Lobes of the thymus

Heart

Lung

LOCATION AND GROSS ANATOMY OF THYMUS

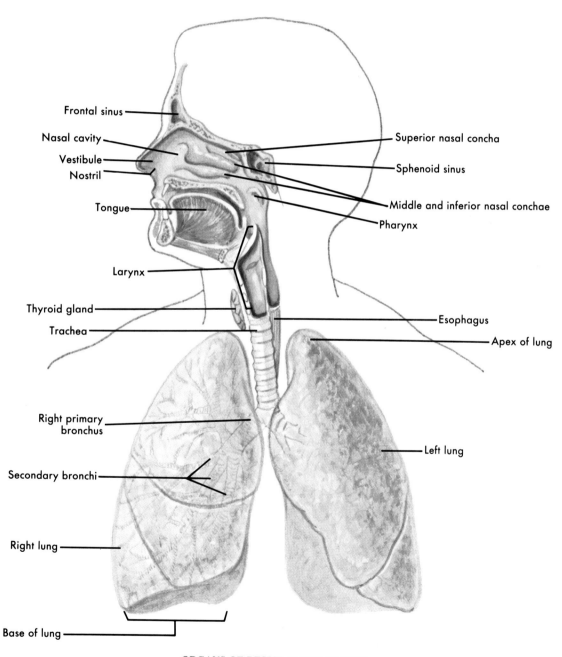

Frontal sinus

Nasal cavity

Vestibule

Nostril

Tongue

Larynx

Thyroid gland

Trachea

Right primary
bronchus

Secondary bronchi

Right lung

Base of lung

Superior nasal concha

Sphenoid sinus

Middle and inferior nasal conchae

Pharynx

Esophagus

Apex of lung

Left lung

**ORGANS OF RESPIRATORY SYSTEM
AND ASSOCIATED STRUCTURES**

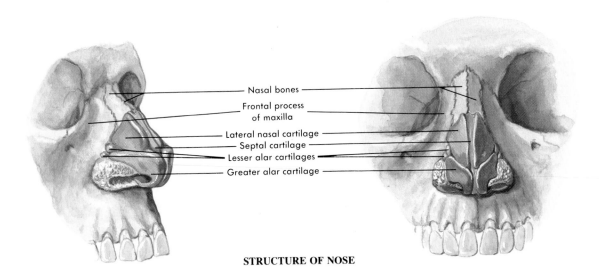

Nasal bones
Frontal process
of maxilla
Lateral nasal cartilage
Septal cartilage
Lesser alar cartilages
Greater alar cartilage

STRUCTURE OF NOSE

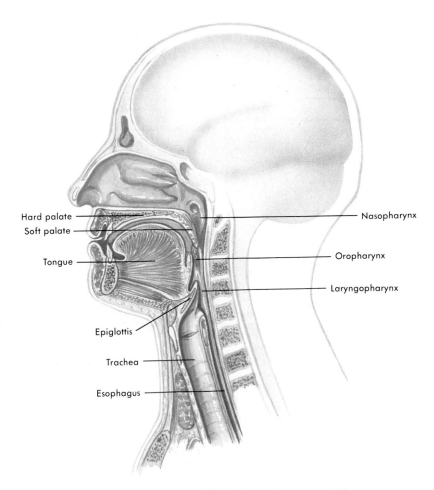

Hard palate
Soft palate
Tongue
Epiglottis
Trachea
Esophagus

Nasopharynx
Oropharynx
Laryngopharynx

STRUCTURES OF NASAL PASSAGES AND THROAT

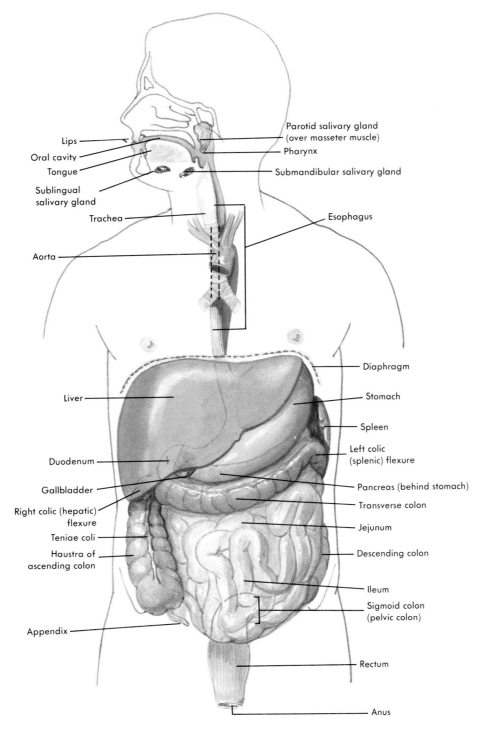

Lips

Oral cavity

Tongue

Sublingual salivary gland

Trachea

Aorta

Parotid salivary gland (over masseter muscle)

Pharynx

Submandibular salivary gland

Esophagus

Liver

Duodenum

Gallbladder

Right colic (hepatic) flexure

Teniae coli

Haustra of ascending colon

Appendix

Diaphragm

Stomach

Spleen

Left colic (splenic) flexure

Pancreas (behind stomach)

Transverse colon

Jejunum

Descending colon

Ileum

Sigmoid colon (pelvic colon)

Rectum

Anus

**ORGANS OF DIGESTIVE SYSTEM AND
SOME ASSOCIATED STRUCTURES**

A-11

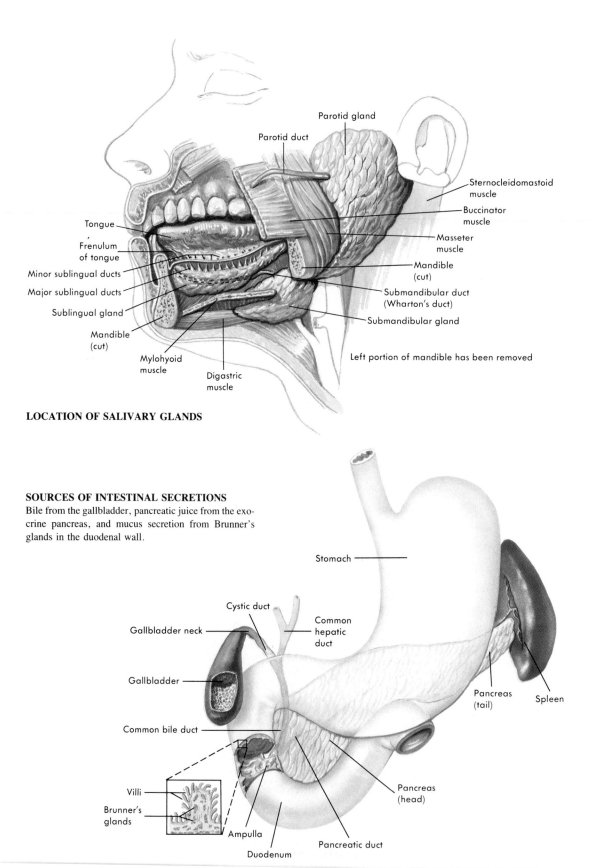

Parotid gland

Parotid duct

Sternocleidomastoid muscle

Buccinator muscle

Tongue

Masseter muscle

Frenulum of tongue

Minor sublingual ducts

Mandible (cut)

Major sublingual ducts

Submandibular duct (Wharton's duct)

Sublingual gland

Submandibular gland

Mandible (cut)

Left portion of mandible has been removed

Mylohyoid muscle

Digastric muscle

LOCATION OF SALIVARY GLANDS

SOURCES OF INTESTINAL SECRETIONS

Bile from the gallbladder, pancreatic juice from the exocrine pancreas, and mucus secretion from Brunner's glands in the duodenal wall.

Stomach

Cystic duct

Common hepatic duct

Gallbladder neck

Gallbladder

Pancreas (tail)

Spleen

Common bile duct

Pancreas (head)

Villi

Brunner's glands

Ampulla

Pancreatic duct

Duodenum

A-12

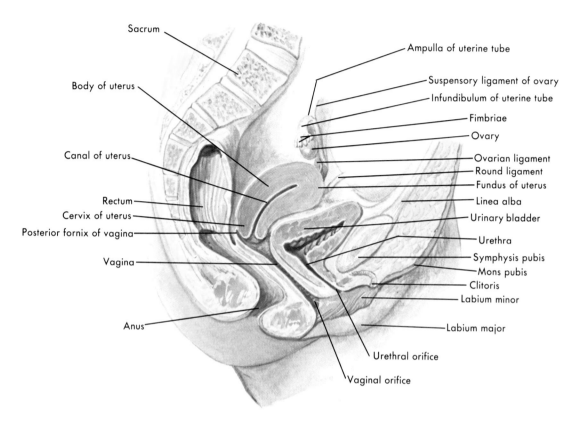

Sacrum

Body of uterus

Canal of uterus

Rectum

Cervix of uterus

Posterior fornix of vagina

Vagina

Anus

Ampulla of uterine tube

Suspensory ligament of ovary

Infundibulum of uterine tube

Fimbriae

Ovary

Ovarian ligament

Round ligament

Fundus of uterus

Linea alba

Urinary bladder

Urethra

Symphysis pubis

Mons pubis

Clitoris

Labium minor

Labium major

Urethral orifice

Vaginal orifice

**FEMALE REPRODUCTIVE ORGANS AND
ASSOCIATED STRUCTURES**

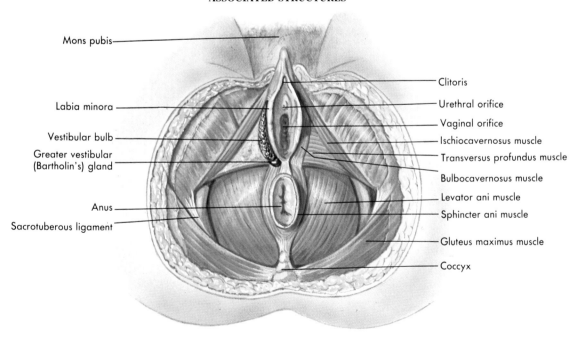

Mons pubis

Labia minora

Vestibular bulb

Greater vestibular
(Bartholin's) gland

Anus

Sacrotuberous ligament

Clitoris

Urethral orifice

Vaginal orifice

Ischiocavernosus muscle

Transversus profundus muscle

Bulbocavernosus muscle

Levator ani muscle

Sphincter ani muscle

Gluteus maximus muscle

Coccyx

FEMALE PERINEUM

A-13

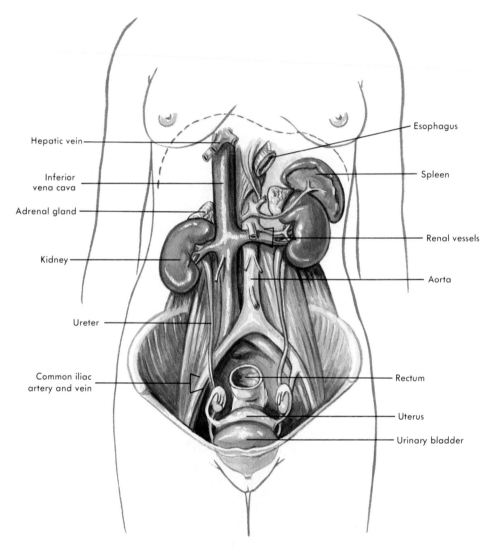

Hepatic vein

Inferior
vena cava

Adrenal gland

Kidney

Ureter

Common iliac
artery and vein

Esophagus

Spleen

Renal vessels

Aorta

Rectum

Uterus

Urinary bladder

URINARY SYSTEM AND SOME ASSOCIATED STRUCTURES

Hearing

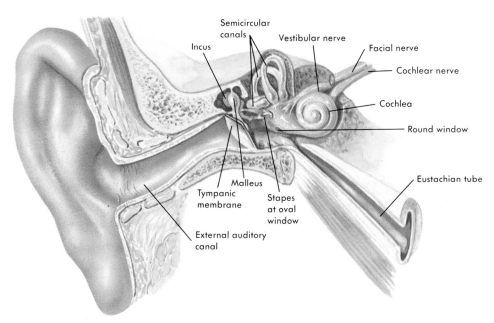

GROSS ANATOMY OF THE EAR IN FRONTAL SECTION

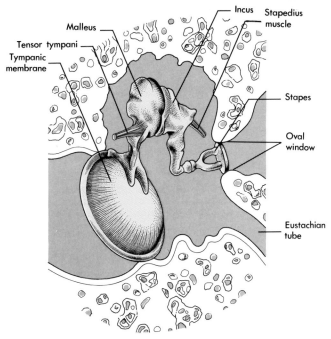

IMPEDENCE-MATCHING COMPONENTS OF INNER EAR

Sight

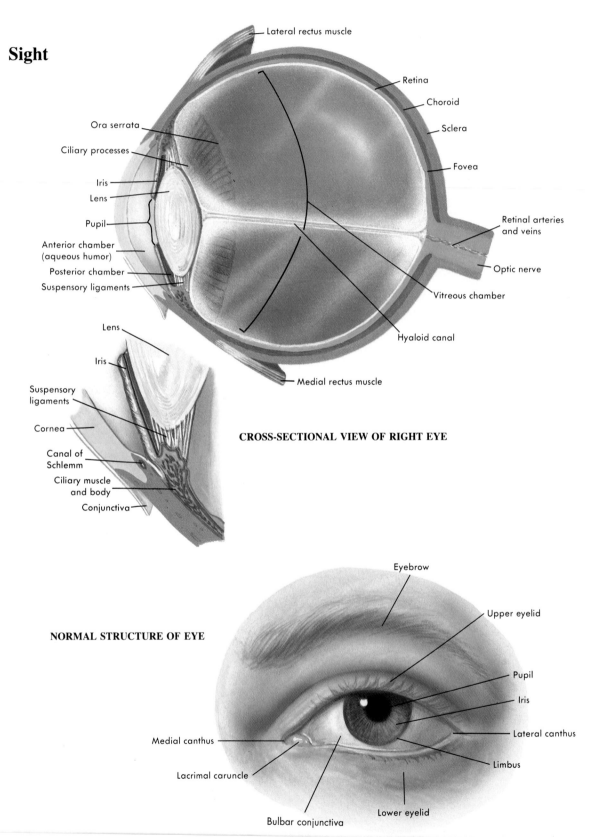

Lateral rectus muscle

Retina

Choroid

Sclera

Fovea

Ora serrata

Ciliary processes

Iris

Lens

Pupil

Retinal arteries
and veins

Anterior chamber
(aqueous humor)

Optic nerve

Posterior chamber

Suspensory ligaments

Vitreous chamber

Hyaloid canal

Medial rectus muscle

Lens

Iris

Suspensory
ligaments

Cornea

CROSS-SECTIONAL VIEW OF RIGHT EYE

Canal of
Schlemm

Ciliary muscle
and body

Conjunctiva

NORMAL STRUCTURE OF EYE

Eyebrow

Upper eyelid

Pupil

Iris

Lateral canthus

Medial canthus

Limbus

Lacrimal caruncle

Bulbar conjunctiva

Lower eyelid

Learning Medical Terminology

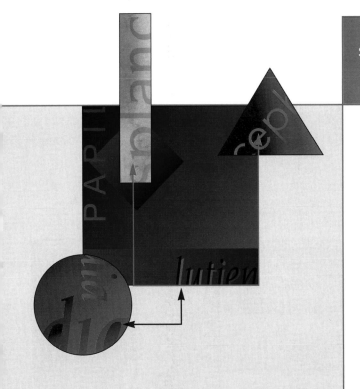

The Basic Foundation of Medical Terminology

This is the first of the five sections of *Learning Medical Terminology*. This section contains four chapters to introduce the student to the basic foundation of medical language.

Chapter 1 is a brief introduction to the separate parts of words, with examples to help the student understand the construction of medical terms.

Chapter 2 presents the initial step in building and learning the vocabulary. The most essential components of the language, prefixes and suffixes, are conveniently arranged in chart form with meanings and examples.

Chapter 3 is the second step in building the vocabulary by the addition of the roots and combining forms that relate to the structures of the body. The chapter is divided into two sections, external and internal anatomy, arranged in chart form, with pronunciations and identification of the specific body parts.

Chapter 4 is the third step in the development of the foundation. It contains descriptive words, roots and combining forms, divided into separate sections. These sections cover actions, conditions, characteristics, body fluids and substances, chemicals, and colors. Each section is presented in chart form with meanings clearly shown.

MOTHER GOOSE & GRIMM / By Mike Peters

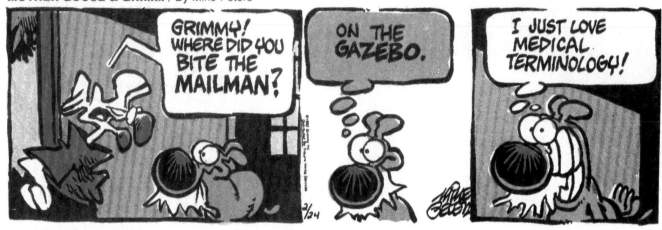

MOTHER GOOSE AND GRIMM / By Mike Peters

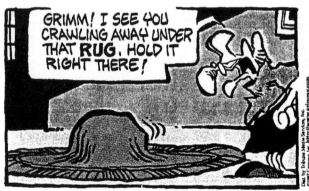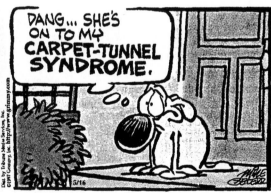

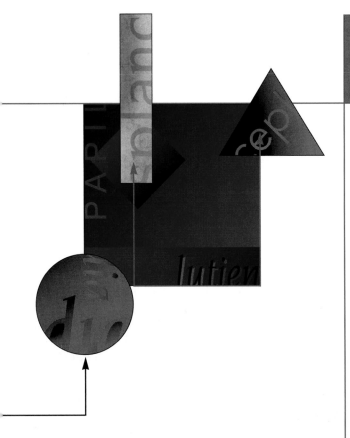

An Introduction to Medical Terminology

This chapter introduces word elements (prefixes, suffixes, and roots and combining forms), their meanings, and ways of combining them to build medical terms. Basic pronunciation rules are presented, with pertinent examples.

OBJECTIVE

The primary objective of this book is to enable you, the student, to learn medical terminology. When first confronted with medical terms, you may be bewildered by their strange spelling and pronunciation. This is understandable when you consider that approximately 75% of these terms are based on either Greek or Latin. New terms are constantly being coined, but most are derivatives of Greek or Latin words. The Greeks were the founders of modern medicine, although Latin has become the universal source of medical language.

When you complete this worktext, you will have a basic, workable vocabulary, applicable to any branch of medicine. You do not need prior knowledge of Greek, Latin, anatomy, or physiology to build a medical vocabulary. The knowledge you do need is presented step by step in this worktext, which will help you to learn, and be comfortable with, medical language.

This is accomplished by:

1. breaking a word apart and identifying its parts (prefix, suffix, and root and combining form).
2. describing the structure and functions of each of the body systems.
3. relating applicable words and their parts to each of the body systems.
4. using illustrations, diagrams, and charts to assist in the learning process.
5. reviewing text material using questions (and answers) throughout and at the end of each chapter.

Most medical terms are a combination of two or more word parts. The identification of a word involves a search for the meaning of each of its parts. When they are translated separately and combined, the parts give the essential meaning of the entire word.

The fundamental method of building a medical vocabulary, as it is outlined in this book, consists of breaking down a word and identifying its parts: prefix, suffix, root or roots, and combining form. A prefix is the beginning part of a word, and a suffix is the end part. A root is the foundation, or basic meaning, of a word and may appear with a prefix, with a suffix, or between a prefix and suffix. Prefixes and suffixes can never stand alone; they must always be attached to a root. For example:

In the word *antisepsis:*

> the **prefix** *anti-* means against;
> the **root** *sepsis* means infection.
> Antisepsis means against infection.

In the word *rhinitis:*

> the **root** *rhin-* means nose;
> the **suffix** *-itis* means inflammation.
> Rhinitis means inflammation of the nose.

A combining form is a root with an added vowel (known as a combining vowel) that connects the root with a suffix or with another root. For example:
In the word *glycohemia:*

> the **root** *glyc-* means sugar or sweet;
> when we add the **combining vowel** *o* to glyc-,
> it becomes the **combining form** *glyco-;*
> the **root** *hem-* means blood;
> the **suffix** *-ia* means state or condition.
> Glycohemia means sugar in the blood.

Some words contain more than one root, each of which retains its basic meaning. These are called compound words and are very common in medicine. *Glycohemia,* just shown, is an example of a compound word. Another example of a compound word is *osteoarthritis.* The combining form *osteo-* comes from the root *oste-,* which means bone; the root *arthr-* means joint or joints; and the suffix *-itis* means inflammation. Therefore, the compound word *osteoarthritis* means inflammation of the bone joints.

SPECIFIC SUGGESTIONS FOR LEARNING MEDICAL TERMINOLOGY

The identification of prefixes, suffixes, and roots of words pertaining to anatomy is the first step in building a medical vocabulary. The next step is to learn to recognize the most common roots referring to conditions, actions, characteristics, body fluids, body substances, chemicals, and colors. This will help you to understand anatomic structures, diseases, procedures, and other descriptive terms by simply breaking each word into its components, defining the components separately, and then combining them to discover the meaning of the word as a whole. If you practice analyzing medical words that you see or hear, you will find, in time, that you are able to define words at a glance, much the same as you would learn a foreign language.

It is possible to memorize some medical words without regard to a breakdown of their components, but you cannot memorize the entire medical dictionary. Although most medical terms can be learned easily from their components, there is no way to use components to analyze those terms that are derived from proper names. Use your medical dictionary when you do not recognize a term that bears a proper name, when you cannot arrive at a definition by analysis, or when the meaning is not clear. This book does not pretend to break down all medical terms into components, but it does give you the key to analysis by listing more than 500 specific roots and combining forms of the type you will find in the majority of medical words. Treat each medical word as if it were a puzzle you were attempting to solve, and you will see how enjoyable and rewarding it will be to define the word without reference to a medical dictionary.

Pronunciation of Medical Terms

Medical terms are hard to pronounce, especially if you have never heard them spoken. Here are some shortcuts you will find helpful:

> *ch* is sometimes pronounced like *k*.
> Examples—chromatin, chronic

ps is pronounced like *s*.
Examples—psychiatry, psychology

pn is pronounced with only the n sound.
Examples—pneumonia, pneusis

c and *g* are given the soft sounds of *s* and *j*, respectively, before *e*, *i*, and *y*.
Examples—generic, giant, cycle, cytoplasm

c and *g* have a hard sound before other letters.
Examples—cast, cardiac, gastric, gonad

ae and *oe* are pronounced *ee*.
Examples—fasciae, coelom

i at the end of a word is pronounced *eye* (to form a plural).
Examples—alveoli, glomeruli, fasciculi

es at the end of a word is often pronounced as a separate syllable.
Examples—stases (stay′seez), nares (nah′reez)

To help in pronunciation, the phonetic spelling of words is used, where necessary, in the glossaries.

Plurals

The plural of most English words is formed by adding *s* or *es*, but in medical terms the plural may be formed by changing the ending. Some common medical plurals include **ae** or **ata** for the singular **a**, **a** for the singular **um**, **i** for the singular **us**, and **es** for the singular **is**. Some examples are:

ae, as in fasciae (singular—*fascia*)
ata, as in adenomata (singular—*adenoma*)
a, as in crania (singular—*cranium*)
i, as in glomeruli (singular—*glomerulus*)
es, as in pelves (singular—*pelvis*)

Spelling

Rules for pronunciation and the formation of plurals are essential for spelling, but it is very important that you consult a medical dictionary if you are not sure. Phonetic spelling has no place in medicine. Some terms sound alike but are spelled differently. For example, the *ileum* is a part of the intestinal tract, but the *ilium* is a pelvic bone. A misspelled word may lead to the wrong meaning, creating confusion and possibly an incorrect diagnosis.

▲ EXERCISES   AN INTRODUCTION TO MEDICAL TERMINOLOGY

Exercise 1.1   *List the four principal parts of a medical word.*

1. _____   3. _____

2. _____   4. _____

Exercise 1.2   *Identify the place and/or purpose of the four parts listed in Exercise 1.1.*

1. _____

2. _____

3. _____

4. _____

Exercise 1.3   *Matching*

_____ **1.** -ia   **A.** inflammation
_____ **2.** anti-   **B.** nose
_____ **3.** -itis   **C.** blood
_____ **4.** -sepsis   **D.** joint
_____ **5.** rhin-   **E.** bone
_____ **6.** glyc-   **F.** against
_____ **7.** oste-   **G.** infection
_____ **8.** hem-   **H.** state or condition
_____ **9.** arthr-   **I.** sugar

Exercise 1.4   *For the following statements, indicate T for true or F for false in the space provided.*

_____ **1.** *Ps* and *pn* are pronounced with a silent *p*.
_____ **2.** Phonetic spelling is acceptable in medical language.
_____ **3.** The medical dictionary is an unimportant tool.
_____ **4.** The letters c and *g* always have a hard sound.
_____ **5.** Like English, the plurals of medical terms always end in *s* or *es*.

CROSSWORD PUZZLE   CHAPTER 1

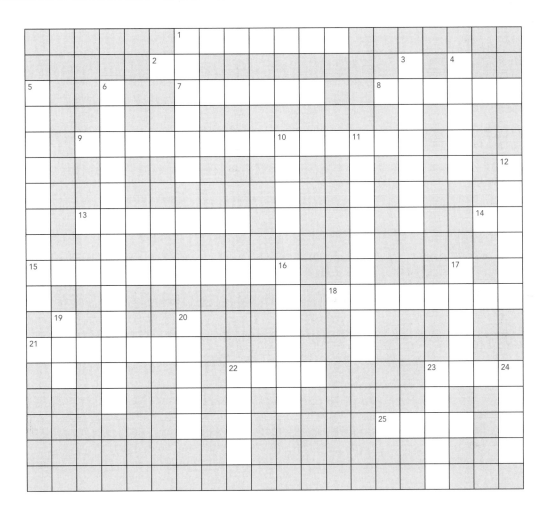

ACROSS

1. Many roots relate to the _____ of the body

2. The plural suffix of fascia

7. Beginning word part

8. Founders of modern medicine

9. A word part

13. Science related to the study of the parts of the body

14. A suffix meaning state or condition

15. Words that come from proper names or other words

18. A type of visual aid to assist in learning

21. Type of dictionary

22. A root meaning nose

23. A prefix meaning against

25. Means bone

DOWN

1. Infection

3. First

4. Opposite of teach

5. Words with more than one root

6. Phonetic sounding out of a word

10. Means sugar or sweet

11. Learning medical terminology is the _____ of this text

12. Additional visual aids to assist in learning

16. Ending word part

17. Source of medical language

19. Means blood

20. Part of intestinal tract that sounds like a pelvic bone

22. A foundation word part

23. A root meaning joint

24. Inflammation

HIDDEN WORDS PUZZLE

Can you find the 20 words hidden in this puzzle? All hidden words puzzles have words running from top to bottom, left to right, and diagonally downward.

CHARACTERISTICS

CONDITIONS

VOCABULARY

PHONETIC

ANALYZE

PRONUNCIATION

FOUNDATION

DIAGNOSIS

SINGULAR

MEDICAL

TERMINOLOGY

PHYSIOLOGY

DIAGRAMS

SPELLING

COLORS

COMPONENTS

SUBSTANCES

LANGUAGE

ACTIONS

DEFINE

```
W P V F C R P B M J E Q A X T E J B T H B F W
D W O K J O E E K X W U C I X Y N O I O Q P E
Q F A W S I L B E C X G T N B Y O S N M G Z W
M H R S Y M T O P J N V I D N Q R B M T R F Q
E O N E P P L W R H L L O E A S P U X V W G Z
D I A G R A M S Q S O A N S L N A V P V U I R
I F G C O N D I T I O N S E B R P A D T I Y X
C T K V N D Q P V N U G E P F M U I H G Q P K
A E E I U Q Y V O G N U P T E F W P J A I X B
L L S S N O K Q T U O A L W I L L O L X M H C
D T W C C O H D D L Q G R Z N C L O Q G S L U
S O C U I H C K A A U E P A E S F I Q J X F C
V G D R A F A O F R Q G K A D L E A N O F E J
M N X X T E R M I N O L O G Y N P R G J S U
N L Q O I B Y F A P U V I D E O W N F D F P X
E V Y N O Q A T J C O X B G I X N T I N Y R A
L V U T N W N X C B T N V Q Z K S L V M V A I
U E W S X X D L H O R E E V D K L I C H E O P
H R I L V H A C X F X N R N F I W T M A K M X
D Y J V E Z I F Q D C O H I T H A N A L Y Z E
N H G J W W S J W E F S Z A S S P G D F O T M
V B N X N C G M B F O U N D A T I O N X P B R
M D E M W S E I E I Q B P H Y S I O L O G Y L
T F M C J Y U S E N W S M M L P X C M T S Z Y
G H F G R E H D B E K T T G I W Q W S U N I Q
G W Y O E F C D V O C A B U L A R Y X X H T S
L G Q X S L I M J Q N N O N M J G C K G Y X Q
G B U G A B X M S D K C G H A I C Z K S E E Y
G P G W I C Y K Q Q B E E R U T U U V B B A K
T W U I F Y M T W J E S I N M X Y I I D N L V
```

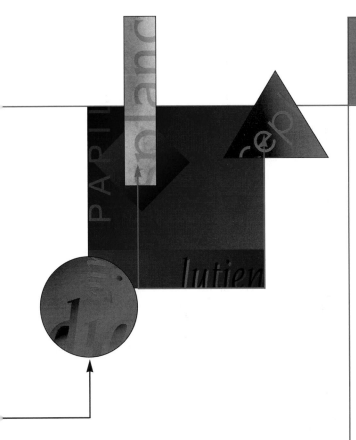

Building a Medical Vocabulary

In this chapter the student becomes familiar with prefixes (the beginnings of words) and suffixes (the endings of words), by means of definitions and word examples. These word parts are listed alphabetically in chart form to enhance learning.

STEP 1: PREFIXES AND SUFFIXES

This chapter and the next two chapters present the basic building blocks of a medical vocabulary. Your ability to break down medical terms into their separate parts or to recognize a complete word, depends on your learning of the roots and combining forms that appear in medical terms and the prefixes and suffixes that alter or modify the meaning and usage of a term.

By learning the meanings of the word parts given in these chapters, you will find that you can define most of the medical words in subsequent chapters. The meanings of the word parts presented in these chapters will generally *not* be repeated; however, these chapters can be used for reference whenever you do not recognize the meaning of a word part.

Prefixes

A prefix consists of one or more syllables placed at the beginning of a word. A prefix never stands alone. It is placed in front of a verb, adjective, or noun to modify its meaning. Most prefixes are parts of words in ordinary language and do not specifically refer to medical terminology. However, many prefixes do occur frequently in medical language, and studying them is an important first step in learning medical terms. The principal prefixes used in medical terminology are given in Table 2-1.

TABLE 2.1 PREFIXES

Prefix	Meaning	Examples
a-, an-	without, lack of, not	Aphasia (without speech) Anemia (lack of blood)
ab-	away from	Abductor (leading away from) Aboral (away from mouth)
ad-	toward, to, near	Adductor (leading toward) Adrenal (near the kidney)
ambi-	both	Ambidextrous (ability to use both hands equally)
amphi-	on both sides, double	Amphibious (living on land or in water) Amphithymia (dual mental state of depression and elation)
ampho-	both	Amphogenic (producing young of both sexes)
ana-	up, toward, apart	Anatomy (to cut apart) Anacatharsis (vomiting up)
ante-	before, in front of, forward	Antecubital (before elbow) Anteflex (to bend forward)
anti-	against, opposing	Antisepsis (against infection) Anticarious (against cavities)
ap-, apo-	separation from, derived from	Apobiosis (death of a part) Apophysis (outgrowth of bone)
aut-, auto-	self	Autoanalysis (self-analysis) Autoerotism (sexual self-love)
bi-	two, double, twice	Bifocal (two foci) Biarticulate (double joint)
cata-	down, under, lower, against	Catabolism (breaking down) Catalepsy (reduced movement)
circum-	around	Circumflex (winding around) Circumarticular (around joint)

TABLE 2.1 PREFIXES—cont'd

Prefix	Meaning	Examples
co-,* com-,† con-	with, together	Commissure (coming together) Conductor (leading together)
contra-	opposed, against	Contralateral (opposite side) Contraception (prevention of conception)
de-	down, from	Dehydrate (remove water from) Decay (break down)
di-	two, twice	Dicephalous (having two heads) Dichromic (having two colors)
dia-	between, through, apart, across, completely	Diapedesis (ooze through) Diaphragm (wall across) Diagnosis (complete knowledge)
dis-	apart, free from	Disinfection (infection) Dissect (cut apart) Disarticulation (separation at a joint)
dys-	difficult, bad, painful	Dyskinesis (difficult motion) Dyspepsia (bad digestion) Dyspareunia (painful coitus)
e-, ec-, ex-	out of, from, away from	Enucleate (remove whole from) Ectopic (out of place) Exostosis (outgrowth of bone)
ect, ecto-, exo-	outer, outside, situated on	Ectal (on the suface) Ectoderm (outer skin) Ectocytic (outside of cell) Exogenic (originating outside)
em-,‡ en-	in	Empyema (pus in) Encranial (in the cranium)
end-, endo-, ent-, ento-	within, inner	Endaural (within the ear) Endocranial (within cranium) Entiris (inner eye color) Entocele (internal hernia)
ep-, epi-	upon, on, over	Epicostal (upon a rib) Epidermis (outer skin layer) Eponychia (infection over the nail bed)
eu-	normal, good, well, healthy	Eucrasia (normal health) Euplastic (healing well)

*co- before a vowel.
†com- before b, m, and p.
‡em- before b, m, and p.

Continued

TABLE 2.1 PREFIXES—*cont'd*

Prefix	Meaning	Examples
extra-, extro-	*outside of, beyond, outward*	Extraoral (outside of mouth) Extroversion (turning inside out)
hemi-	*half*	Hemiepilepsy (epilepsy on one side of body) Hemilingual (half of tongue)
hyper-	*excessive, above, beyond*	Hyperactive (overactive) Hypertension (above normal blood pressure)
hyp-, hypo-	*under, deficient, beneath*	Hypalgia (reduced pain sense) Hypothyroidism (deficiency of thyroid activity)
im-,* in-	*in, into, within*	Implant (insert into) Injection (forcing fluid into)
im-,* in-	*not*	Immature (not mature) Involuntary (not voluntary)
infra-	*below, beneath*	Infraorbital (beneath eye) Infracostal (below rib)
inter-	*between*	Intercostal (between ribs) Internodal (between nodes)
intra-	*within*	Intracardiac (within heart) Intraocular (within the eye)
intro-	*into, within*	Introversion (turning inward) Introrsus (turned in)
mes-, meso-	*middle*	Mesencephalon (midbrain) Mesonasal (middle of nose)
meta-	*change, beyond*	Metachrosis (color change) Metabasis (disease changes)
micr-, micro-	*small*	Micracoustic (faint sounds) Microbe (minute organism)
mult-, multi-	*many*	Multiarticular (many joints) Multiform (many shapes)
neo-	*new, recent*	Neoblastic (new tissue growth) Neonatal (newborn)

*im- before *b*, *m*, and *p*.

TABLE 2.1 PREFIXES—*cont'd*

Prefix	Meaning	Examples
pan-	*all, entire*	Panacea (cure-all) Pantalgia (entire body pain)
para-	*beside, beyond, after*	Paracardiac (beside the heart) Paracyesis (pregnancy outside the uterus)
per-	*through, excessive*	Permeable (may pass through) Peracute (excessively sharp)
peri-	*around*	Periosteum (around bone) Peribulbar (around eye bulb)
poly-	*many, much, excessive*	Polycystic (many cysts) Polydipsia (excessive thirst)
post-	*after, behind*	Postoperative (after surgery) Postocular (behind the eye)
pre-, pro-	*before, in front of*	Prenatal (before birth) Project (throw forward)
pseud-, pseudo-	*false*	Pseudarthrosis (false joint) Pseudocyesis (false pregnancy)
re-	*again, backward*	Reflex (bend back) Regurgitation (vomiting)
retro-	*backward, behind*	Retrograde (going backward) Retrolingual (behind tongue)
semi-	*half*	Semiconscious (partly aware) Seminormal (half normal)
sub-	*under, beneath*	Subcutaneous (under the skin) Subungual (beneath the nail)
super-, supra-	*above, superior, excess*	Superactivity (overactivity) Suprarenal (above kidneys)
sym-,* syn-	*together, with*	Symmelia (fusion of limbs) Synclinal (bent together)
trans-	*across, through*	Transection (cut across) Transaortic (through aorta)
ultra-	*beyond, excess*	Ultravirus (very small virus) Ultrasonic (beyond upper limit of human hearing)

*sym- before *b*, *m*, *p*, and *ph*.

REVIEW 2.A

PREFIXES

Complete the following:

1. A prefix _____never_____ stands alone.

2. The prefix *ante-* means _____before_____ .

3. A prefix meaning two or twice is _____bi_____

_____ .

4. A prefix meaning around is _____circum_____

_____ or _____ .

5. A prefix for half is _____hemi_____ or

_____semi_____ .

6. *Super-* has a similar meaning to the prefix

_____supra_____ .

7. The prefix *sym-* is used before _____b, m, p,_____
_____and ph_____ .

8. The prefix for false is _____pseud_____ .

9. The prefix *pan-* means _____all, entire_____ .

10. The prefixes *mes-* and *meso-* mean _____
_____middle_____ .

Matching

D	**1.** a-, an-	**A.**	self
H	**2.** ambi-, ampho-	**B.**	difficult, bad
G	**3.** contra-	**C.**	apart, free from
B	**4.** dys-	**D.**	without, lack of, not
F	**5.** ep-, epi-	**E.**	below, beneath
A	**6.** aut-, auto-	**F.**	upon, on, over
J	**7.** multi-	**G.**	opposed, against
C	**8.** dis-	**H.**	both
I	**9.** infra-	**I.**	normal
E	**10.** eu-	**J.**	many

Suffixes

A suffix consists of one or more syllables placed at the end of a word. Like a prefix, a suffix never stands alone. Suffixes are added to the roots of words to modify their meanings. To make pronunciation easier, the last letter or letters of the root may be changed before adding the suffix. For this purpose, two general rules may be followed:

1. The last vowel of the root may be changed to another vowel. Usually, but not always, an *o* or another vowel may be inserted between the root and a suffix that begins with a consonant. This vowel is known as a *combining vowel.* For example:

In the word *cardiology:*
   to the *root cardi-* meaning heart,

the *combining vowel o* is added, producing the *combining form cardio-,* to which is added the *suffix -logy,* which means study of. Cardiology means study of the heart.

2. When a suffix begins with a vowel, the last vowel of the root may be dropped before adding the suffix. For example:

In the word *carditis:*
the *ending vowel i* of
   the *root cardi-* is dropped before adding
   the *suffix -itis,* which means inflammation. Carditis means inflammation of the heart.

Most suffixes are in common use, but some are specific to medical language. The most common suffixes encountered are listed in Table 2-2, with those used in ordinary language in *italics.*

TABLE 2.2 SUFFIXES

Suffix	Meaning	Examples
-ac, -al, -ic, -ous, -tic	pertaining to, relating to	Cardiac (pertaining to the heart) Neural (pertaining to nerve) Hemorrhagic (relating to bleeding) Delirious (relating to mental disturbance) Acoustic (pertaining to sound)
-algia, -dynia	pain	Neuralgia (pain in nerves) Mastodynia (pain in breast)
-ate, -ize	use, subject to	Impregnate (to make pregnant) Visualize (use imagination)
-cele	protrusion (hernia)	Cystocele (bladder hernia) Rectocele (rectal protrusion into vagina)
-centesis	surgical puncture to remove fluid	Paracentesis (from a body cavity) Thoracentesis (from chest cavity)
-cle, -cule, -ole, -ola, -ule, -ulum, -ulus	small	Follicle (little bag) Molecule (small mass) Arteriole, arteriola (small artery) Nodule (small node) Ovulum (small egglike structure) Homunculus (small man)
-cyte	cell	Leukocyte (white blood cell) Erythrocyte (red blood cell)
-ectomy	cutting out	Lobectomy (of a lobe) Appendectomy (of the appendix)
-emesis	vomit	Hematemesis (vomiting blood) Hyperemesis (excessive vomiting)
-emia	blood condition	Leukemia (malignant blood disease) Anemia (lack of red blood cells)
-ent, -er, -ist, -or	person or agent	Recipient (one who receives) Examiner (one who examines) Oculist (eye physician) Donor (one who donates)
-esis, -ia, -iasis, -ism, -ity, -osis, -sis, -tion, -y	state or condition	Paresis (partial paralysis) Anesthesia (loss of sensation) Psoriasis (skin condition) Priapism (persistent erection) Acidity (excess acid) Narcosis (drugged state) Inhalation (inhaling) Therapy (treatment condition)

Continued

TABLE 2.2 SUFFIXES—cont'd

Suffix	Meaning	Examples
-form, -oid	*resembling, shaped like*	Fusiform (spindle shaped) Ovoid (egg shaped)
-genesis	*beginning process, origin*	Pathogenesis (origin of disease) Homogenesis (young same as parent)
-gram, -graphy	*recording, written record*	Mammogram (x-ray film of breast) Cardiography (heart action record)
-graph	*instrument that records*	Cardiograph (heart action) Encephalograph (brain function)
-ible, -ile	*capable, able*	Flexible (capable of bending) Contractile (able to contract)
-ites, -itis	*inflammation*	Tympanites (drumlike swelling of abdomen) Adenitis (inflammation of a gland)
-logy	*science, study of*	Biology (science of life) Histology (study of tissues)
-oma	*tumor*	Carcinoma (malignant growth) Sarcoma (cancerous tumor)
-penia	*deficiency of, lack of*	Glycopenia (sugar in tissues) Leukopenia (white blood cells)
-pexy, -pexis	*fixation, storing*	Nephropexy (of floating kidney) Glycopexis (glycogen in liver)
-phagia, -phagy	*eating, devouring*	Geophagia (eating dirt or clay) Aerophagy (swallowing air)
-phobia	*abnormal fear or intolerance*	Acrophobia (fear of heights) Photophobia (fear of light)
-plasty	*surgical shaping or formation*	Rhinoplasty (nose formation) Otoplasty (external ear)
-pnea	*breathing*	Apnea (absence of breathing) Dyspnea (difficult breathing)
-ptosis	*prolapse, downward displacement*	Proctoptosis (prolapse of anus) Nephroptosis (prolapse of kidney)
-rrhage, -rrhagia	*excessive flow*	Hemorrhage (excessive blood flow) Metrorrhagia (abnormal menses)
-rrhaphy	*suturing in place*	Herniorrhaphy (repair of hernia) Osteorrhaphy (wiring of bone)

TABLE 2.2 SUFFIXES—*cont'd*

Suffix	Meaning	Examples
-rrhea	flow or discharge	Rhinorrhea (nasal discharge) Galactorrhea (breast milk)
-rrhexis	rupture	Enterorrhexis (intestinal rupture) Metrorrhexis (rupture of uterus)
-scope	instrument for examining	Microscope (minute objects) Cystoscope (urinary bladder)
-scopy	act of examining	Microscopy (minute objects) Cystoscopy (urinary bladder)
-stomy	surgical opening	Colostomy (colon to body surface) Gastrostomy (into stomach)
-tome	instrument for	Cystotome (cutting into bladder) Neurotome (dissecting nerves)
-tomy	cutting, incision	Cystotomy (of urinary bladder) Phlebotomy (incision of vein)

REVIEW 2.B

SUFFIXES

Complete the following:

1. A suffix __never__ stands alone.

2. A suffix is added to a root to __modify__ its meaning.

3. A suffix meaning pain is __algia__.

4. A suffix for protrusion is __cele__.

5. State or condition may be indicated by several suffixes, two of which are __ia__ and __sis__.

6. A suffix meaning instrument that records is __graph__.

7. The suffixes -*ites* and -*itis* mean __inflammation__.

8. The suffix __oma__ means tumor.

9. The suffix for prolapse or downward displacement is __ptosis__.

10. The suffix -*phobia* means __abnormal fear__.

Matching

__G__ 1. -al, -ic
__J__ 2. -ectomy
__F__ 3. -penia
__E__ 4. -scopy
__B__ 5. -emesis
__A__ 6. -centesis
__H__ 7. -stomy
__I__ 8. -logy
__D__ 9. -rrhage, -rrhagia
__C__ 10. -form, -oid

A. surgical puncture
B. vomit
C. resembling, shaped like
D. excessive flow
E. act of examining
F. deficiency of, lack of
G. pertaining to
H. surgical opening
I. science of, study of
J. cutting out

EXERCISES   BUILDING A MEDICAL VOCABULARY

Step 1: Prefixes and Suffixes

The following exercises constitute an additional opportunity to review and use the preceding prefixes and suffixes. As in the review questions, the answers are provided in an appendix. To make the best use of these exercises, if you find that you cannot answer a given question, we strongly suggest that you look it up in the preceding text material. You should use the answers provided only to check your accuracy and not as a short route to completion of the exercises.

Exercise 2.1   *In the blank following each pair of prefixes and suffixes, indicate whether their meaning is the same or opposite.*

1. dys-
   eu- __Opposite__

2. ecto-
   endo- __Opposite__

3. semi-
   hemi- __Same__

4. hyper-
   hypo- __Same__

5. -algia
   -dynia __Same__

6. a-
   an- __Same__

7. circum-
   peri- __Same__

8. -iasis
   -osis __(scribbled out)__

9. bi-
   di- __Same__

10. -ectomy
    -rrhaphy __Opposite__

11. -ac
    -al __Same__

12. anti-
    contra- __Same__

13. -ible
    -ile __Same__

14. -gram
    -graphy __Same__

15. ante-
    anti- __Opposite__

Exercise 2.2   *Define the following prefixes.*

1. post- __after, behind__
2. dys- __difficult, bad, painful__
3. a- __without, Lack of, not__
4. infra- __below, beneath__
5. retro- __backward, beneath__
6. endo- __within, inner__
7. inter- __between__
8. para- __beside, beyond, after__
9. ambi- __both__
10. cata- __down, under, Lower, against__

Exercise 2.3   *Define the following suffixes.*

1. -ate _____use, subject to_____
2. -genesis _____beginning process, origin_____
3. -itis _____inflammation_____
4. -oma _____tumor_____
5. -phobia _____abnormal fear or intolerance_____

6. -cele _____protrusion_____
7. -logy _____science, study of_____
8. -tome _____instrument for_____
9. -rrhea _____flow or discharge_____
10. -phagia _____eating, devouring_____

Exercise 2.4   *Matching*

K	1. -cyte	A. blood condition
L	2. -ic	B. away from
M	3. hemi-	C. instrument
I	4. -ptosis	D. rupture
J	5. con-	E. between, through
A	6. -emia	F. breathing
B	7. ab-	G. upon, on, over
O	8. -emesis	H. resembling, shaped like
N	9. auto-	I. prolapse
D	10. -rrhexis	J. with, together
E	11. dia-	K. cell
C	12. -scope	L. pertaining to
H	13. -oid	M. half
G	14. epi-	N. self
F	15. -pnea	O. vomit

CROSSWORD PUZZLE

ACROSS

1. Before birth
5. Ability to use both hands equally
9. Suffix meaning small
13. Prefix meaning not
15. Beneath the eye
16. Prefix meaning without
17. Prefix meaning out of
18. Suffix meaning blood condition
20. Prefix meaning up or apart
21. Prefix meaning under or beneath
22. Prefix meaning difficult
23. Prefix meaning new
24. Prefix meaning separation from

DOWN

1. Suffix meaning fixation
2. Prefix meaning away from
3. Prefix meaning in
4. Prefix meaning two or twice
5. Against infection
6. Prefix meaning down or from
7. Suffix meaning state or condition
8. Under the skin
10. Cut across
11. Pain in nerves
12. Not voluntary
14. Excessive thirst
19. Suffix for resembling

HIDDEN WORDS PUZZLE

```
V I U S F I A U H X L X L I C S D A F J M I J W A P C J D B
W W Y I S L H P H Y U I O O Y V X V Q C D S U K U X X E O V
W I B V Q Z J Z C I P T W L S K N V V M J G H R Q E M N G J
I C L G L I D N C J G E N C T N O J G D O Y Y Y Q K X O P P
J E H H I G R P D W W R R V O V A M F X N E U L C I E B T E
D B F T E P I D E R M I S T C V I Q X G R J Y X S K O G O P
Z Y A Y I M R W W Z Q F R S E G L I B U H I Q L H P D I X I
I C S N V D O M Y I R D P E L N F R N O P Y S M O D J E Y U
Y V S P E N T R I N T R O V E R S I O N R R G E I T L P B L
X T V N E S S S R F Y D Q M F D E I N M P C J B B P J G Y S
S M O D F P T R F H F A J M F V M X O E Q M E Y T S Y G G T
S M Y F U P S H E M A T E M E S I S B N C Y W X J K U W Q O
P R U S L O J I E L K G O U I D C N L R E H R W A R U V O N
B B H Y V W J N A S B D E N T J O L J V D E C A Y C R A P O
K B C H D W N O E E I E W R W G N N L E D M A N E M I A Z D
Q F M N R J L P Q M O A X C V T S E O V C L R P J M J T E U
M L H P M D W L D B L I S N G D C P U R I T D R G G X T P L
O Y U I C Q I A L O O E F I M C I P W R S U I M M A T U R E
L Q V J F M H S I Q G I J P Q B O N M Y A M A O E U P C F O
E H G P O O B T S S Y D N U V M U F I Q K L C Y N V D F C K
W T C O F V C Y B E O L J Y N O S L C Q Z X G K T U E X P N
V V I Y R V V G W P C T U F T F B V U J Y G O I P B D S Q N
D R F V F N S J Q N I T H D N B W F Z O V Y W S A F T D P D
```

Can you find the 20 words hidden in this puzzle? All hidden words puzzles have words running from top to bottom, left to right, and diagonally downward.

SEMICONSCIOUS	EPIDERMIS	DECAY
RHINOPLASTY	BIOLOGY	HEMATEMESIS
DYSPEPSIA	NODULE	CYSTOCELE
IMMATURE	INTROVERSION	NEURALGIA
ANEMIA	HEMORRHAGE	DISSECT
HYPERTENSION	INJECTION	DONOR
ANESTHESIA	CARDIAC	

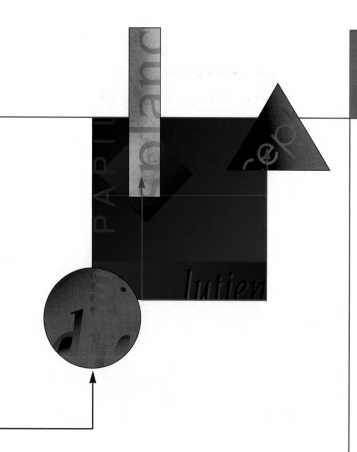

Adding to the Foundation

In this chapter the student is presented with lists of roots and their combining forms, grouped according to relationship to external or internal anatomy. External anatomy refers to any visible part of the body, and internal anatomy refers to organs, bones, and other tissues within the body.

STEP 2: ROOTS AND COMBINING FORMS

This chapter consists of extensive lists of roots and combining forms pertaining to the structure of the body (anatomy). You will remember that a root is the foundation or basic meaning of a word. A combining form is a root with an added combining vowel, attaching the root to a suffix or another root. Table 3-1 relates to external body structure (that which can be seen with the naked eye). Each root is listed alphabetically with its pronunciation and associated body part. Each combining form is divided by a slash mark (/) separating the root and the combining vowel, which is usually, but not always, an *o*.

External Anatomy

TABLE 3.1 EXTERNAL ANATOMY

Root/combining form	Pronunciation	Body part
blephar/o-	blef'ahr-o	Eyelid or eyelash
brachi/o-	bra'ke-o	Arm
bucc/o-	buk'o	Cheek
canth/o-	kan'tho	Either corner of the eye
capit/o-	kap'it-o	Head
carp/o-	karp'o	Wrist
cephal/o-	sef'al-o	Head
cervic/o-	ser'vik-o	Neck (also refers to necklike projection of the cervix uteri, which is internal anatomy)
cheil/o-, chil/o-	kile'o	Lip
cheir/o-, chir/o-	ki'ro	Hand
cili/o-	sil'ee-o	Eyelid, eyelash, or small hairlike processes
cor/e-, cor/o-	kor'ee, kor'o	Pupil of eye
dactyl/o-	dak'til-o	Finger usually, sometimes toe
dent/i-, dent/o-	dent'ee, dent'o	Tooth or teeth
derm/a-, derm/o- dermat/o-	derm'a, derm'o, derm'at-o	Skin
dors/i-, dors/o-	dor'see, dor'so	Posterior or back
faci/o-	fa'she-o	Face
gingiv/o-	jin'jiv-o	Gums
gloss/o-	glos'o	Tongue
gnath/o-	nath'o	Jaw
irid/o-	ir'id-o	Iris of eye
labi/o-	lay'be-o	Lip, especially lips of mouth
lapar/o-	lap'ahr-o	Loin or flank; sometimes abdomen
later/o-	lat'er-o	Side

Continued

Root/combining form	Pronunciation	Body part
lingu/o-	ling'wo	Tongue
mamm/a-, mamm/o-	mam'ah, mam'o	Breast
mast/o-	mast'o	Breast
mel/o-	mel'o	Limb
nas/o-	naze'o	Nose
occipit/o-	ock-si'pit-o	Back of head
ocul/o-	ock'ule-o	Eye
odont/o-	oh-dont'o	Tooth or teeth
om/o-	oh'mo	Shoulder
omphal/o-	om'fah-lo	Navel or umbilicus
onych/o-	on'ik-o	Nail or nails
ophthalm/o-	of-thal'mo	Eye or eyes
or/o-	or'o	Mouth
ot/o-	oh'toe	Ear
papill/o-	pah-pill'o	Nipple or nipple-shaped projection
phall/o-	fal'o	Penis
pil/o-	pile'o	Hair
pod/o-	pod'o	Foot or foot-shaped part
rhin/o-	rine'o	Nose
somat/o-, somatic/o-	sew-mat'o, sew-mat'ik-o	Body
steth/o-	steth'o	Chest
stom-, stomat/o-	sto'mah-toe	Mouth
tal/o-	tal'o	Ankle or anklebone
tars/o-	tahr'so	Instep of foot or eyelid edge
thel/o-	theel'o	Nipple
thorac/o-	the'rah-ko	Chest or thorax
trachel/o-	trake'el-o	Neck or necklike structure
trich/o-	trik'o	Hair or hairlike structure
ventr/i-, ventr/o-	ven'tree, ven'tro	Front of body, belly

REVIEW 3.A

EXTERNAL ANATOMY ROOTS AND COMBINING FORMS

Complete the following:

1. *Blepharo-* and *cilio-* mean ___eyelid___ .

2. The combining forms for head are ___capit/o-___ and ___cephal/o-___ .

3. A combining form for hair is ___pil/o-___ .

4. A combining form for lip is ___cheil/o-___ .

5. *Rhino-* and *naso-* both refer to ___nose___ .

6. Two combining forms for breast are ___mamm/a-,o___ and ___mast/o-___ .

7. *Cervico-* and *trachelo-* mean ___neck___ .

8. A combining form for mouth is ___or/o-___ _____ .

9. *Ophthalmo-* and ___ocul/o-___ are combining forms for eye.

10. *Stetho-* and ___thorac/o-___ are combining forms for chest.

Matching

__G__	1. carpo-	A.	tongue
__I__	2. derma-, dermo-, dermato-	B.	pupil of eye
__H__	3. brachio-	C.	ear
__A__	4. glosso-	D.	back of head
__J__	5. ventri-, ventro-	E.	foot
__C__	6. oto-	F.	cheek
__B__	7. core-, coro-	G.	wrist
__D__	8. occipito-	H.	arm
__E__	9. podo-	I.	skin
__F__	10. bucco-	J.	front of body or belly

Internal Anatomy

Table 3-2 relates to internal body structure (that which is inside the body). Each root is listed alphabetically, with its pronunciation and associated body part. The combining form is divided with a slash mark (/) separating the root and the combining vowel, which is usually, but not always, an *o*.

TABLE 3.2 INTERNAL ANATOMY

Root/combining form	Pronunciation	Body part
aden/o-	ad'e-no	Gland
adren/o-	ad-re'no	Adrenal gland
angi/o-	an'je-o	Vessel, usually a blood vessel
arteri/o-	ar-te're-o	Artery
arteriol/o-	ar-te're-o"lo	Arteriole

Continued

TABLE 3.2 INTERNAL ANATOMY—*cont'd*

Root/combining form	Pronunciation	Body part
arthr/o-	ar'throe	Joint
atri/o-	a'tree-o	Atrium or upper heart chamber
balan/o-	bal'ah-no	Glans penis or glans clitoridis
bronch/i-, bronch/o-	brong'ke, brong'ko	Bronchus
bronchiol/o-	brong'ke-olo	Bronchiolus
cardi/o-	kar'de-o	Heart
cerebell/o-	ser"e-bel'o	Cerebellum part of brain
cerebr/i-, cerebr/o-	ser'e-bri, ser'e-bro	Cerebrum part of brain
choledoch/o-	ko-lee'dok-o	Common bile duct
chondr/i-, chondr/io-, chondr/o-	kon'dree, kon'dree-o, kon'dro	Cartilage
chord/o-	kor'do	Cord (vocal or spermatic)
cleid/o-	kli'do	Clavicle (collar bone)
colp/o-	kol'po	Vagina
cost/o-	kos'to	Rib
cyst/i-, cyst/o-	sis'ti, sis'to	Bladder, cyst, sac
cyt/o-	si'to	Cell
duoden/o-	du"o-de'no	Duodenum section of intestine
encephal/o-	en-sef'ah-lo	Brain
enter/o-	en'ter-o	Intestine
episi/o-	e-peez'e-o	Vulva
fibr/o-	fie'bro	Fibers
gastr/o-	gas'tro	Stomach
gli/o-	glee'o	Neuroglia, or gluey substance
hepat/ico-, hepat/o-	he-pat'i-ko, he-pat'o	Liver

TABLE 3.2 INTERNAL ANATOMY—*cont'd*

Root/combining form	Pronunciation	Body part
hist/o-	his'to	Tissue
hyster/o-	his'ter-o	Uterus
ile/o-	ill'e-o	Ileum section of intestine
ili/o-	ill'e-o	Ilium (upper part of hip bone)
jejun/o-	je-joo'no	Jejunum section of intestine
kerat/o-	ker'ah-to	Horny tissue (and cornea of eye)
laryng/o-	lah-ring'go	Larynx (voice box)
lien/o-	li'en-o	Spleen
lymph/o-	lim'fo	Lymphatic vessels, lymphocytes
mening/o-	me-ning'go	Membranes covering brain and spinal cord
metr/a-, metr/o-	me'trah, me'tro	Uterus
myel/o-	my'el-o	Bone marrow or spinal cord
my/o-	my'o	Muscle
myring/o-	mi-ring'o	Eardrum
nephr/o-	nef'ro	Kidney
neur/o-	nu'ro	Nerve, nerves, nervous system
oophor/o-	o-of'or-o	Ovary
orchi/o-, orchi/do-	or'ke-o, or'ki-do	Testis, testes
osche/o-	os'ke-o	Scrotum
oss/eo-, oss/i-, ost/e-, ost/eo-	os'se-o, os'see, os'tee, os'tee-o	Bone or bones
palat/o-	pal'ah-to	Palate (roof of mouth)
pharyng/o	fah-ring'go	Pharynx (throat)
phleb/o-	fleb'o	Vein or veins
phren/i-, phren/ico-, phren/o-	fren'ee, fren'i-ko, fren'o	Diaphragm, mind

Continued

TABLE 3.2 INTERNAL ANATOMY—*cont'd*

Root/combining form	Pronunciation	Body part
pleur/o-	ploor'o	Pleura, rib (or side)
pneum/a-, pneum/o-, pneum/ato-, pneum/ono-	nu'mah, nu'mo, nu-mat'o, nu-mon'o	Lungs, respiration (air, breath)
proct/o-	prok'to	Rectum or anus
pulm/o-	pull'mo	Lungs
pyel/o-	pi'el-o	Pelvis of kidney
rachi/o-	ra'ke-o	Spine
rect/o-	rek'to	Rectum
ren/i-, ren/o-	ren'i, ren'o	Kidney
sacr/o-	sa'kro	Sacrum
salping/o-	sal-ping'go	Fallopian or eustachian tube
sarc/o-	sar'ko	Flesh, muscular substance
splanchn/i-, splanchn/o-	splank'ni, splank'no	Viscera, splanchnic nerve
splen/o-	splen'o	Spleen
spondyl/o-	spon'di-lo	Vertebra, spinal column
stern/o-	stern'no	Sternum (breastbone)
tend/o-, ten/o-, tenont/o-	ten'doe, ten'o, ten'on-toe	Tendon
thym/o-	thi'mo	Thymus gland
thyr/o-	thi'ro	Thyroid gland
trache/o-	tra'ke-o	Trachea
ureter/o-	u-re'ter-o	Ureter (kidney to bladder tube)
urethr/o-	u-re'thro	Urethra (bladder to outside)
vas/o-	vaz'o	Vessel or duct
ven/e-, ven/i-, ven/o-	vene'eh, vene'ee, vene'o	Vein or veins
vesic/o-	ves'i-ko	Bladder, blister
viscer/o-	vis'er-o	Viscera

REVIEW 3.B

INTERNAL ANATOMY ROOTS AND COMBINING FORMS

Complete the following:

1. The combining form for gland is _aden/o_.
2. A combining form for uterus is _hyster/o_.
3. *Ileo-* is the combining form meaning _intestine_
4. *Gastro-* is the combining form meaning
   stomach.
5. The combining form for common bile duct is
   choledoch/o.
6. *Pneuma-* or *pulmo-* refers to _lungs_
7. The combining form for spleen is
   splen/o.
8. *Osteo-* refers to _bone_.
9. A combining form for vein is _phleb/o_.
10. *Cleido-* is a combining form meaning
    clavicle.

Matching

_F_ 1. urethro-
_I_ 2. procto-
_G_ 3. tracheo-
_A_ 4. splanchni-
_H_ 5. sarco-
_D_ 6. myelo-
_B_ 7. rachi-
_J_ 8. kerato-
_E_ 9. myo-
_C_ 10. reni-

A. viscera
B. spine
C. kidney
D. bone marrow or spinal cord
E. muscle
F. urethra
G. trachea
H. flesh
I. rectum or anus
J. horny tissue

EXERCISES   ADDING TO THE FOUNDATION

Step 2: Roots and Combining Forms

The following exercises provide further opportunities for learning the roots and combining forms presented in this chapter. Once again, we urge you to consult the answers only after you have completed the exercises.

Exercise 3.1

In the blank following each pair of roots or combining forms, indicate whether their meaning is similar or different.

1. blepharo-
   facio- _differnt_
2. angio-
   vas- _Same_
3. capito-
   cephalo- _Same_
4. lieno-
   ileo- _different_
5. oculo-
   ophthalmo- _Same_
6. oro-
   oto- _different_
7. talo-
   tarso- _Same_

8. rhino-
   naso- _Same_
9. splanchno-
   viscero- _Same_
10. pilo-
    tricho- _Same_
11. myo-
    myelo- _different_
12. linguo-
    glosso- _Same_
13. odonto-
    dento- _Same_
14. reno-
    nephro- _Same_

15. coro-
    irido- _different_
16. phlebo-
    veno- _Same_
17. rachio-
    spondilo- _different_
18. colpo-
    hystero- _different_
19. omphalo-
    papillo- _different_
20. stetho-
    thoraco- _Same_

Exercise 3.2

Fill in the combining form for each of the following body parts.

1. cartilage _chondr/i_
2. bladder or blister _cyst/i_
3. membranes covering brain and spinal cord
   mening/o
4. fibers _fibr/o_
5. common bile duct _choledoch/o_
6. tendon _tend/o_
7. lip _labi/o_
8. eye _ocul/o_
9. wrist _carp/o_
10. finger _dactyl/o_

11. nose _rhin/o_
12. muscle _myo_
13. horny tissue _kerato_
14. kidney pelvis _____
15. larynx _laryngo_
16. thyroid gland _thyro_
17. breast _mamma_
18. ankle _talo_
19. body _somato_
20. ear _oto_

Exercise 3.3   *Define the following roots and combining forms.*

1. bucco- Cheek
2. cheilo- lip
3. dactylo- fingers/toes
4. latero- side
5. onycho- nails

6. gnatho- Jaw
7. somato- body
8. omo- Shoulder
9. stomato- mouth
10. podo- foot

Exercise 3.4   *Matching*

D 1. brachio-
K 2. cantho-
J 3. carpo-
B 4. gingivo-
G 5. derma-
H 6. melo-
A 7. occipito-
L 8. talo-
F 9. trachelo-
I 10. ventro-
E 11. thelo-
C 12. cephalo-

A. back of head
B. gums
C. head
D. arm
E. nipple
F. neck
G. skin
H. limb
I. front of body or belly
J. wrist
K. either corner of the eye
L. ankle

CROSSWORD PUZZLE — CHAPTER 3

ACROSS

1. Heart
3. Finger or toe
5. Nose
7. Bronchus
9. Mouth
10. Ear
11. Skin
14. Heart
15. Common bile duct
16. Hair
19. Nail(s)
21. Jaw
23. Artery
25. Eardrum

DOWN

1. Angle at ends of eyelid slits
2. Tooth or teeth
4. Cartilage
6. Vertebra or spinal column
7. Arm
8. Neck
12. Pharynx
13. Eyelid or eyelash
17. Duodenum
18. Larynx
20. Vein
21. Gums
22. Liver
24. Shoulder

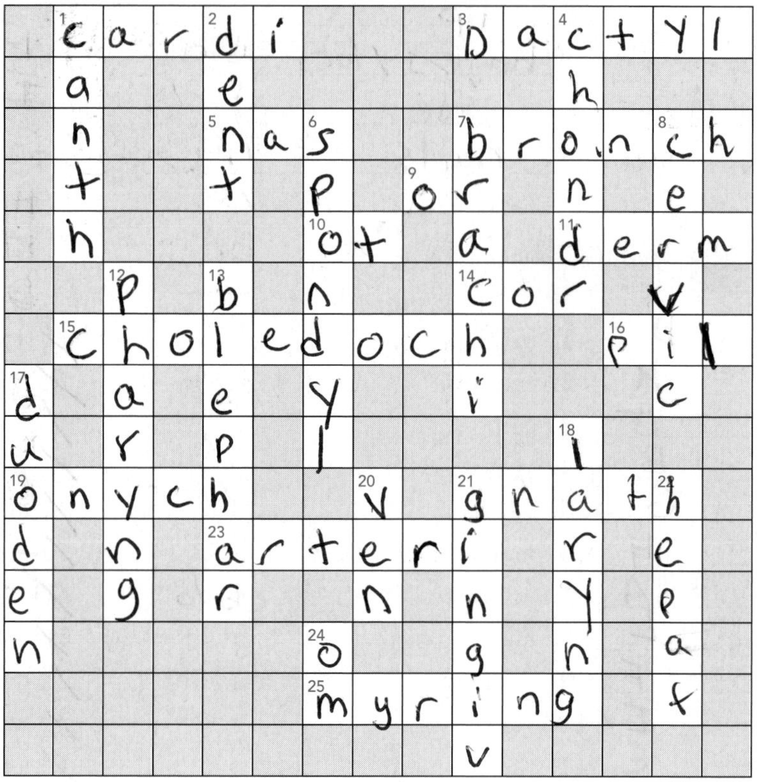

HIDDEN WORDS PUZZLE   CHAPTER 3

Can you find the 20 words hidden in this puzzle? All hidden words puzzles have words running from top to bottom, left to right, and diagonally downward.

ENCEPHAL

DACTYL

HEPAT

CARP

LABI

BRACHI

CLEID

LINGU

COST

NAS

CERVIC

GASTR

SOMAT

CYST

OSS

CHONDR

GNATH

ADEN

DERM

MY

```
I  D  Y  N  H  W  B  L  P  H  C  A  F  S  I  U
I  H  I  D  E  R  M  Y  U  I  V  N  R  Z  J  W
J  A  J  G  P  X  J  Y  V  I  W  H  A  O  J  R
P  O  N  N  A  D  E  N  J  U  D  O  W  Y  R  E
P  N  D  A  T  S  M  S  D  V  I  V  J  W  R  R
C  O  S  T  S  D  T  B  P  E  C  L  D  H  T  O
T  S  S  H  X  C  E  R  V  I  C  W  I  Q  O  D
U  W  S  C  L  D  A  C  T  Y  L  T  W  U  Y  Y
P  U  R  R  U  E  N  C  E  P  H  A  L  I  Y  M
S  F  Z  U  X  I  I  H  N  N  X  B  A  F  G  G
Y  Q  R  B  X  D  C  I  S  O  M  A  T  S  B  F
V  B  T  O  M  F  K  S  L  I  N  G  U  B  R  I
S  T  I  X  Y  E  A  R  Q  U  H  D  D  N  Q  R
Q  G  Z  C  H  B  S  C  C  M  C  A  R  P  E  P
C  X  R  S  A  U  G  P  Y  L  Y  G  B  J  X  T
Y  M  H  W  F  O  D  I  N  Z  S  B  J  D  Y  V
B  E  Z  P  K  L  I  E  F  R  T  S  V  X  S  L
```

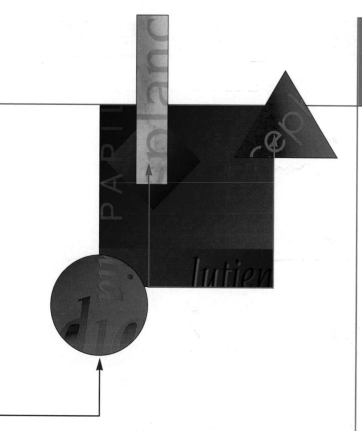

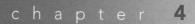

Completing the Foundation

This chapter presents five additional lists of roots and their combining forms, grouped as verbs, adjectives, body fluids, body substances and chemicals, and colors.

STEP 3: ADDITIONAL ROOTS AND COMBINING FORMS

The following lists of roots and combining forms relate to action or description. Table 4-1 lists verbal (verb-based) roots and combining forms that show an activity, a condition, or an action. Each combining form is divided by a slashmark (/) between the root and its combining vowel.

TABLE 4.1 VERBAL ROOTS AND COMBINING FORMS

Root/combining form	Meaning	Examples
audi/o-	hearing	Audiometer (hearing test device) Audiology (study of hearing)
bio-	life	Biology (study of living things) Biogenesis (origin of life)
caus-, caut-	burn	Causalgia (burning pain) Cautery (device to scar or burn)
clas-	break	Osteoclasis (surgical fracture) Clastothrix (splitting of hair)
-duct-	lead	Abduct (lead away from) Duct (tube leading to or from)
-ectas-	dilate	Phlebectasia (dilation of veins) Venectasia (dilation of veins)
-edem-	swelling	Cephaledema (swelling of head) Edematous (swollen)
-esthes-	sensation	Anesthesia (without sensation) Esthesiogenic (producing sensation)
fiss-	split, cleft	Fissure (a cleft or groove) Fissile (capable of being split)
-flect-, flex-	bend	Anteflect (bend forward) Flexion (bending)
gen/o-	producing	Genesis (origin or beginning) Genophobia (fear of sexuality)
-iatr/o-	treatment	Geriatrics (treatment of aging) Pediatrics (treatment of children)
kin/e-, kin/o-	movement, motion	Kinetogenic (producing movement) Kinomometer (motion measurer)
ly/o-, lys/o-	dissolve	Lyotropic (readily soluble) Lysogen (producing dissolution)
morph/o-	form, structure, shape	Amorphous (no definite form) Polymorphic (many forms)
-op/ia	vision	Myopia (nearsightedness) Hyperopia (farsightedness)
opt/ico-, opt/o-	seeing	Opticokinetic (eye movements) Optometer (device for refraction)

Continued

TABLE 4.1 VERBAL ROOTS AND COMBINING FORMS—*cont'd*

Root/combining form	Meaning	Examples
phag/o-	eating	Phagomania (food craving) Phagophobia (fear of eating)
phan/ero-	visible, manifest	Phanerosis (becoming visible) Phantasm (unreal mental image)
-phas-	speech	Aphasia (loss of speech functions) Dysphasia (difficulty in speaking)
phil-	affinity, love for	Philanthropy (love of mankind) Philoneism (love of change)
-plegia	paralysis	Hemiplegia (one-sided paralysis) Paraplegia (paralysis of lower trunk and legs)
-poiesis	formation, production	Hemopoiesis (blood cell formation) Leukopoiesis (white blood cell production)
schist/o-, schiz/o-	split, cleft, division	Schistocystis (bladder fissure) Schizonychia (splitting of nails)
spasm/o-	spasm	Spasmogenic (causing spasm) Spasmolysis (relieving spasm)
-stasis	standing still, stoppage	Epistasis (stoppage of a flow) Hemostasis (stoppage of blood flow)
top/o-	place, location	Topalgia (localized pain) Toponarcosis (localized anesthesia)
troph/o-	nourishment, food	Trophism (nutrition) Dystrophy (defective nutrition)

R E V I E W   4 . A

VERBAL ROOTS AND COMBINING FORMS

Complete the following:

1. Verb-based roots show an activity, an action, or a(n) _____Condition_____ .

2. The combining form *audi-* means _____ hearing _____ .

3. The combining form _____ -estas _____ means dilate.

4. The combining form *caus-* means _____ burn _____ .

5. The combining form for speech is _____ -phas _____ .

6. The combining form _____ phag _____ means eating.

7. _____ phil _____ means love for or affinity.

8. The combining form for standing still is _____ Stasis _____ .

9. _____ top _____ means place or location.

10. The combining form meaning treatment is _____ iatr _____ .

Matching

D	1. -duct-	A.	break
G	2. phanero-	B.	sensation
J	3. optico-	C.	movement
H	4. -edem-	D.	lead
I	5. fiss-	E.	dissolve
B	6. esthes-	F.	formation
E	7. lyso-	G.	visible
A	8. clas-	H.	swelling
F	9. -poiesis	I.	split, cleft
C	10. kine-	J.	seeing

Adjectival Roots and Combining Forms

Table 4-2 lists adjectival (adjective-based) roots and combining forms that describe a quality or character-istic. Each combining form is divided by a slash mark (/) between the root and its combining vowel.

TABLE 4.2 ADJECTIVAL ROOTS AND COMBINING FORMS

Root/combining form	Meaning	Examples
ankyl/o-	bent, crooked, stiff, fixed	Ankyloglossia (tongue-tie) Ankylosis (stiff or fixed joint)
brachy-	short	Brachydactylia (short fingers) Brachygnathous (receding underjaw)
brady-	slow	Bradycardia (slow heartbeat) Bradypepsia (slow digestion)
brev/i-	short	Brevicollis (short neck) Breviflexor (short flexor muscle)
cel-, coel-	hollow, cavity	Celiac (of the abdominal cavity) Coelom (body cavity of embryo)
cry/o-	cold	Cryotherapy (treatment using cold) Cryoanesthesia (freezing body part)
crypt/o-	hidden	Cryptorchidism (undescended testis) Cryptomnesia (subconscious memory)
dextr/o-	right, right side	Dextrocardia (heart on right side) Dextromanual (right handed)
dipl/o-	double, twice	Diplocoria (double pupil in eye) Diplopia (double vision)
dolich/o-	long	Dolichocephalic (long head) Dolichoderus (long neck)
eso-	within, inward	Esophoria (crossed eye) Esodeviation (a turning inward)
eury-	wide, broad	Eurysomatic (thickset body) Eurycephalic (unusually broad head)
glyc/o-	sugar, sweet	Glycemia (glucose in the blood) Glycogeusia (sweet taste)
hapl/o-	simple, single	Haploid (single chromosome set) Haplopathy (uncomplicated disease)
heter/o-	other, different	Heterocellular (of different cells) Heterohypnosis (induced by another)
hom/eo-, hom/o-	same, alike	Homeomorphous (similar shape) Homozygous (having identical genes)

TABLE 4.2 ADJECTIVAL ROOTS AND COMBINING FORMS—*cont'd*

Root/combining form	Meaning	Examples
hydr/o-	wet, water	Hydremia (excess water in blood) Hydroadipsia (absence of thirst)
is/o-	equal, alike	Isocellular (having similar cells) Isocoria (equal sized pupils)
lei/o-	smooth	Leiodermia (smooth, glossy skin) Leiotrichous (smooth hair)
lept/o-	slender, small, thin	Leptodactylous (slender fingered) Leptodermic (thick skinned)
lev/o-	left, to the left	Levoduction (eyes turn left) Levorotation (turning to the left)
macr/o-	large	Macrencephaly (having large brain) Macrobiosis (long life)
mal-	ill, bad	Malady (illness) Malaise (general discomfort)
malac/o-	soft, softening	Malacia (softening) Malacotomy (incision of soft parts)
meg/a-, meg/alo-, meg/aly-	large, oversized	Megalgia (severe pain) Megalomania (grandiose delusions) Hepatomegaly (enlarged liver)
mi/o-	less, decrease	Miopragia (decreased activity) Miosis (contraction of pupil)
necr/o-	death	Necrophobia (fear of death) Necropsy (autopsy)
olig/o-	few, little	Oligomenorrhea (scanty menses) Oligosymptomatic (few symptoms)
opisth/o-	backward, behind, dorsal	Opisthocheilia (recession of lips) Opisthoporeia (walking backward)
orth/o-	straight, normal, correct	Orthodontics (straightening teeth) Orthograde (walking erect)
oxy-	sharp, quick	Oxyesthesia (overly acute senses) Oxyrhine (sharp-pointed nose)
pachy-	thick	Pachyderma (abnormally thick skin) Pachyonychia (overly thick nails)
pale/o-	old, primitive	Paleogenetic (originated in past) Paleologic (primitive reasoning)

Continued

TABLE 4.2 ADJECTIVAL ROOTS AND COMBINING FORMS—cont'd

Root/combining form	Meaning	Examples
platy-	flat, wide	Platyglossal (wide, flat tongue) Platycephaly (flattened skull)
ple/o-	more	Pleonexia (excessive greediness) Pleonosteosis (excess bone growth)
poikil/o-	irregular, varied	Poikiloderma (mottled skin) Poikilothermic (cold blooded)
-scler/o-	hardness	Sclerosis (hardening) Arteriosclerosis (artery hardening)
scoli/o-	twisted, crooked	Scoliokyphosis (curvature of spine) Scoliosis (crooked spine)
sinistr/o-	left, to the left	Sinistrocular (left eyed) Sinistromanual (left handed)
sten/o-	narrow	Stenosed (narrowed, contracted) Stenostomia (narrow oral cavity)
stere/o-	solid, three-dimensional	Stereoscopic (solid appearance) Stereopsis (three-dimensional vision)
tachy-	rapid, fast	Tachyphagia (bolting one's food) Tachylogia (rapid speech)
tel/e-, tel/o-	distant, end	Telalgia (pain from another area) Telencephalon (end brain)
therm/o-	heat	Thermogenic (producing heat) Thermolabile (destruction by heat)
xer/o-	dry	Xerochilia (dry lips) Xerostomia (dry mouth)

REVIEW 4.B

ADJECTIVAL ROOTS AND COMBINING FORMS

Complete the following:

1. Adjectival roots and combining forms describe _a quality or characteristic_.

2. The combining form _brachy_ means short.

3. The combining form meaning double is _diplo_.

4. The combining form *dolicho-* means _long_.

5. The combining *eury-* means _wide_.

6. *Hetero-* means _different_.

7. *Homeo-* means _same_.

8. A combining form meaning large is _macro_.

9. The combining form *necro-* means _death_.

10. The combining form _tachy_ means rapid or fast.

Matching

F	1. thermo-	A.	thick
J	2. steno-	B.	left
I	3. mal-	C.	simple, single
H	4. sclero-	D.	cold
A	5. pachy-	E.	slow
G	6. malaco-	F.	heat
C	7. haplo-	G.	soft
B	8. levo-	H.	hardness
E	9. brady-	I.	ill, bad
D	10. cryo-	J.	narrow

Additional Terms

Tables 4-3 through 4-5 list a number of additional terms used in medical language. Collectively, these terms complete the basic foundation for learning medical terminology. They are presented as words, roots, and combining forms, in separate charts relating to body fluids, body substances and chemicals, and colors. Each combining form is divided by a slash mark (/) between the root and its combining vowel.

TABLE 4.3 BODY FLUIDS

Word, root/combining form	Meaning
aqua, hydr/o-	water
chol/e-, chol/o-	bile
chyle	milky fluid (product of digestion)
dacry/o-, lacrima	tears
galact/o-, lac	milk
hem/a-, hemat/o-, hem/o-	blood
hidr/o-, sudor	sweat
lymph/o-	lymph
mucus	secretion of mucous membranes
myx/o-	mucus
plasma	fluid portion of blood
ptyal/o-	saliva
pus	liquid product of inflammation
py/o-	pus
sangui-, sanguin/o-	blood, bloody
serum	clear portion of blood fluid
sial/o-	saliva, salivary glands
ur/e-, ur/ea-, ur/eo-, ur/in-, ur/ino-, ur/o-	urine or urea

TABLE 4.4 BODY SUBSTANCES AND CHEMICALS

Word, root/combining form	Meaning
adip/o-	fat
amyl/o-	starch
cerumen	earwax
collagen	fibrous protein of connective tissue, cartilage, bone, and skin
ele/o-, ole/o-	oil
ferrum	iron
glyc/o-, scchar/o-, sacchar/i-	sugar
hal/o-	a salt
heme	iron-based, pigment part of hemoglobin
hormone	body-produced chemical substance
hyal/o-, hyalin	glassy, translucent substance
lapis	stone
lip/o-, lipid	fat, fatty acids
lith/o	stone or calculus
mel/i-	honey or sugar
natrium	sodium
petrous	stony hardness
sal	salt
sebum	sebaceous gland secretion

TABLE 4.5 COLORS

Word, root/combining form	Meaning
albus	white
chlor/o-, chloros	green
chrom/o-	color (as compared to no color)
cirrhos	orange-yellow
cyan/o-	blue
erythr/o-	red
leuc/o-, leuk/o-	white
lutein	saffron yellow
melan/o-	black
poli/o-	gray (relating to gray matter of the nervous system)
rhod/o-	red
ruber, rubor	red, redness
xanth/o-	yellow, yellowish

R E V I E W   4 . C

BODY FLUIDS, BODY SUBSTANCES AND CHEMICALS, AND COLORS

Complete the following:

1. A word meaning water is ___agua___ .

2. The combining form for mucus is _____
   ___Myxlo___ .

3. The combining form for pus is _____
   ___Pylo___ .

4. The clear portion of blood fluid is _____
   ___serum___ .

5. The combining form *hidro-* means _____
   ___sweat___ .

6. A combining form for milk is _____
   ___galactlo___ .

7. The word ___cerumen___ means earwax.

8. A combining form for fat is ___lipid___ .

9. The combining form for blue is _____
   ___cyanlo___ .

10. The combining form for black is _____
    ___melanlo___ .

Matching

___G___ 1. rubor   A. stony hardness

___E___ 2. leuko-   B. saliva

___J___ 3. polio-   C. sugar

___I___ 4. meli-   D. salt

___H___ 5. chole-   E. white

___A___ 6. petrous   F. iron

___C___ 7. glyco-   G. red

___B___ 8. ptyalo-   H. bile

___D___ 9. sal   I. honey or sugar

___F___ 10. ferrum   J. gray

EXERCISES   COMPLETING THE FOUNDATION

The following exercises provide a review of the foundation material from Chapters 2, 3, and 4. The word parts are not necessarily clustered according to use, as was done in the preceding exercises. Approach the exercises as a challenge. You may find it necessary to look back through Chapters 2 and 3, as well as this chapter, to locate answers. Once more, try to avoid using the answers in Appendix G, except as a final check.

Exercise 4.1

In the blank following each pair of words, roots or combining forms, indicate whether their meaning is the same or opposite.

1. myxo-
    mucus _____Same_____

2. macro-
    -megaly _____Same_____

3. lepto-
    pachy- _____Opposite_____

4. levo-
    dextro- _____opposite_____

5. erythro-
    rhodo- _____Same_____

6. homeo-
    iso- _____Same_____

7. sinistro-
    levo- _____Same_____

8. hydro-
    xero- _____Opposite_____

9. leuko-
    albus _____Same_____

10. hema-
    sangui- _____Same_____

Exercise 4.2

This exercise will help you to learn to break medical words into their component parts to define them. Define each component and then define the word. Do not define those suffixes following a slash mark (/).

1. Postocular:
    post _____behind_____
    ocul/ar _____eye_____

2. Aphasia:
    a _____without_____
    phas/ia _____speech_____

3. Proctoptosis:
    procto _____anus_____
    ptosis _____prolapse_____

4. Microscope:
    micro _____small_____
    scope _____to examine_____

5. Oophorectomy:
    oophor _____ovary_____
    ectomy _____excision_____

6. Hematopoiesis:
    hemato _____blood_____
    poiesis _____formation_____

7. Endocardium:
    endo _____within_____
    cardi/um _____heart_____

8. Intercostal:
    inter _____between_____
    cost/al _____ribs_____

9. Paraurethral:
    para _____near_____
    urethr/al _____urethra_____

10. Osteomalacia:
    osteo _____bone_____
    malac/ia _____softening_____

11. Xerostomia:

xero _dry_

stom/ia _mouth_

12. Schizonychia:

schiz _division_

onych/ia _nail_

13. Diplopia:

dipl _double_

opia _vision_

14. Pleomorphism:

pleo _many_

morph/ism _forms_

_____

_____

15. Hydronephrosis:

hydro _water_

nephr _kidney_

osis _condition_

16. Retrocervical:

retro _behind_

cervic/al _neck_

17. Leukorrhea:

leuko _white_

rrhea _flow_

18. Leiomyoma:

leio _smooth_

my _muscle_

oma _tumor_

| **Exercise 4.3** | *Fill in the appropriate word, root, or combining form.* |

1. Bile _chol/e-_

2. Sweat _hidr/o-_

3. Saliva _ptyal/o-_

4. Iron _heme_

5. Fluid portion of blood _plasma_

6. Salt _sal_

7. Sugar _glyco_

8. Oil _ele/o-_

9. Starch _amyl/o-_

10. Sebaceous gland secretions _Sebum_

CROSSWORD PUZZLE

CHAPTER 4

ACROSS

1. Meaning of therm
4. Root for black
7. Root for formation
8. Root for salt
11. Meaning of the root *ptyal*
13. Chemical substance produced by the body
15. Meaning of the root *mal*
16. Word meaning lead away from
20. Root meaning paralysis
21. Root meaning break
22. Root meaning form, shape, structure
23. Root meaning smooth

DOWN

2. Root meaning hearing
3. Root meaning stone
5. Root meaning dilate
6. A cleft or groove
8. Root meaning hardness
9. Root meaning milk
10. Root meaning twisted or crooked
12. Word for earwax
13. Root for wet or water
14. Root for standing still
17. Meaning of the root *chrom*
18. Meaning of the root *pachy*
19. Root meaning fast
20. Root for eating
22. Root meaning less or decrease

HIDDEN WORDS PUZZLE

CHAPTER 4

Can you find the 20 words hidden in this puzzle? All hidden words puzzles have words running from top to bottom, left to right, and diagonally downward.

PLEGIA

BREV

FISS

SIAL

HEM

BRADY

CHOL

FLEX

STEN

KIN

MELAN

CLAS

LITH

BIO

LIP

AMYL

CYAN

PHAS

CRY

OP

Y	E	C	R	Y	S	F	K	K	L	X	I	U	M
S	I	A	L	K	Z	P	T	L	I	P	V	T	Z
V	Q	M	S	A	M	Y	L	C	T	N	K	B	D
E	Y	V	F	I	S	S	O	E	H	E	M	T	W
G	C	H	I	D	D	G	K	K	G	O	E	D	G
S	P	K	Y	Z	U	U	X	C	W	I	L	X	C
Y	D	Q	E	P	A	S	F	W	B	R	A	D	Y
X	D	J	J	P	H	A	S	L	R	I	N	N	A
F	N	U	U	S	H	X	S	T	E	N	O	P	N
L	C	O	C	G	O	Z	N	Z	V	X	D	X	E

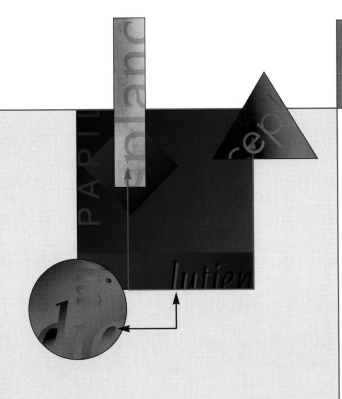

The Body Shell and Its Supports

This is the second of the five sections of *Learning Medical Terminology.* This section contains four chapters introducing the student to the language of the body structure and the systems that support, move, and protect it.

Chapter 5 acquaints the student with the six branches of science that deal with the study of the body, the basic structure of the body, and the terms used to describe directions, planes, positions, and regions of the body. Beginning with this chapter, a glossary of medical terminology (Related Terms list) relating to the material in the text will be found in each chapter.

Chapter 6 describes the skeletal system and its function as a supporting framework for the body.

Chapter 7 describes the muscular system and how it produces movement of the body in conjunction with the skeletal system.

Chapter 8 describes the integumentary system and its many functions.

Drawings within the chapters illustrate the principal anatomic parts for that chapter. In addition, there are color plates at the front of the text that provide more vivid detail.

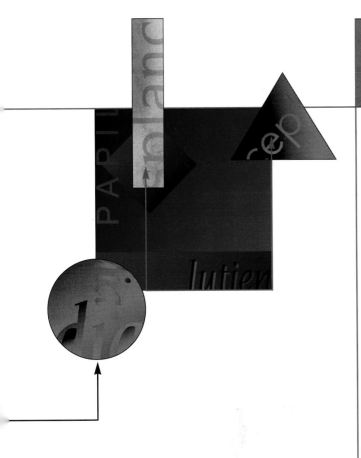

Understanding the Body and Its Structure

A jokester once said that the human body is a remarkably intricate and complex apparatus manufactured by the unskilled labor of two workers.

This chapter describes the basic structures of the human body, their characteristics and composition, and descriptive anatomic terms are introduced.

STUDY OF THE BODY

Six branches of science deal with the study of the body. They are anatomy, physiology, pathology, embryology, histology, and biology:

Anatomy, which literally means cutting apart, is the study of the structure of the body and the relationship of its parts. It derives its name from the fact that the structure of the human body is learned mainly from dissection.

Physiology is the study of the normal functions and activities of the body.

Pathology is the study of the changes caused by disease in the structure or functions of the body.

Embryology is the study of the origin and development of an individual organism. After conception, the period from the second through the eighth week is called the embryonic stage. After this, the developing organism is referred to as the fetus.

Histology is the microscopic study of the minute structure, composition, and function of normal cells and tissues.

Biology is the study of all forms of life.

It's a FACT

There are more than 50 trillion cells in the average adult body.

53

BASIC STRUCTURE

The human body may be compared to a machine, its many parts working together to promote good health, growth, and life itself. It is a combination of organs and systems supported by a framework of muscles and bones, with an external covering of skin for protection.

The *cell* is the smallest unit of life from which tissues, organs, and systems are constructed (*cyt-* is the root for cell). Cells similar in structure and function form a mass called a *tissue.* Groups of different tissues combine to form an *organ* of the body (for example, the liver, heart, or lungs), each of which performs a special function. The organs are grouped into *systems* for the purpose of performing specific and more complicated functions.

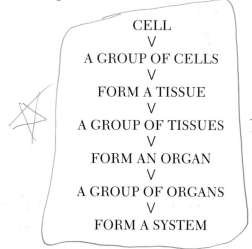

CELL
V
A GROUP OF CELLS
V
FORM A TISSUE
V
A GROUP OF TISSUES
V
FORM AN ORGAN
V
A GROUP OF ORGANS
V
FORM A SYSTEM

The body is maintained by a process called *metabolism* (*meta-* means change; *bolus* refers to mass; *-ism* means condition). Metabolism is the sum total of the process of *anabolism* (*ana-* means building up) and *catabolism* (*cata-* means breaking down). When metabolism ceases, the organism dies.

All living matter is irritable and excitable; it reacts to stimulation. With appropriate stimulation, nerve cells conduct impulses; muscle cells contract; and gland cells secrete substances.

CELLS

Understanding the structure and function of the body begins with the smallest unit of life, the cell. Specialized cells carry out the functions of growth, secretion, excretion, irritability, nutrition, and reproduction. They are activated by mechanical, chemical, or nervous stimulation.

Composition of Cells

Each cell of the body is enclosed by a membrane called the *plasma membrane.* This membrane protects the internal structure of the cell and regulates the passage of materials in and out of the cell. Inside the membrane is a jellylike substance, *cytoplasm,* surrounding a centrally located body, the *nucleus* (Figure 5.1).

The cytoplasm contains *fibers* that provide a lattice type of framework for the cell and also contains huge numbers of *organelles* (little organs) outside the nucleus, including the following:

The *endoplasmic reticulum* is a network of canals consisting of smooth and rough portions. The smooth portion manufactures carbohydrates and some fats. Attached to the rough portion are thousands of granules called *ribosomes,* made up of ribonucleic acid *(RNA).* The ribosomes make proteins before passing them on to the Golgi apparatus.

The *Golgi apparatus* consists of vesicles, or small sacs, believed to manufacture carbohydrates and combine them with protein in a closed globule that is secreted by the cell.

The *mitochondria* are microscopic sacs with enzyme molecules attached to their membranous walls. These enzymes are considered to be the "power plants" of the cell, supplying its energy.

The *lysosomes* are membranous closed sacs containing enzymes capable of digesting large molecules and particles for use by the cell. They also protect the cell by digesting invading bacteria by *phagocytosis* (*phago-* means eating).

The nucleus, enclosed in a membrane called the *nuclear membrane,* is a spheroid (round), centrally located body, that is highly specialized, regulating growth and reproduction. It contains deoxyribonucleic acid *(DNA)* molecules, which form the *genes* that determine heredity. During cell division, the DNA molecules become short and rodlike and are then called *chromosomes.*

There are 46 chromosomes (23 pairs) in all human cells, with the exception of mature sex cells, which only have half this number (23). At conception, the mature male and female reproductive (sex) cells unite, each contributing a chance combination of 23 chromosomes out of innumerable possible combinations. This explains why no two individuals are alike, except in the case of identical twins.

The *nucleolus* is a round body within the nucleus, consisting mainly of RNA. Its function is to combine RNA with protein to form the ribosomes.

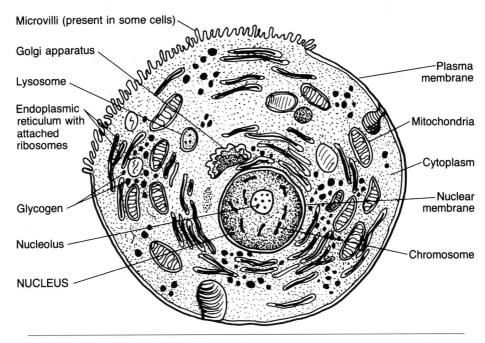

Figure 5.1 Diagram of a cell showing cellular structures, as seen with the electron microscope.

R E V I E W   5 . A

Complete the following:

1. The six branches of science that deal with the study of the body are _Anatomy_ , _physiology_, _pathology_, _Embryology_, _Histology_ , and _Biology_ .

2. The smallest unit of life is _the cell_ .

3. The body is maintained by a process called _methabolism_ .

4. Specialized cells are activated by _mechanical_ _chemical_ , or _nervous_ stimulation.

5. The _genes_ determine heredity.

6. There are _23_ chromosomes in a mature sex cell.

7. The nucleus regulates _growth_ and _reproduction_ .

8. Cells similar in structure and function form a(n) _mass called a tissue._

9. All living matter is _irritable_ and _excitable_ .

10. The membrane enclosing each cell of the body is the _nuclear_ membrane.

TISSUES

Tissues are groups of specialized cells that are similar in structure and function but have different characteristics in accordance with their function. The basic types of tissue are *epithelial, connective, muscle,* and *nervous.*

Epithelial Tissue

Epithelial tissue (*epi-* means upon, on, or over) is found throughout the human body. It makes up the outer covering of external and internal body surfaces such as the skin; mucous membranes; serous membranes; and the lining of the digestive, respiratory, and urinary tracts.

The main functions of epithelial tissue are to protect, absorb, and secrete. For example, the skin protects underlying structures; other types allow substances to pass through them and serve as absorbing tissue (lungs and intestines) or secreting tissue (mucous membranes and glands).

A special type of epithelial tissue called *endothelium* (*endo-* means within or inner) lines the heart, blood and lymph vessels, and other serous body cavities. *Mesothelium* (*meso-* means middle), another type of epithelial tissue, covers the surface of serous membranes (pleura, pericardium, and peritoneum).

There are various types of epithelial tissue, classified according to the number of layers of cells:

Simple epithelial tissue has one layer of cells.
Stratified epithelial tissue has three or more layers of cells.
Pseudostratified epithelial tissue has one layer of cells but appears to have more.

Epithelial tissue is also classified according to the shape of the surface layer of the cells:

Squamous cells have a flat appearance.
Cuboidal cells have a cubelike appearance.
Columnar cells resemble columns.
Transitional cells vary from squamous to cuboidal because they are found only in the urinary tract and change appearance according to the amount of pressure to which they are subjected.

Three types of epithelial tissue are illustrated in Figure 5.2. All types are composed largely or entirely of cells that undergo *mitosis* (cell division) for the replacement of old or damaged cells.

Connective Tissue

Connective tissue, the most widespread tissue, props and shapes the body, holds organs in place, and con-

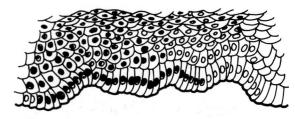

Stratified squamous epithelium

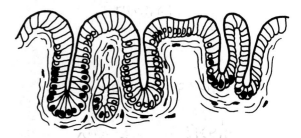

Simple columnar epithelium

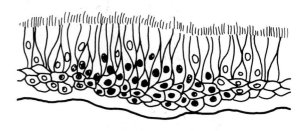

Pseudostratified ciliated columnar epithelium

Figure 5.2 Types of epithelial tissue.

nects body parts to each other (Figure 5.3). The main types of connective tissue are:

bone—hard and unbendable (supports and protects the body).
cartilage—firm, but bendable (found throughout the body).
dense fibrous—strong, bendable (mostly tendons and ligaments).
areolar (loose, ordinary)—elastic, stretchable, weblike network of fibers and cells providing support for internal organs.
adipose—fatty tissue (pads and protects organs, stores excess fat, and insulates against body heat loss).
hematopoietic—specialized connective tissue that forms both red and white blood cells. (See also Chapters 6 and 17.)
blood—although liquid, classified as connective tissue; is found in the blood vessels (Chapter 9).

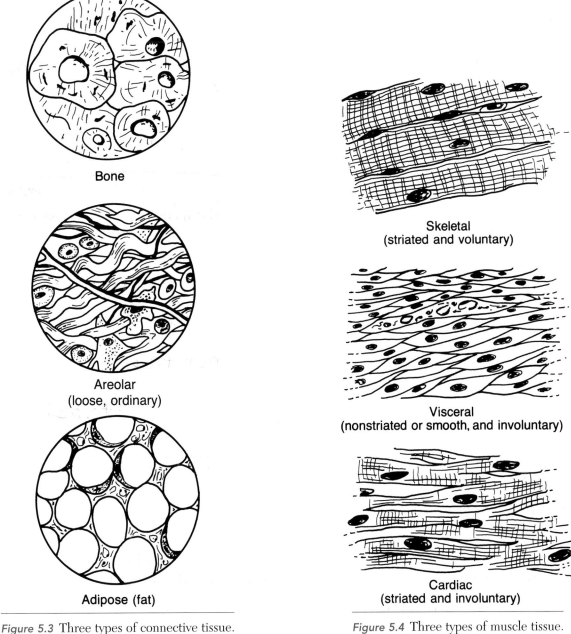

Bone

Areolar
(loose, ordinary)

Adipose (fat)

Figure 5.3 Three types of connective tissue.

Skeletal
(striated and voluntary)

Visceral
(nonstriated or smooth, and involuntary)

Cardiac
(striated and involuntary)

Figure 5.4 Three types of muscle tissue.

Muscle Tissue

There are three types of muscle tissue: *skeletal*, which is striated (striped) and voluntary (movable at will); *visceral*, which is nonstriated (smooth) and involuntary; and *cardiac*, which is striated but involuntary. Skeletal muscles move bones. Visceral muscles are located in the walls of hollow internal structures (blood vessels, intestines, and the uterus). Cardiac muscle makes up the heart (Figure 5.4).

The main function of muscle tissue is to contract. Muscle cells are long and slender and are called fibers. The fibers decrease in length and increase in thickness during contraction of a muscle.

Nervous Tissue

Nervous tissue is composed of nerve cells called *neurons*, which consist of *dendrites*, *cell bodies*, and *axons*, and supporting tissue between the cells to keep them in position (Figure 5.5). The supporting structure of nervous tissue is called *neuroglia* (*neuro-* means nerve; *-glia* means glue). Nervous tissue is the most highly specialized tissue in the body, requiring more oxygen and more nutrition than any other body tissue (Chapter 15).

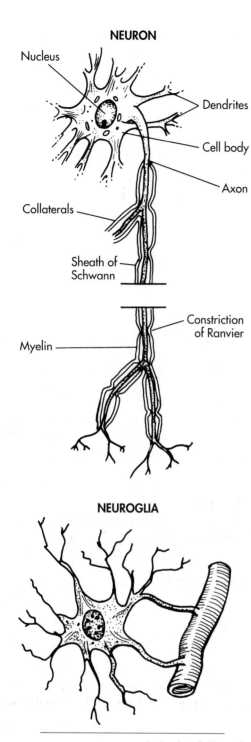

NEURON

Nucleus

Dendrites

Cell body

Axon

Collaterals

Sheath of Schwann

Constriction of Ranvier

Myelin

NEUROGLIA

Figure 5.5 Structure of nerve cells.

REVIEW 5.B

Complete the following:

1. The basic types of tissue are <u>epithelial</u>, <u>connective</u>, and <u>muscle</u>.

2. The most widespread tissue in the body is <u>Epithelial</u> tissue.

3. Three types of epithelial tissue classified by numbers of layers of cells are <u>simple</u>, <u>stratified</u>, and <u>pseudostratified</u>.

4. The three types of muscle tissue are <u>cardiac</u>, <u>skeletal</u>, and <u>visceral (smooth)</u>.

5. <u>neuroglia</u> is the supporting structure of nervous tissue.

6. <u>hematopoietic</u> tissue is found in bone marrow.

7. Striated means <u>striped</u>.

8. The main functions of epithelial tissue are to <u>protect</u>, <u>absorb</u>, and <u>secrete</u>.

9. A type of cell varying from squamous to cuboidal is a(n) <u>transitional</u> cell.

10. Nervous tissue is composed of nerve cells called <u>neurons</u>.

ORGANS

In the body, groups of cells form tissues, and similar tissues form organs (for example, the heart, lungs, liver, and kidneys). Organs, although they act as individual units, do not function independently; several combine to form a system, with each system having a special function.

SYSTEMS

A system is a combination of organs that performs a particular function. The systems of the body and their functions are:

skeletal—framework of the body, supporting organs and furnishing a place of attachment for muscles.

muscular—permits motion/movement of the body.

integumentary—includes skin, hair, nails, and sweat and sebaceous glands; covers and protects the body, aids in temperature regulation, and has functions in sensation and excretion.

cardiovascular—transports the blood.

lymphatic—retrieves plasma and tissue fluids and has a role in the immune system.

respiratory—absorbs oxygen and discharges carbon dioxide.

gastrointestinal—digests and absorbs food and excretes waste.

genitourinary—reproduction and urine excretion.

endocrine—manufactures hormones.

nervous with the *special senses*—processes stimuli and enables the body to act and respond.

immune—protects the body from invading organisms and disease.

TUMORS

The term *tumor* or *neoplasm* (*neo-* means new; *-plasm* means formation) refers to the development of abnormal new tissue. Normal cells in a tissue, organ, or system interact with each other to regulate growth, cell reproduction, structure, and size. *Genes* are the basic units of heredity. In the cell nucleus, DNA in the form of inherited genes is the source of this regulation. One type of gene, called an *oncogene,* promotes cell reproduction and growth; another type of gene, called a *tumor suppressor gene* inhibits or suppresses cell growth. Tumors arise from *mutations* (changes) to either or both of these two major types of genes. Oncogenes may be stimulated to produce excessive growth. Tumor suppressor genes may be inactivated and unable to restrain or inhibit cell growth and proliferation. Normal cells have limited life cycles for reproduction built into their genetic makeup and are also subject to internal and intercellular controls that keep them in place in the tissue or organ. Cell death may occur at the end of the normal life cycle or by suicide (*apoptosis*) prematurely triggered by external agents (*apo-* means separation from; *-ptosis* means dropping). Cells that live beyond their normal time, continuing to reproduce excessively, form tumors.

Tumors may be *benign* (noncancerous) or *malignant* (cancerous). Benign tumors are *hyperplasias* (overgrowths) of cells that do not invade or establish new tumors or *metastases* (singular—*metastasis*; *meta-* means beyond; *-stasis* means standing) in other tissues or organs. *Malignant tumors* (cancers), by contrast, are characterized by the tendency of tumor cells to break away from the *primary site* (original tumor) and *metastasize* (invade) to *secondary sites* (other tissues or organs of the body), usually via the circulatory and lymphatic systems. Cancers may develop from inherent genetic flaws, from natural, internally produced chemicals, and from environmental agents that damage genes or directly stimulate tumor growth. These agents include viruses, bacteria, parasites, sunlight, x-rays, and chemical *carcinogens* (*carcino-* means cancer; *-gen* means producing) such as benzene, formaldehyde, tobacco, and alcohol.

Grading and Staging of Malignant Tumors

For diagnostic and treatment purposes, malignant tumors are described by *grade* (extent of growth and development) and *stage* (degree of spread).

There are four grades. *Grade I* has the best survival rate, *grade II* is more life threatening, *grade III* has an even poorer prognosis, and *grade IV* has the worst survival rate.

Staging is based on the extent of metastasis, most commonly described by the *TNM* system developed by the American Joint Committee for Cancer Staging and End Results Reporting. *T* refers to tumor, *N* refers to lymph node involvement, and *M* refers to extent of metastasis, with numerical subscripts from 0 to 4 indicating degree of severity in each category. For example $T_1 N_0 M_0$ describes a small tumor with no lymph node involvement and no metastasis; $T_2 N_2 M_1$ describes a larger tumor with lymph node involvement and metastasis.

Other systems of classification are described in the list of Related Terms in Chapters 8 and 11 on the integumentary system and the gastrointestinal system.

Common Metastases

Although all the factors in metastasis of cancer cells are not known, the lymphatic and circulatory systems are known to be involved. For example, the circulation of blood to the lungs provides a common site for metastases from the skin and other organs; blood from the intestines goes to the liver, a common metastatic site for colorectal cancers; and prostate cancer usually metastasizes to the bones. Specific malignancies within the individual systems will be found in the appropriate list of Related Terms.

DIRECTIONS, ANATOMIC PLANES, AND POSITIONS

A number of anatomic terms are used in describing the body and determining direction. The terms listed in the following section refer to the anatomic position, with the body standing erect and the arms hanging to the side, palms facing forward (Figure 5.6). A plane refers to a flat surface formed by an imaginary sectioning of the body in the anatomic position.

Directions

anterior—ventral (or front) surface of the body.
posterior—dorsal (or back) surface of the body.
medial—nearer to or toward the midline.
lateral—farther from the midline or to the side of the body.
internal—inside.
external—outside.
proximal—nearer to the point of origin or closer to the body.

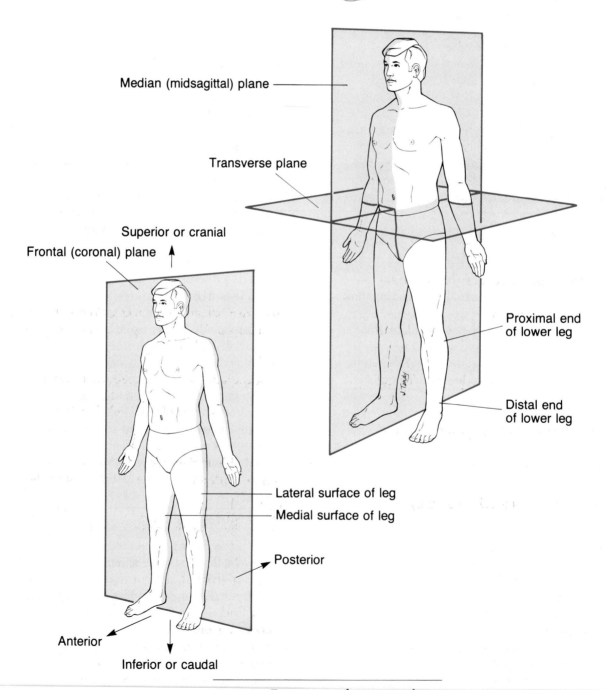

Median (midsagittal) plane

Transverse plane

Superior or cranial

Frontal (coronal) plane

Proximal end of lower leg

Distal end of lower leg

Lateral surface of leg

Medial surface of leg

Posterior

Anterior

Inferior or caudal

Figure 5.6 Directions and anatomic planes.

distal—away from the point of origin or away from the body.

superior—above.

inferior—below.

cranial—toward the head.

caudal—toward the lower end of the body (*cauda* means tail).

Anatomic Planes

frontal (coronal) plane—a section through the side of the body, passing at right angles to the median plane and dividing the body into anterior and posterior portions.

median (midsagittal, midline) plane—a section that passes from the front to the back through the center of the body and divides the body into right and left equal portions.

sagittal plane—a section parallel to the long axis of the body, or parallel to the median plane, dividing the body into right and left unequal parts.

transverse plane—a horizontal section passing at right angles to both the frontal and median planes and dividing the body into cranial and caudal parts.

Anatomic Positions

Numerous terms describe anatomic positions. Some of the more frequently used ones are listed below:

erect—standing position.

Fowler's—head of bed raised, knees elevated.

knee-chest (genupectoral)—kneeling, with chest resting on same surface.

lateral recumbent (Sims')—lying on left side with right thigh and knee drawn up.

prone—lying face down.

Trendelenburg's—inclined position with head lower than body and legs.

supine (dorsal)—lying flat on back.

Body Regions (Figure 5.7, A and B)

Head

auricular—around the ears.

buccal—the cheeks.

infraorbital—immediately below the eyes.

mental—the chin.

occipital—back part of the head.

orbital—around the eyes.

submaxillary—either side of the submental, below the ramus of the mandible.

submental—below the chin.

supraorbital—above the eyebrows.

Thorax and abdomen

axillary—axilla (armpit) and its borders.

clavicular—on either side of the sternum (breastbone), extending the length of the clavicle (collarbone).

epigastric—area within the costal (rib) arch, located in the median part of the abdomen.

hypochondriac—right and left areas on either side of the epigastric region.

hypogastric—in the lower abdomen between the inguinal regions, lying between and below the iliac spines.

infraclavicular—below the clavicle.

inguinal (iliac)—triangular area on either side of the hypogastric region.

lateral abdominal (lumbar)—on either side of the umbilical region.

mammary—breasts, on either side of the chest between the third and sixth ribs, extending below the lower margins of the pectoralis major muscles on either side.

pubic—the central portion of the hypogastric region, above the pubis.

sternal—over the front of the sternum.

subinguinal—just below the inguinal region.

supraclavicular—above the clavicle.

umbilical—medial abdominal region, above the hypogastric region.

Posterior trunk

coxal—just below the lumbar regions in the back and lateral abdominal regions on either side; bordered by gluteal regions (area over the buttocks).

infrascapular—below the scapulae (shoulder blades), extending down to the last ribs.

interscapular—part of the medial region of the back, between the scapulae, on either side of the vertebral column.

lumbar—immediately below the infrascapular region, extending down to the crest of the ilium.

medial region of back—central zone of the back, extending from the neck as far down as the base of the sacrum.

nuchal—back of the neck beginning just below the occipital (back of head) region, extending down to the spine of the seventh cervical vertebra.

sacral—area over the sacrum at the base of the medial region.

scapular—areas on either side, covering the scapula.

suprascapular—areas on either side above the scapular region, extending to the curve of the neck.

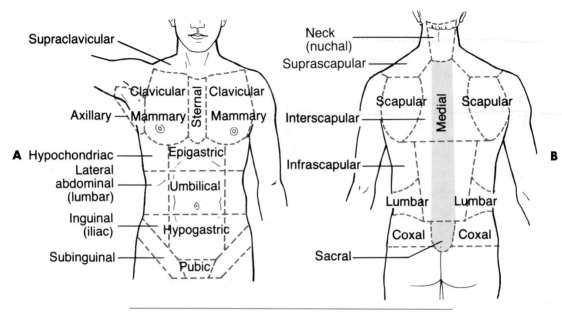

Figure 5.7 Body regions. **A,** Anterior view. **B,** Posterior view.

REVIEW 5.C

Complete the following:

1. The systems of the body are Skeletal, Muscular, integumentary, Cardiovascular, lymphatic, respiratory, gastrointestinal, genitourinary, endocrine, nervous, immune.

2. A type of gene promoting cell reproduction and growth is the Oncogene.

3. A cancerous tumor is a(n) malignant tumor.

4. *Cranial* means toward the head.

5. *Distal* is the opposite of Proximal.

6. The four anatomic planes of the body are frontal, median, Sagittal, and transverse planes.

7. *Prone* means lying face down.

8. The Interscapular region is between the scapulae on either side of the vertebral column.

9. auricular refers to the region around the ears.

10. Several Organs combine to form a system.

11. The *genupectoral* is also called the Knee-Chest position.

12. The framework of the body is formed by the Skeletal system.

Beginning with this chapter, a Related Terms list (word list with definitions), with phonetic pronunciation guides, will be found in each chapter to help the student understand the terms that relate to the preceding material. Each list is organized according to its text, with some review material and some additions, including anatomic terms, diseases, conditions, procedures, and other descriptive terms.

■ RELATED TERMS UNDERSTANDING THE BODY AND ITS STRUCTURE

adipose tissue (ad'i-pos) fatty connective tissue such as that found in the buttocks and abdominal walls.

apoptosis (a-po-toe'sis) cell suicide or self-destruction.

areolar tissue (ah-re'o-lar) type of connective tissue consisting of stretchable, weblike networks of fibers and cells providing support for internal organs.

axon (ak'son) essential conducting part of a nerve fiber.

benign not progressive or invasive, opposite of malignant.

bony tissue dense connective tissue that forms the skeletal framework of the body.

carcinogen (kar-sin"o-jen) a cancer-producing agent.

cardiac muscle tissue heart muscle.

cartilage (kar'ti-lij) firm, elastic, somewhat dense connective tissue that forms many parts of the skeleton.

cell body that part of a neuron containing the nucleus.

centrosome (sen'tro-som) area of cell cytoplasm near the nucleus, containing centrioles (minute cells), which play an important part in mitosis (cell division).

chromosomes (kro'mo-somz) rodlike bodies in the nucleus, composed mainly of DNA and containing the genes, which transmit the hereditary codes.

collaterals small side branches of an axon.

columnar epithelium (ko-lum'nar ep"i-the'le-um) cells arranged in one layer, resembling columns.

connective tissue forms the framework of the body, holds organs in place, and connects body parts to each other.

cuboidal epithelium surface layer of cells, having a cubelike appearance.

cytoplasm (si'to-plazm") jellylike substance of a cell, within the plasma membrane, surrounding the nucleus.

dense fibrous tissue strong, pliant connective tissue of the body, found where organs are subjected to stress or strain.

dendrite part of a neuron that conducts impulses toward the cell body.

deoxyribonucleic acid (DNA) (de-ok'se-ri"bo-nu-kle'ic) large molecule that is the main constituent of chromosomes.

endothelium (en"do-the'le-um) layer of simple squamous cells lining the inner surfaces of the circulatory organs and serous body cavities.

enzyme (en'zim) protein able to catalyze (speed up or change) chemical reactions in living cells.

epithelium (ep"i-the'le-um) epithelial tissue covering the external and internal body surfaces.

gene basic DNA molecule that is responsible for heredity.

Golgi (gol'je) apparatus cellular component of the cytoplasm, believed to condense substances before they leave the cell as secretions.

inorganic matter mineral.

invertebrate (in-ver"te-brate) division of the animal kingdom, including all organisms with no backbone.

involuntary muscle tissue muscle tissue that cannot be controlled at will; types are visceral (nonstriated, smooth), and cardiac (striated, striped).

lysosomes (li'so-somz) microscopic membranous sacs in the cytoplasm that contain enzymes capable of phagocytosis (ingestion and digestion for nutrition and protection of the cell).

malignant cancerous, opposite of benign in relation to tumor.

mesothelium (mes"o-the'le-um) epithelial tissue covering the serous membranes that line the abdominal and chest cavities.

metabolism (me-tab'o-lizm) sum of all physical and chemical processes by which living organisms are maintained.

metastasis (me-tas′tah-sis) invasion of malignant cells from a primary site to a secondary site.

mitochondria (mi′to-kon′dre-ah) component of the cytoplasm, containing enzymes that are considered to be the source of supply of energy for the cell (also called *chondriosomes*).

mitosis (mi-to′sis) process of cell division.

molecule (mol′e-kul) chemical combination of two or more atoms that form a specific chemical substance (DNA and RNA are molecules).

mutation transformation or change in genes, often resulting in growth pattern changes in cells.

neoplasm abnormal tissue growth, tumor.

nervous tissue tissue composing nerves and nerve centers.

nucleolus (nu-kle′o-lus) spherical body within the nucleus, composed mainly of RNA and some protein (plural, *nucleoli*).

nucleus (nu′kle-us) spheroid body in the cell, containing the chromosomes and nucleoli (plural, *nuclei*).

oncogene (ong′ko-jean) cell gene responsible for growth; mutation stimulates overgrowth or tumor.

organic matter animal and vegetable (living) matter.

phagocytosis (fag″o-si-to′sis) ingestion and digestion of particulate matter by cells.

primary site original site of tumor formation in a tissue or organ.

ribonucleic acid (RNA) (ri″bo-nu-kle′ik) a nucleic acid, similar to DNA, that relates to the function of the ribosomes.

ribosomes (ri′bo-somz) organelles (tiny organs) in the cytoplasm, attached to the endoplasmic reticulum, that build and transmit proteins.

secondary site cancer (malignancy) that has invaded from a primary site.

squamous epithelium (skwa′mus) flat epithelial cells arranged in one or more layers.

stratified epithelium cells arranged in three or more layers; may be columnar or squamous.

striated (stri′at-ed) striped.

transitional epithelium a tissue made up of cells varying from squamous to cuboidal according to the amount of pressure to which they are subjected.

tumor suppressor gene cell gene that inhibits or suppresses cell growth and reproduction.

vertebrate (ver″te-brate) division of the animal kingdom comprising all animals that have a vertebral column or backbone, including mammals, reptiles, fish, and birds.

voluntary muscle tissue striated muscle tissue that can be controlled at will (also called skeletal muscle).

EXERCISES   UNDERSTANDING THE BODY AND ITS STRUCTURE

Exercise 5.1   *Complete the following:*

1. Specialized cells that are similar in structure and functions are assembled into a(n) ___tissue___ .
2. Groups of different tissue are combined to form a(n) ___organ___ .
3. For the purpose of performing specific functions, the organs are grouped into a(n) ___system___ .
4. The smallest unit of life and the building block for tissues, organs, and systems is called a(n) ___cell___ .
5. The body is maintained by a process called ___metabolism___ .
6. A special type of epithelial tissue, called ___endothelium___ , lines the heart, blood and lymph vessels, and other serous body cavities.
7. The most highly specialized tissue in the body is ___nervous___ tissue.
8. Cells arranged in three or more layers are called ___stratified epithelial tissue___ .
9. The connective tissue of the body making up tendons and ligaments is called ___dense fibrous___ .
10. The number of chromosomes in a human cell is ___46___ .
11. The original site of a tumor is known as a(n) ___primary___ site.
12. The spread of tumor cells to other areas is known as ___metastasis___ .

Exercise 5.2   *Matching*

C ___ **1.** neoplasm	**A.** face down
G ___ **2.** mutation	**B.** head
F ___ **3.** ventral	**C.** new formation
E ___ **4.** distal	**D.** standing up
B ___ **5.** cranial	**E.** ends of fingers
L ___ **6.** caudal	**F.** front
A ___ **7.** prone	**G.** changes
K ___ **8.** supine	**H.** right and left epigastric area
D ___ **9.** erect	**I.** either side of umbilical region
H ___ **10.** hypochondriac	**J.** breast area of chest
I ___ **11.** lateral abdominal	**K.** face up
J ___ **12.** mammary	**L.** lower end of body

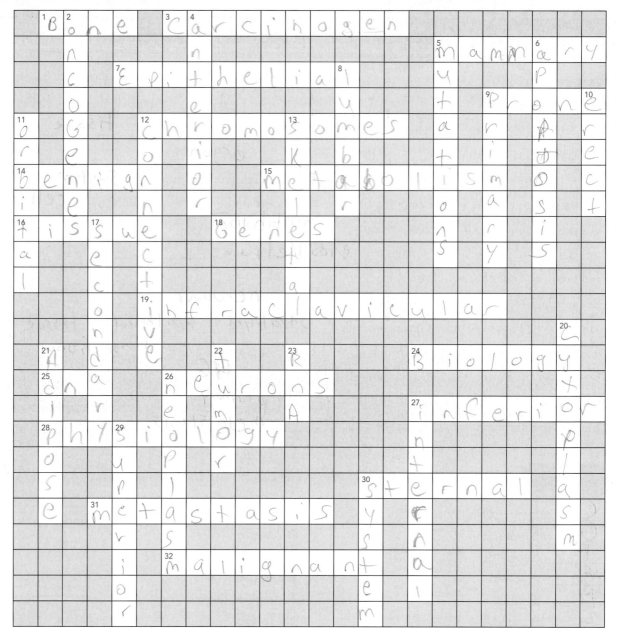

ACROSS

1. Type of hard connective tissue
3. Cancer-producing agent
5. Breast
7. One of four basic types of tissue
9. Face down
12. 23 pairs in each cell
14. Noncancerous
15. Process by which the body is maintained
16. Formed by a group of cells
18. Basic units of heredity
19. Below the clavicles
24. Study of all forms of life
25. These molecules become chromosomes during cell division
26. Nerve cells
27. Below
28. Study of the body's normal functions and activities
30. Area over breastbone
31. Invasion of cancerous tumors
32. Cancerous

DOWN

2. Promote cell reproduction and growth
4. Ventral or front surface of body
5. Changes
6. Cell death
8. Region between scapula and ilium
9. Original tumor site
10. Standing position
11. Region around the eyes
12. Another of four basic tissue types
13. Voluntary striped muscle tissue
17. Location of metastasis
20. Jellylike substance of cells
21. Fatty tissue
22. May be benign or cancerous
23. Ribonucleic acid
26. Development of abnormal new tissue
27. Inside
29. Above
30. Formed by a group of organs

HIDDEN WORDS PUZZLE   CHAPTER 5

Can you find the 20 words hidden in this puzzle? All hidden words puzzles have words running from top to bottom, left to right, and diagonally downward.

HEMATOPOIETIC

EPITHELIAL

PATHOLOGY

NERVOUS

MUSCLE

CHROMOSOMES

METABOLISM

POSITIONS

NUCLEUS

PLANES

CONNECTIVE

PHYSIOLOGY

ANATOMY

REGIONS

BLOOD

EMBRYOLOGY

HISTOLOGY

BIOLOGY

TISSUES

CELL

```
J O Q D U Y N R T U F J O A B Q V L K Y T H H A Q
O R J F L X R R I C A B F P X T M T V I G E Q X R
P E Y W F D D M S H N N G N U C L E U S Q P F L J
R T X T J N N U S X A V T E L Y W G Q B F Y T C Y
F N K H O T W R U F T Q F R B H H F R R T X X N N
X B H W O V X E E K O M Q V Y I A P U M T O I Y S
W L C H R O M O S O M E S O D S P C L U O A H P L
C O N N E C T I V E Y R N U J T T K S A R I Y F I
E O D B M M G V V Y P H Y S I O L O G Y D G N M C
L D B K B K A C J V F I S J F L G N S I R D M U D
L A D A R I M T Y V M E T A B O L I S M X R R E W
Z B H Y Y T G S O E C W E H W G R A W U D Z D V V
J O H P O T I N T P G F K E E Y M E O H T B C H F
N K Q O L K D L K L O M U S C L E L G J M B N U K
W O F R O A X Y O A R I O K B U I P K I S V R M J
M S E N G R N D F U S Q E T Z I P A T H O L O G Y
X A Z P Y P V E I J I W V T C N O L L X R N E D E
Q W S J I D L E S C Q N K H I K S L O J K N S W M
X N M D X W O Z J R E E D W H C I B O X H X Y X F
O S V J Y L H O Z S K G X F Q X T U W G V Y H H N
L K M O Q X M X N T Y U H P B V I Q B K Y Y Y O V
V S D V I M U H M P W X J V V M O T O X L I T X X
U W Y S T F V W G H K E Y U G Z N P L R R L I C S
C K A L P I H W U I Q A Y O E B S K Q N D W L W E
```

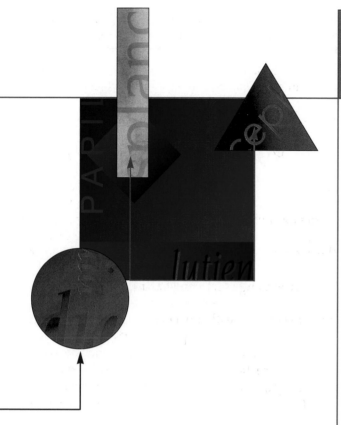

The Skeletal System

the framework of the body

This chapter describes the bones of the body, which make up the skeleton, and the ways in which they connect and are moved, relative to structure, classification, and location.

SKELETON

The skeleton is the jointed framework, made up of 206 bones, that supports and gives shape to the body. This framework helps to protect vital and delicate organs from external injury and furnishes attachment points for muscles, ligaments, and tendons, making movement possible. Bones store mineral salts, and some bones contain the hematopoietic (blood cell–forming) red bone marrow.

The study of bone is called *osteology* (*oss-* and *ost-* are roots meaning bone).

Composition of Bone

Bone (*osseous* tissue), a specialized form of connective tissue, is about 50% water and 50% solid matter. Part of the solid matter consists of inorganic (mineral) salts, which give bone its hardness. When the embryonic skeleton is first formed, it is made of cartilage and fibrous membrane in the shape of bones, which harden and become bone before birth. Because this ossifying process takes up to 25 years to complete, the bones of children are more flexible and less subject to fracture than mature adult bones. The inorganic matter that gives bone its hardness contains higher proportions of lime as the body ages, causing the bones to become brittle and more easily fractured in old age.

Structure of Bone

The bone structure consists of a hard outer shell called *compact bone tissue* and an inner, spongy, latticelike structure called *cancellated* or *cancellous bone*. The dense compact bone is thick in the midshaft to avoid bending under stress and tapers to paper thinness at the ends. When a long bone in an adult is sectioned longitudinally, the *medullary cavity* (innermost part) of the *diaphysis* (shaft) is seen to be filled with yellow marrow, which stores fat. The yellow marrow has replaced red marrow, which is hematopoietic (blood cell–forming) tissue containing

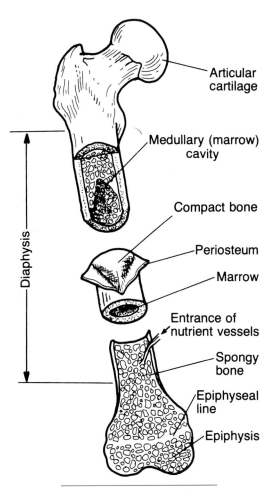

Figure 6.1 Structure of bone.

red blood cells in various stages of growth (Figure 6.1). In the adult, red marrow has mostly disappeared, except for that found in spaces in cancellated bone such as the flat bones of the skull, pelvis, vertebrae, ribs, and sternum and the upper ends of the shafts of the humerus and femur.

The surfaces of bone, with the exception of the cartilage-covered articular surfaces, are covered by a tough, fibrous, vascular membrane called the *periosteum,* which is very thick except where muscles are attached to the bone. The outer layer is vascular, and the inner layer in the growing bone is lined with *osteoblasts* (immature bone cells). The deposition of bone from this layer of osteoblasts on the surface of the shaft provides for growth of bone and for repair when a bone is fractured. The periosteum also provides a confining membrane for the bone. It contains numerous blood vessels that enter the canals of the bone to supply it with nutrients. If the periosteum is removed, the bone is deprived of its nutrition and dies. Periosteum is regenerative, except in the skull, where, if a section is removed, a plate must be used to fill the gap. Numerous nerves in the periosteum account for the pain experienced after an injury to a bone.

Arteries that nourish bone tunnel into the medullary (bone marrow) cavity and make *anastomoses* (connections) with the numerous blood vessels of the periosteum. The bones have a poor capillary network but have many minute arterioles. Venous blood of the marrow and bone is returned to the circulation by numerous large veins that leave the bone by *foramina* (openings) at the extremities.

Growth of Bone

The long bones grow in length at the junctions of the *epiphyses* (ends of the developing bones) and the *diaphyses* (shafts) and grow in thickness, through the activity of the osteoblasts, in the deep layers of the periosteum. Growth of the long bones is produced by the growth of cartilage followed by deposits of bone to the diaphyses along the epiphyseal line. Growth of bone is controlled by a hormone secreted by the anterior lobe of the pituitary gland.

Growth of bone is precisely balanced by the teamwork of the osteoblasts and *osteoclasts* (large phagocytic cells). The osteoblasts produce bony tissue, and the osteoclasts eat away bony tissue in the medullary cavity, preventing the bone from becoming too thick. Healthy bone is constantly being broken down, reabsorbed, and repaired, but the process slows down with increasing age.

CLASSIFICATION OF BONES

Bones are classified according to their shape—long, flat, short, and irregular. The *femur* (bone between the hip joint and the knee) and the *humerus* (bone between the shoulder and the elbow) are examples of long bones. The short bones are those of the *carpals* (wrist) and *tarsals* (ankle bones). The flat bones are those of the *sternum* (breastbone), *scapula* (shoulder blade), and *pelvis.* The *vertebrae* are examples of irregular bones.

The skeleton of the human body (Figures 6.2 and 6.3) is divided into two main parts, *axial* and *appen-*

dicular. The axial skeleton has 80 bones and forms the vertical axis of the body. These bones include the 28 bones of the *skull*, the *hyoid* bone (U-shaped bone located in the neck), the *vertebral column, ribs,* and *sternum.* The appendicular skeleton is made up of the 126 bones that support the extremities: *clavicle, scapula, humerus, radius, ulna, carpals, metacarpals, phalanges* (fingers), *pelvic girdle, femur, patella, tibia, fibula, tarsals, metatarsals,* and *phalanges* (toes).

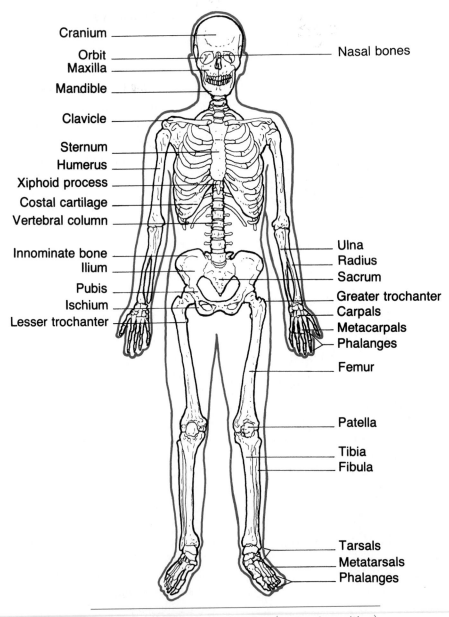

Figure 6.2 Skeleton, anterior view (anatomic position).

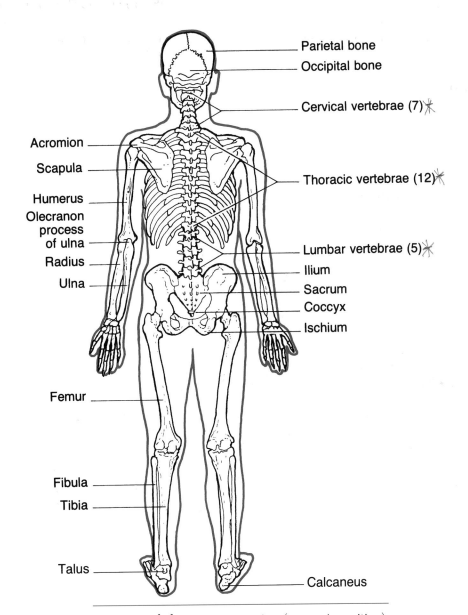

Figure 6.3 Skeleton, posterior view (anatomic position).

REVIEW 6.A

Complete the following:

1. The skeleton is made up of ___206___ bones.

2. The shaft of long bones is called the ___ ___diaphysis___.

3. Bone marrow is contained in the ___ ___medullary___ cavity of long bones.

4. The outer membrane covering bones is called ___periosteum___.

5. Immature bone cells are called ___osteoblasts___

6. Bones are classified according to shapes, which are ___long, flat, short, irregular___.

7. The humerus is an example of a(n) ___ ___long___ bone.

8. The carpals and tarsals are classified as ___ ___short___ bones.

9. The two main parts of the skeleton are the ___axial___ and the ___appendicular___.

10. The U-shaped bone in the neck is called the ___hyoid___ bone.

Structural Descriptive Terms of Bones

canal—tunnel.
condyle—rounded projection.
crest, crista—high ridge.
facet—small, smooth area.
foramen—(plural, foramina) opening or hole.
fossa, fovea—basinlike depression.
head—rounded eminence or projection.
line—low ridge.
meatus—passage or opening.
process—any projection.
sinus—cavity or channel.
spine—sharp projection.
sulcus—open, ditchlike groove.
suture—seam.
trochanter—broad, flat process.
tubercle—small, rounded eminence.
tuberosity—protuberance (swelling or knob).

AXIAL SKELETON

Skull

The skull includes two major segments, the *cranium* (brain case) and the facial framework. There are 8 bones in the cranium, 14 in the face, and 6 *ossicles* (small bones) in the ears (Figure 6.4). The skull protects the brain and the organs of special sense—hearing, sight, taste, and smell. All the bones of the skull are immobile except the *mandible* (lower jawbone).

The bones of the skull are united by *sutures* (seams). In the newborn there are membranes covering two areas where bony tissue has not yet formed, leaving soft spots called *fontanels* (little fountains). The *coronal suture* separates the *frontal bone* from the two *parietal bones* and leaves a membrane-covered, diamond-shaped area called the *anterior fontanel,* which can be seen rising and falling with the heartbeat of the infant. At the age of 10 to 18 months this fontanel closes. The *occipital fontanel,* located at the back of the head, closes by 2 months of age. The sutures, which initially are joined by cartilage to permit the growth of the brain, ossify by about 25 years of age.

Within the bones of the skull and the face are hollows called *sinuses,* which lessen the bone weight, provide resonating chambers for the voice, and moisten and warm incoming air.

Cranial bones

The *frontal* bone forms the forehead and helps form the *orbits* (eye sockets) and the front part of the cranial floor. The two cavities within this bone are called the *frontal sinuses.* The *coronal suture* separates the frontal from . . .

Two *parietal* bones, forming the roof of the skull and upper part of each side, that are separated from each other by the *sagittal suture.* These bones are separated from . . .

The *occipital* bone by the *lambdoid suture.* The occipital bone forms the back of the skull as well as the base. In the base is a large opening, the *foramen magnum* (meaning large hole or opening), for the passage of the spinal cord from the skull into the spine.

Two *temporal* bones form part of the cranial floor and the lower part of the sides. These bones

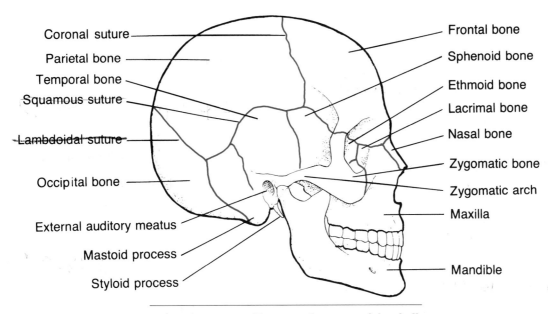

Figure 6.4 Principal bones and sutures of the skull.

contain the middle and inner ear structures and the *mastoid sinuses.*

The *sphenoid,* a butterfly-shaped bone at the base of the skull, extends laterally to support parts of the orbits and forms the lateral walls of the skull. It contains the *sphenoid sinuses.*

The *ethmoid* bone lies in front of the sphenoid but behind the nasal bones of the face, forming the front of the base of the skull, the medial walls of the orbits, and part of the roof and lateral walls of the nose. It contains the *ethmoid sinuses.*

Facial bones

Two *maxillary* bones form the upper jaw, nose, orbits, and roof of the mouth. Located within these bones are the *maxillary sinuses,* which connect with the nose.

Two *zygomatic* or *malar* bones (cheekbones) have chewing muscles attached to them.

Two *lacrimal* bones located at the inner corners of the eyes form bony channels through which tear ducts drain into the nasal cavity.

Two *nasal* bones form the upper part of the bridge of the nose.

The *vomer* is the thin, flat bone that forms the lower part of the nasal septum. (The tip of the nose and the nostrils are composed of cartilage.)

Two *inferior nasal conchae (turbinates)* are ledges that form the side and lower wall of each nasal cavity.

Two *palatine* bones form the posterior portion of the hard palate and the sides of the nasal cavity.

The *mandible,* which forms the lower jaw, is the only movable bone in the skull and is the largest and strongest bone of the face.

Hyoid Bone

The *hyoid* bone is a **U**-shaped bone in the neck. It does not form a joint with any other bone. It is located above the larynx and below the mandible and is suspended from the temporal bones by ligaments. It serves for the insertion of muscles of the tongue (hyoglossus) and floor of the mouth (mylohyoid and geniohyoid).

Vertebral Column

The vertebral or spinal column (backbone) is made up of 24 *vertebrae* (plural of *vertebra*), the *sacrum,* and the *coccyx.*

The vertebral column shelters the spinal cord, supports the skull and thorax, lends stiffening to the trunk, anchors the pelvic girdle, and provides attachment points for many of the main muscles. It is made up of:

The seven *cervical* (neck) vertebrae, the first of which is the *atlas,* which supports the skull and rotates on the second cervical vertebra, the *axis;*

The 12 *thoracic* (chest) vertebrae, to which the ribs are attached;

The five *lumbar* (lower back) vertebrae, which support the lower trunk;

The *sacrum,* which is a triangular bone, formed by the fusion of five vertebrae, to which the pelvic girdle is attached;

The *coccyx* (tailbone), located at the extreme tip of the vertebral column, is the result of fusion of several rudimentary vertebrae.

Each vertebra has a **body** (anterior portion) and an **arch** (posterior portion). The body bears the weight, and the arch helps to form the canal that houses the spinal cord. Between the vertebrae are **intervertebral disks,** which are made up of cartilage and serve as shock absorbers, or cushions (see Figures 6.2 and 6.3).

Ribs

There are twelve pairs of ribs, which are flat, curved bones attached posteriorly to the thoracic portion of the vertebral column. The first seven pairs are known as the **true ribs** because of their connection to the sternum by **costal** (referring to ribs) cartilages. The remaining five pairs are called **false ribs,** with the eighth, ninth, and tenth pairs joined to the cartilage of the seventh rib, and the eleventh and twelfth pairs, the so-called **floating ribs,** unattached anteriorly. The ribs form the chest wall and protect the heart and lungs.

Sternum

The **sternum** (breastbone) is a flat, sword-shaped bone, located in the midline of the chest, to which are attached the two **clavicles** (collar-bones), one on each side, and the anterior ends of the first seven pairs of ribs.

The thoracic vertebrae, the ribs and costal cartilages, and the sternum make up the thoracic cage, the bony structure that protects vital organs of the chest and allows it to expand and contract during **respiration** (breathing).

REVIEW 6.B

Complete the following:

1. An opening or passage in bone is called a(n) __meatus__ .

2. A sharp projection is called a(n) __spine__ .

3. All skull bones are immobile except for the __mandible__ .

4. __Sutures__ unite the bones of the skull.

5. The butterfly-shaped bone at the base of the skull is the __sphenoid__ bone.

---

6. The zygomatic (malar) bones are also called __cheek bones__ .

7. The spinal column is made up of vertebrae, __sacrum__ , and __coccyx__ .

8. The three groups of vertebrae in the spinal column are the __cervical__ , __thoracic__ , and __lumbar__ .

9. There are __12__ pairs of ribs.

10. The cushions of cartilage between the vertebrae are known as __inter-vertebral disks__ .

APPENDICULAR SKELETON

Upper Extremities

The bones of the upper extremities are:

The two **clavicles** (collarbones), flat bones attached, one on each side, to the scapulae laterally, and to the sternum anteriorly, forming the **sternoclavicular joint;**

The two **scapulae** (shoulder blades), large triangular bones at the back of the thorax, one on each side, which form the shoulder girdle together with the clavicles;

The two **humerus** bones, long bones, one in each arm, extending from the shoulder to the elbow, articulating (joining) with the scapula at the shoulder and the ulna and radius at the elbow;

The two **ulna** bones, medial long bones of the forearms, forming the elbow joints by articulation with the humerus bones at the **olecranon processes** (Figure 6.5);

The two **radius** bones, lateral long bones of the forearms, articulating with the ulna at both ends, the humerus at the elbow, and some wrist bones to form the wrist joint.

The **wrists** (see Figure 6.5), composed of eight small, irregularly shaped **carpal** bones in two rows. The proximal row has four carpals, articulating with the radius and ulna.

Beginning on the radial side, these are:

> **scaphoid** or **navicular** (boat shaped)
> **lunate** or **semilunar** (crescent shaped)
> **triquetrum** or **pyramidale** (wedge shaped)
> **pisiform** or **lentiform** (pea shaped)

The distal row of four carpals, on the radial side are:

trapezium or *greater multangular*
trapezoid or *lesser multangular*
capitate (rounded head)
hamate (hooklike)

The *hands* (see Figure 6.5) are made up of:

metacarpals, five long bones that articulate with the carpals, forming the palm of the hand, and articulating with the . . .
phalanges (finger bones), long bones forming the knuckle joints. Each finger has three phalanges, except for the thumb, which has two.

Lower Extremities

The bones of the lower extremities include those of the hip, thigh, leg, ankle, and foot (see Figures 6.2, 6.3, and 6.6).

The *pelvic girdle* (two *innominate bones*—hip bones) consists of three pairs of bones that fuse early in life into one solid, irregular bone. This girdle connects to the sacrum and coccyx and forms a basinlike structure that supports the trunk, affords an attachment for the lower limbs, and protects the lower abdominal organs. These three pairs of bones that fuse are:

the *ilium,* uppermost and largest pair, flaring to the side;
the *ischium,* lowest, strongest, and posterior pair;
the *pubis,* most anterior pair, meets at the *symphysis pubis,* a cartilaginous joint.

The *femur* (thighbone), the longest bone in the body, articulates with the *acetabulum* (hip socket) at the proximal end and with the *tibia* (a lower leg bone) at the distal end. The *greater* and *lesser trochanters* are two processes on the femur, for attachment of muscles. The *lateral* and *medial condyles,* two bony prominences at the lower end of the femur, articulate with the tibia and *patella.*

The *patella* (kneecap) is a small, flat bone (resembling a thick saucer), overlapping the distal end of the femur and proximal end of the tibia, and protecting the knee joint.

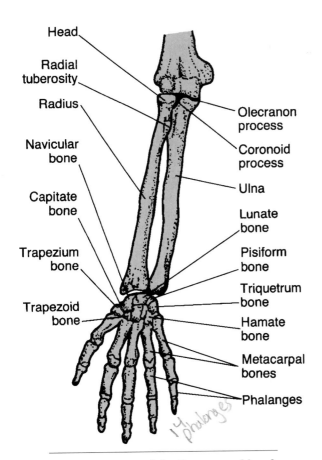

Figure 6.5 Bones of the forearm and hand.

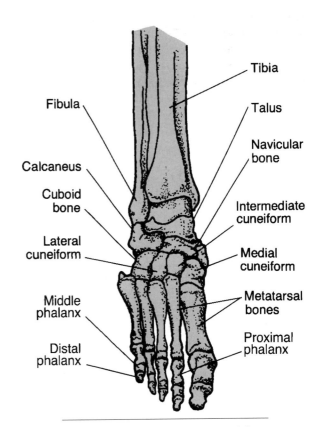

Figure 6.6 Bones of the ankle and foot.

The *tibia* (shinbone) is the larger, more weight-bearing and medially placed bone of the two lower leg bones, articulating at its proximal end with the femur and at its distal end with the *fibula* and the *talus,* the ankle joint bone, forming the bony prominence on the inside of the ankle, the *medial malleolus.*

The *fibula* (splint bone) is a long, slender, lateral bone, articulating on the proximal end with the tibia and at the distal end with the tibia and talus, forming the bony prominence on the outside of the ankle, the *lateral malleolus.*

The *tarsals* (anklebones) are seven short bones, resembling those of the wrist in structure and function, which articulate with the tibia and fibula.

The *talus (astragalus)* forms the ankle joint with the tibia and fibula.

The *calcaneus,* the largest tarsal, forms the heel.

The *navicular* or *scaphoid* has a boat shape.

The *cuneiforms,* three wedge-shaped bones, form the arch of the foot and are numbered from the medial side:

medial cuneiform—largest of the three;
intermediate cuneiform—smallest of the three;
lateral cuneiform.

The *cuboid* has a cube shape.

The *foot* bones resemble those of the hands, having:

Five *metatarsals,* forming the foot, and articulating with the *tarsals* and the *phalanges,* with the first metatarsal (on the big toe side) being the heaviest and the most weight bearing;

Fourteen *phalanges,* with structure and arrangement similar to those of the fingers, the great toe having two and the others three each.

JOINTS

The term applied to the study of the joints is *arthrology* (*arthr-* means joint). A joint is an articulation between bones, or bones and cartilage, that is held in place by ligaments of connective tissue and may or may not permit motion between them.

Joints are classified according to the degree of movement they permit and their tissue structure; there is a direct relationship between these two classifications.

1. Degree of movement:
   synarthroses—allow no movement.
   amphiarthroses—allow slight movement.
   diarthroses—freely permit movement.

2. Tissue structure:
   fibrous (synarthroses) joints contain fibrous tissue that unites bones and permits no movement. An example of this type is found in the sutures of the skull.
   cartilaginous (amphiarthroses) joints contain cartilage that connects the bones and permits slight movement. Examples of this type are found in the vertebrae and the symphysis pubis.
   synovial (diarthroses) joints are freely movable, the most numerous, and the most complex in the body. They have six characteristic structures:

   (1) *joint capsule*—forms a covering around the articulating ends of the bones, holding them to each other.
   (2) *synovial membrane*—lines the joint capsule and secretes synovial fluid lubricating opposing surfaces of the bones.
   (3) *joint cavity*—space between the opposing surfaces of bones of the joint.
   (4) *articular cartilage*—thin covering of cartilage that cushions the articulating bone surfaces.
   (5) *ligaments*—cords of white, dense fibrous tissue that help to bind the bones together.
   (6) *articular disks*—pads of cartilage between articulating surfaces in some synovial joints.

The movable joints are further divided into subtypes (Figure 6.7):

hinge joints—those that permit movement in only one direction, as in the elbow and the knee.

ball-and-socket joints—the round head of one bone fits into a cuplike cavity of another, permitting movement in different directions, as in the joint of the femur and the hipbone.

gliding joints—the least movable of this group, in which the adjacent bone surfaces glide upon each other to permit movement, such as that of the wrists and ankles.

pivot (rotary) joints—one bone pivots around a stationary bone, such as the axis and atlas (cervical vertebrae).

condyloid (knuckle) joints—the oval head of one bone fits into a shallow depression in another, such as the union between the radius and the carpal bones.

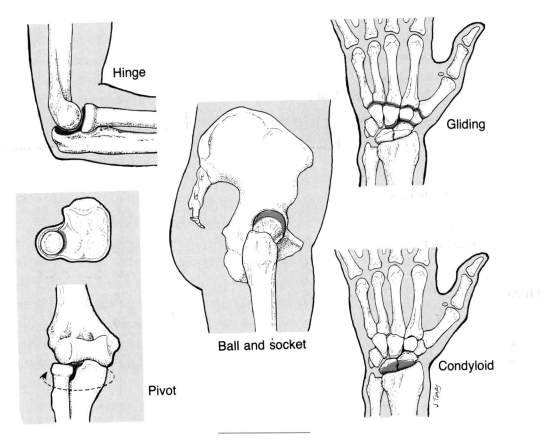

Figure 6.7 Joints.

Not all joints can perform all the movements listed. The immovable joints are incapable of performing any of them. Of the freely movable joints, only the ball-and-socket can perform all the movements listed. The hinge joints are able to perform only flexion and extension. The slightly movable joints can perform rotation.

TYPES OF MOVEMENT

The following are descriptive terms for defining the different types of motion:

flexion—bending at a joint, as the forearm or elbow.
extension—straightening, or unbending, of a joint; this movement is the opposite of flexion.
abduction—movement that draws a body part away from the midline of the body, such as the extension of the arms straight out from the shoulders.
adduction—movement that draws the body part toward the midline of the body, such as returning the extended arms.

rotation—movement that turns a body part on its own axis; for example, the turning of the head.
pronation—turning down or downward; for example, turning the palm of the hand downward.
supination—turning upward; for example, turning the palm upward.
eversion—turning outward.
inversion—turning inward.
circumduction—a movement describing a circle, such as with an outstretched arm.

BURSAE

The *bursae* are sacs of connective tissue lined with synovial membrane and filled with synovial fluid. Synovial fluid relieves pressure between moving parts. Bursae become inflamed (bursitis) in areas such as the patella (housemaid's knee) and the olecranon process (tennis elbow).

REVIEW 6.C

Complete the following:

1. The collarbones are called _Clavicles_ .
2. The shoulder blades are called _Scapulae_ .
3. The long bones of the arm are the _humerus_ _ulna_ , _ulna_ , and _radius_ .
4. The eight carpal bones are located in the _wrist_ .
5. The pelvic girdle is formed by the _ilium_ , _ischium_ , and _pubis_ .
6. The patella is the _kneecap_ .

7. The seven ankle bones are called _tarsals_ .
8. Fibrous joints allow _no_ movement, cartilaginous joints allow _slight_ movement, and synovial joints allow _free_ movement.
9. The most movable type of joint in the body is the _ball-and-socket_ joint.
10. The bending of a joint is called _flexion_ .

RELATED TERMS   THE SKELETAL SYSTEM THE FRAMEWORK OF THE BODY

ANATOMY

Bones

acetabulum (as″e-tab′u-lum) a cup-shaped socket in the hip joint (plural—*acetabula*).

acromion (ak-kro′me-on) outward extension of the spine of the shoulder blade forming the point of the shoulder (also called *acromial process*).

anastomosis (ah-nas″to-mo′sis) joining of blood vessels or other tubular structures (plural—*anastomoses*).

astragalus (as-trag′ah-lus) anklebone (also called *talus*).

atlanto- combining form referring to the *atlas.*

atlas (at′las) first cervical vertebra.

axis second cervical vertebra.

calcaneus (kal-ka′ne-us) heel bone (also called *calcaneum*).

calvaria (kal-va′re-ah) skull cap.

capitate (kap′i-tat) a bone of the wrist.

carpus (kar′pus) any wrist bone.

clavicle (klav′i-k′l) collarbone.

coccyx (kok′siks) tailbone of the spinal column.

condyle (kon′dile) a rounded projection at the end of an articulating bone (such as the tibia or humerus).

coronal suture suture formed by the frontal bone with the two parietal bones.

cubitus (ku′bi-tus) the forearm.

cuboid cube-shaped bone on the outer side of the tarsus, between the calcaneus and the metatarsals.

cuneiforms (ku-ne′i-formz) three wedge-shaped bones in the foot.

diaphysis (di-af′i-sis) central part of the bone shaft.

epicondyle (ep′i-kon′dile) a projection on a bone above its condyle.

epiphysis (e-pif′i-sis) end part of developing bone.

ethmoid bone of the skull behind the nose and between the orbits.

femur (fee′mur) thighbone.

fibula (fib′u-lah) outer and smaller of the two lower leg bones.

fontanel, fontanelle (fon-tah-nel′) unossified areas (soft spots) of the cranium of an infant.

foramen magnum (fo-ray'men) large opening in the occipital bone at the base of the skull connecting the cranial cavity to the vertebral canal.

frontal bone bone forming the forepart of the cranium.

hamate (hah'mate) a bone of the wrist (also called *unciform*).

haversian canals (ha-ver'shan) network of canals in compact bone that contain blood and lymph vessels, nerves, and connective tissue (named after their discoverer).

humerus (hu'mer-us) upper arm bone.

hyoid (hi'oid) U-shaped bone located at the base of the tongue just above the thyroid cartilage.

ilium (il'e-um) pelvic bone.

incus (ing'kus) middle ossicle of the ear (resembling an anvil).

innominate (i-nom'i-nat) hipbone, including the ilium, ischium, and pubic bones (pelvic bones).

ischium (is'ki-um) pelvic bone.

lacuna (lah-ku'nah) a space (plural—*lacunae*).

lacrimal (lak'ri-mal) bone lying within medial angle of the orbit.

lambdoid suture (lam'doid) suture separating the occipital and parietal bones of the cranium.

lamella (lah-mel'ah) thin plate of bone (plural—*lamellae*).

lamina (lam'i-nah) thin plate or layer.

lentiform (len'ti-form) pea-shaped bone of the wrist (also called *pisiform*).

lunate (lu'nat) crescent-shaped bone of the wrist (also called *semilunar*).

malar (ma'lar) cheek bone (also called *zygomatic*).

malleolus (mal-lee'o-lus) medial and lateral prominences on either side of the ankle joint.

malleus (mal'e-us) largest, hammer-shaped bone of the ossicles of the ear, attached to the tympanic membrane (eardrum).

mandible (man'di-b'l) lower jawbone.

manubrium (mah-nu'bre-um) uppermost portion of the sternum (plural—*manubria*).

mastoid process (mas'toid) process of the temporal bone located behind the ear (sometimes referred to as the *mastoid bone*).

metacarpal (met"ah-kar'pal) one of five bones of the hand.

metaphysis (me-taf'i-sis) area of spongy bone between the epiphyseal plate and diaphysis of long bone.

metatarsal (met"ah-tar'sal) foot bones between ankles and toes.

navicular (nah-vik'u-lar) boat-shaped bone of wrist or foot.

occipital (ok-sip'i-tal) bone forming back of skull.

olecranon (o-lek'rah-non) curved process of the ulna at the elbow.

ossein (os'e-in) organic content of bone.

ossicle (os'ik-ul) any small bone.

osteoblast (os'te-o-blast) bone-forming cell.

osteoclast (os'te-o-klast) remodeling cell of bone.

osteocyte (os'te-o-site) bone cell (also called *osseous cell*).

osteogenesis (os"te-o-jen'e-sis) production of bone.

palate (pal'at) irregular bones forming a separation between the oral and nasal cavities.

parietal (pah-ri'e-tal) two bones forming the lateral surfaces of the cranium.

patella (pah-tel'ah) kneecap.

pelvic girdle arch formed by the innominate bones.

periosteum (per"e-os'te-um) membrane covering bone.

phalanges (fa-lan'jez) bones of toes or fingers (singular—*phalanx*).

pisiform (pi'si-form) pea-shaped bone of the wrist (see *lentiform*).

pubis pubic bone (also called *os pubis*).

pyramidale (pi-ram"i-da'le) wedge-shaped bone at the inner side of the wrist (also called *os triquetrum*).

radius (ra'de-us) forearm bone.

sacrum (sa'krum) wedge-shaped bone of spinal column, just above the coccyx.

sagittal suture (saj'i-tal) suture between the parietal bones.

scaphoid (skaf'oid) boat-shaped bone of wrist or foot (see *navicular*).

scapula (skap'u-lah) shoulder blade (plural—*scapulae*).

semilunar crescent-shaped, carpal bone (also called *lunate*).

sesamoid (ses'ah-moid) any small flat bone embedded in a tendon or joint capsule. (The patella is the largest sesamoid in the body.)

shoulder girdle formed by clavicle and scapula.

sphenoid (sfe'noid) wedge-shaped bone at the base of the skull.

squamous suture (skwa'mus) suture between the parietal and temporal bones on the lateral side of the cranium and between the lower lateral portions of the occipital and temporal bones.

stapes (sta'pez) stirrup-shaped, innermost auditory ossicles.

sternum (ster'num) breastbone. The body of the sternum is called the *gladiolus* (glah-di'o-lus); the process at the lower end is called the *xyphoid* (zif'oid) *process;* and the uppermost portion is called the *manubrium.*

styloid process (sti'loid) projection on the distal end of the radius and the ulna.

substantia spongiosa ossium (sub-stan'she-ah spon"je-o'sah) inner spongy layer of bone.

symphysis pubis (sim'fi-sis) cartilaginous joint between pubic bones.

talus (ta'lus) anklebone (see *astragalus*).

tarsals (tar'salz) seven short bones of the ankle.

temporal two irregular bones forming the sides and base of the skull.

tibia (tib'e-ah) larger of the two lower leg bones (shinbone).

trapezium (trah-pe'ze-um) wrist bone on the radial side.

trapezoid (trap'e-zoid) bone of the wrist.

triquetrum (tri-kwe'trum) wedge-shaped bone of the wrist (also called *pyramidale*).

trochanter (tro-kan'ter) greater and lesser processes for attachment of muscles of the femur.

turbinate (tur'bi-nat) bone on lower side of nasal cavity (also called *concha nasalis*).

ulna (ul'nah) forearm bone.

unciform (in'si-form) see *hamate* bone.

vertebra (ver'ta-brah) spinal column bone (plural—*vertebrae*).

vomer (vo'mer) thin, flat bone forming lower part of nasal septum.

zygomatic (zi'go-mat'ik) cheek bone, or *malar* bone.

Cartilage

alar (a'lar) winglike; greater and lesser cartilages of the nose.

articular thin layer of hyaline cartilage on joint surfaces.

bursae synovial fluid-filled connective tissue sacs.

calcified cartilage containing calcium or calcareous matter.

costal cartilage attaching ribs to the sternum and other ribs.

elastic cartilage that is more flexible and elastic than hyaline cartilage.

epiphyseal (ep"i-fiz'e-al) cartilage between epiphysis and diaphysis.

hyaline (hi'a-lin) flexible, glassy, translucent cartilage.

nasal cartilage of the nose.

semilunar interarticular cartilage of the knee joint.

septal cartilage of the nose.

sternal cartilage connecting ribs to the sternum.

Joints and Related Anatomic Terms

acromioclavicular junction between acromion and clavicle.

amphiarthroses (am"fe-ar-thro'sez) slightly movable joints.

arthrology study of joints.

articulation (ar-tik"u-la'shun) junction between bones.

atlantoaxial joint between atlas and axis.

ball-and-socket joint round head of one bone fits into cavity of another, permitting movement in different directions.

calcaneoastragaloid (kal-ka"ne-o-ah-strag'ah-loid) junction between calcaneus and astragalus.

calcaneocuboid (kal-ka"ne-o-ku'boid) junction between calcaneus and cuboid bone.

calcaneofibular (kal-ka"ne-o-fib'u-lar) junction between calcaneus and fibula.

calcaneonavicular (kal-ka"ne-o-nah-vik'u-lar) junction between calcaneus and navicular bone (also called *calcaneoscaphoid*).

calcaneotibial (kal-ka"ne-o-tib'e-al) junction between calcaneus and tibia.

carpometacarpal (kar"po-met"ah-kar'pal) junction between carpus and metacarpal bone.

costosternal junction of ribs with sternum.

costovertebral junction of ribs with vertebrae.

coxal referring to the hip joint.

cubital referring to elbow joint.

cuboidonavicular junction between cuboid and navicular.

cuneocuboid (ku″ne-o-ku′boid) junction between cuneiform and cuboid.

cuneoscaphoid (ku″ne-o-skaf′oid) junction between cuneiform and scaphoid (also called *cuneonavicular*).

diarthroses (di″ar-thro′sez) freely movable joints.

hinge joint movement permitted in only one plane, as in the elbow.

hip joint articulation of femur with pelvic bones.

humeroradial (hu″mer-o-ra′de-al) junction between humerus and radius.

humeroscapular (hu″mer-o-skap′u-lar) articulation between humerus and scapula (also called *scapulohumeral*).

humeroulnar (hu″mer-o-ul′nar) articulation between humerus and ulna.

intercarpal articulation between carpal bones.

interphalangeal (in″ter-fah-lan′je-al) articulation between phalanges.

intertarsal articulation between tarsal bones.

knee joint articulation between upper and lower leg bones at knee.

lumbosacral junction between sacrum and lumbar vertebrae.

metacarpophalangeal junction between metacarpus and phalanges.

metatarsophalangeal junction between metatarsus and phalanges.

pivot joint one bone rotates over another.

radiocarpal articulation between carpus and radius.

radioulnar articulation between radius and ulna.

sacrococcygeal junction between sacrum and coccyx.

sacroiliac (sa″kro-il′e-ak) joint between sacrum and ilium.

scapuloclavicular (skap″u-lo-klah-vik′u-lar) junction between scapula and clavicle.

sternoclavicular (ster″no-klah-vik′u-lar) junction between sternum and clavicle (also called *sternocleidal*).

sternocostal junction between sternum and ribs.

synarthroses (sin″ar-thro′sez) immovable joints.

synovial (si-no-ve-al) pertaining to the lubricating fluid secreted by the synovial membrane and contained in joint cavities, bursae, and tendon sheaths.

talocalcaneal articulation between the talus (astragalus) and the calcaneus.

talofibular articulation between the talus and fibula.

talonavicular (ta″lo-nah-vik′u-lar) articulation between talus and navicular (scaphoid) bone (also called *taloscaphoid*).

tarsometatarsal articulation between tarsals and metatarsals.

temporomandibular (tem″po-ro-man-dib′u-lar) articulation between mandible and temporal bone.

tibiofibular articulation between tibia and fibula at ankle and knee.

tibiotarsal articulation between tibia and tarsal bones.

PATHOLOGIC CONDITIONS

Inflammation and Infections

Inflammations are characterized by pain, heat, redness, and swelling and may be accompanied by exudations. *Inflammation* is a condition resulting from injury to tissues, but not all inflammations are infections. *Infection* is an invasion of the body by pathogenic microorganisms to which tissues react. The term *infection* is generally applied to invasion by bacteria, viruses, protozoa, and helminths. These terms will be used in this sense throughout the book.

arthritis (ar-thri′tis) acute or chronic inflammation of one or more joints, characterized by pain and stiffness.

Brodie's abscess (bro′dez) chronic, latent infection in cancellous bone, with a small inflammatory focus.

bursitis (ber-si′tis) inflammation of a bursa.

caries (ka′re-ez) decay or death of bone, with chronic inflammation of the periosteum.

chondritis (kon-dri′tis) inflammation of a cartilage.

coxitis inflammation of a hip joint (also called *coxarthritis*).

epiphysitis (e-pif′i-si′tis) inflammation of the epiphysis of a bone, or of the cartilage separating it from the bone.

metatarsalgia (met″ah-tar-sal′je-ah) a neuralgia in the region of the metatarsal caused by a foot abnormality, or an osteochondrosis of the heads of the metatarsal bones (also called *Morton's disease, Morton's toe, Morton's neuralgia,* or *Morton's foot*).

osteitis (os″te-i′tis) inflammation of bone.

osteoarthritis (os″te-o-ar-thri′tis) degenerative joint disease affecting articular cartilages and the synovial membranes.

osteochondritis (os"te-o-kon-dri'tis) inflammation of bone and cartilage.

osteomyelitis (os"te-o-mi"e-li'tis) inflammation of bone that may involve the periosteum, cancellous tissue, and marrow.

periosteomyelitis (per"e-os"te-o-mi"e-li'tis) inflammation of entire bone.

periostitis (per"e-os-ti'tis) inflammation of the periosteum.

Pott's disease osteitis or caries of the vertebrae, usually tuberculous (also called *tuberculous spondylitis*).

spondylarthritis (spon"dil-ar-thri'tis) arthritis of spine.

spondylitis (spon"di-li'tis) inflammation of spinal column (*ankylosing spondylitis*, a form of arthritis, is also called *Marie-Strümpell disease*).

synovitis (sin"o-vi'tis) inflammation of the synovial membrane of a joint.

tenosynovitis (ten"o-sin"o-vi'tis) inflammation of a tendon and its synovial membrane.

tuberculosis, osseous in the bones and joints, producing arthritis and cold abscess.

Hereditary, Congenital, and Developmental Disorders

achondroplasia (ah-kon"dro-pla'ze-ah) hereditary, congenital disorder involving inadequate formation and growth of long bones and causing a particular form of dwarfism.

acrocephaly (ak"ro-sef'ah-le) malformation of skull due to early closure of sutures, causing a pointed, conical shape (also called *oxycephaly*).

acromegaly (ak"ro-meg'ah-le) enlargement of bones of extremities, fingers, toes, and soft tissue parts of the face, caused by excessive pituitary growth hormone.

amelia (ah-me'le-ah) anomaly characterized by absence of a limb or limbs.

amyoplasia congenita (ah-mi"o-pla'se-ah kon-jen'i-tah) lack of muscle growth and development in the neonate with deformity of most of the joints.

anencephalia (an"en-se-fa'le-ah) developmental anomaly in which the vault of the skull is missing and cerebral hemispheres may be missing or reduced to small masses.

arachnodactyly (ah'rak"no-dak'ti-le) abnormality in length of fingers and toes (also called *Marfan's syndrome, dolichostenomelia,* or *arachnodactylia*).

arthroonychodysplasia (ar"thro-on"e-ko-dis-pla'ze-ah) hereditary malformation of head of radius, absence or hypoplasia of patella, and dystrophy of nails (also called *nail-patella syndrome, onychoosteodysplasia,* or *onychoosteodystrophy*).

cleidocranial dysostosis (kli"do-kra'ne-al dis"os-to'sis) rare hereditary condition characterized by defective ossification of cranial bones, complete or partial absence of clavicles, and other anomalies.

clubfoot congenitally deformed foot (see *talipes*).

clubhand congenitally deformed hand.

coxa valga hip deformity, involving an increase in the angle formed by the axis of the head and neck of the femur, and the axis of the shaft.

coxa vara hip deformity, involving a decrease in the angle formed by the axis of the head and neck of the femur, and the axis of the shaft.

craniofacial dysostosis premature fusion of skull bones, and other anomalies (also called *Crouzon's disease*).

craniorachischisis (kra"ne-o-rah-kis'ki-sis) fissure of skull and spinal column.

craniostosis (kra"ne-os-to'sis) ossification of cranial sutures.

dysostosis (dis"os-to'sis) defective ossification of fetal cartilages.

eccentrochondroplasia (ek-sen"tro-kon"dro-pla'se-ah) disorder of epiphyseal development (also called *Morquio's syndrome*).

enchondromatosis (en'kon-dro-mat-osis) abnormal growth of cartilage in long bones causing distortion in length and thinness, producing fractures (also called *dyschondroplasia* and *Ollier's disease*).

exostosis (ek"sos-to'sis) abnormal bony growth projection.

fibrous dysplasia painful, disabling bone development disorder producing thinning of bone cortex and replacement of marrow with fibrous tissue (either *monostotic,* involving only one bone, or *polyostotic,* involving many bones).

genu recurvatum (je'nu re-kur-va'tum) hyperextensive knee joint.

genu valgum the knees are abnormally close together (knock-knee).

genu varum lower extremities are bent outward (bowleg).

giantism abnormal increase of growth in size and stature (also called *gigantism*).

hallux valgus (hal′uks) big toe bent toward the other toes.

hallux varus big toe displaced away from other toes.

hemimelia (hem″e-me′le-ah) shortening or absence of all or part of the distal half of a limb.

Hurler's syndrome hereditary condition involving deformities of bone and cartilage and producing dwarfism (also called *gargoylism, chondroosteodystrophy,* or *lipochondrodystrophy*).

infantile cortical hyperostosis overgrowth of bones (also called *Caffey's disease*).

Klippel-Feil syndrome reduction in number, or fusion of cervical vertebrae, producing short, thick neck, with limited neck motion.

macrobrachia (mak″ro-bra′ke-ah) abnormally large arms.

macrocephaly (mak″ro-sef′ah-le) abnormally large head.

macrognathia (mak″ro-na′the-ah) abnormally large jaws.

macropodia (mak″ro-po′de-ah) abnormally large feet.

Marfan's syndrome hereditary connective tissue disorder characterized by abnormal length of phalanges and extremities (arachnodactyly), looseness of joints, and also affecting other systems. (Some medical authorities believe that Abraham Lincoln had this condition.)

opisthognathism (o″pis-tho′nah-thizm) receding jaws.

osteogenesis imperfecta disorder in which the bones are extremely brittle and fracture easily (also called *fragilitas ossium*).

osteopetrosis (os″te-o-pe-tro′sis) hereditary disorder resulting in abnormally dense bone that fractures easily (also called *marble bones* or *Albers-Schönberg disease*).

osteopoikilosis (os″te-o-poi″ki-lo′sis) hereditary condition characterized by numerous dense calcified areas in bone which appear as mottled bone in x-ray films.

prognathism (prog′nah-thizm) projecting jaws.

pyknodysostosis (pik′no-dis-os-to′sis) syndrome characterized by dwarfism, late or no closure of fontanels, underdevelopment of lower jaw and phalanges, and bone fragility. (Toulouse-Lautrec is believed to have had this condition.)

scaphocephaly (ska″fo-sef′ah-le) long, narrow skull deformity caused by premature closing of the sagittal suture.

syndactylia (sin″dak-til′e-ah) webbed fingers or toes.

talipes (tal′i-pez) twisted foot *(clubfoot).*

Fractures

closed simple fracture, no open wound on the skin.

Colles' fracture of lower end of radius with the lower fragment displaced posteriorly.

comminuted bone crushed or splintered.

compound open wound caused by the fracture.

double fracture in two places (also called *segmental fracture*).

greenstick one side of the bone broken and the other part bent (also called *hickory-stick fracture*).

impacted one fragment driven into the other.

incomplete continuity of the bone not completely destroyed.

silver-fork fracture of lower end of radius.

splintered bone is splintered into fragments.

transverse bone fractured at right angles to its axis.

Metabolic and Deficiency Diseases

chondromalacia (kon″dro-mah-la′she-ah) softening of cartilage.

osteomalacia (os′te-o-mah-la′she-ah) softening of bone.

osteoporosis (os″te-o-po-ro′sis) abnormal loss of bone density.

renal osteodystrophy bone changes caused by chronic kidney disease in childhood (also called *renal rickets,* or *pseudorickets*).

rickets (rik′ets) condition in which bending and distortion of bone takes place, caused by deficiency of vitamin D in childhood.

scurvy vitamin C deficiency condition producing abnormal formation of bones and teeth, and other clinical symptoms.

Oncology*

chondroblastoma a tumor in a bone epiphysis (also called *Codman's tumor*).

chondrofibroma (kon"dro-fi-bro'mah) tumor with fibrous and cartilaginous tissue.

chondroma tumor of cartilage cells.

chondromatosis (kon"dro-mah-to'sis) multiple chrondromas.

chondromyoma myoma containing cartilaginous elements.

chondromyxoma   (kon"dro-mik-so'mah) myxoma containing cartilaginous elements (also called *chondromyxoid fibroma*).

chondromyxosarcoma† malignancy with fibrous, mucus-like cartilaginous elements.

chondrosarcoma† malignancy made up of cartilaginous elements.

osteoblastoma (os"te-o-blas-to'mah) benign tumor of osteoblasts.

osteochondroma (os"te-o-kon-dro'mah) benign tumor made up of bone and cartilage.

osteoma (os"te-o'mah) bone tissue tumor.

osteosarcoma* (os"te-o-sar-ko'-mah) malignant bone tumor.

osteospongioma (os"te-o-spon"je-o'mah) neoplasm in bone cortex.

synovioma (sin-o"ve-o'mah) synovial membrane tumor involving joint or tendon.

SURGICAL PROCEDURES

allograft surgical removal of cancerous bone and replacement with donor bone.

arthrectomy (ar-threk'to-me) excision of a joint.

arthrocentesis (ar"thro-sen-te'sis) puncture of a joint.

arthrodesis (ar"thro-de'sis) surgical fixation of a joint by fusion of the joint surfaces (also called *artificial ankylosis*).

arthroplasty (ar'thro-plas"te) plastic surgery to reconstruct joints.

arthrotomy (ar-throt'o-me) incision of a joint.

bursectomy (ber-sek'to-me) excision of a bursa.

bursotomy (ber-sot'o-me) incision of a bursa.

capsulorrhaphy (kap'su-lor'ah-fe) suturing of a joint capsule.

capsulotomy incision of a joint capsule.

carpectomy (kar-pek'to-me) excision of all or part of a carpal bone.

chondrectomy (kon-drek'to-me) excision of cartilage.

chondrotomy (kon-drot'o-me) division or dissection of cartilage.

clavicotomy (klav"i-kot'o-me) dividing or cutting of a clavicle.

coccygectomy (kok"se-jek'to-me) excising of the coccyx.

condylectomy (kon"dil-ek'to-me) excising of a condyle (knuckle).

costectomy (kos-tek'to-me) excision or resection of a rib.

coxotomy (kok-sot'o-me) opening the hip joint.

cranioclasis (kra"ne-ok'lah-sis) crushing of the fetal head.

cranioplasty plastic surgery on the skull.

craniotomy any surgical procedure on the cranium.

craniotrypesis (kra"ne-o-tri-pe'sis) trephination of the skull.

laminectomy (lam"i-nek'toe-me) cutting out posterior arch of a vertebra (also called *rachiotomy* or *rachitomy*).

laminotomy (lam"i-not'o-me) division of lamina of a vertebra.

metatarsectomy (met"ah-tar-sek'to-me) excision of metatarsus.

ostearthrotomy (os'te-ar-throt'o-me) excision of articular end of a bone.

ostectomy (os-tek'to-me) excision of all or part of a bone.

osteoclasis (os-te-ok'lah-sis) surgical fracture of a bone for reconstructive purposes.

osteoplasty (os'te-o-plas"te) plastic surgery of bone.

osteorrhaphy suturing or wiring of a bone.

osteotomy (os"te-ot'o-me) cutting of a bone.

pubiotomy (pu"be-ot'o-me) cutting of the pubic bone.

scapulopexy (skap'u-lo-pek"se) fixing of scapula to chest wall or vertebrae.

spondylosyndesis (spon"di-lo-sin'de-sis) spinal fusion.

sternotomy (ster-not'o-me) cutting through the sternum.

---

*Oncology is the study of tumors (*neoplasms*), which may be benign or malignant.
†Indicates a malignant condition.

synchondrotomy (sin"kon-drot'o-me) cartilaginous joint division.

syndesmopexy (sin-des"mo-pek"se) fixation of a dislocation by using the ligaments of the joint.

synosteotomy (sin"os-te-ot'o-me) dissection of the joints.

synovectomy (sin"o-vek'to-me) excision of synovial membrane of a joint.

DESCRIPTIVE AND DIAGNOSTIC TERMS

ankylosis (ang"ki-lo'sis) immobility and consolidation of a joint.

arthralgia (ar-thral'je-ah) pain in a joint or joints (also called *arthrodynia*).

arthrocele (ar'thro-sel) swollen joint.

arthrolithiasis (ar"thro-li'thi-ah-sis) gout.

arthroneuralgia (ar"thro-nu-ral'je-ah) pain of a joint.

arthropathy (ar-throp'ah-the) any joint disease.

arthrosclerosis (ar'thro-skle-ro'sis) hardening or stiffening of a joint.

arthrosis (ar-thro'sis) articulation or disease of a joint.

chondralgia (kon-dral'je-ah) pain in a cartilage (also called *chondrodynia*).

chondroid (kon'droid) resembling cartilage.

chondronecrosis death of cartilage.

chondroporosis (kon"dro-po-ro'sis) formation of spaces in cartilage, which occurs normally during ossification.

coccygodynia (kok"se-go-din'e-ah) pain of the coccyx (also called *coccyalgia* or *coccyodynia*).

coxodynia (kok"so-din'e-ah) pain of the hip (also called *coxalgia*).

hemarthrosis (hem"ar-thro'sis) seepage of blood into a joint.

hydrarthrosis (hi"drar-thro'sis) fluid in a joint cavity.

kyphosis (ki-fo'sis) humpback.

lordosis (lor-do'sis) curvature of the spine (swayback).

lumbago (lum-ba'go) lumbosacral pain.

ostealgia (os"te-al'je-ah) pain in a bone (also called *ostalgia* or *osteodynia*).

osteoclasia (os"te-o-kla'ze-ah) destruction and absorption of bony tissue.

osteodiastasis separation of two bones.

osteodystrophy (os"te-o-dis'tro-fe) defective bone formation.

osteogenetic (os"te-o-je-net'ik) forming bone.

osteoid (os'te-oid) resembling bone.

osteolysis (os"te-ol'i-sis) bone dissolution caused by calcium loss.

osteomalacia (os"te-o-mah-la'she-ah) softening of bones.

osteonecrosis (os"te-o-ne-kro'sis) death of bone.

osteoneuralgia (os"te-o-nu-ral'je-ah) neuralgia of bone.

osteopathy (os"te-op'ah-the) any bone disease.

osteorrhagia (os"te-o-ra'je-ah) bone hemorrhage.

osteosclerosis (os"te-o-skle-ro'sis) abnormal hardening of bone.

scoliosis (sko"le-o'sis) abnormal lateral curvature of spine.

LABORATORY TESTS

arthrography radiography (x-ray), using contrast media to outline soft tissue structures in a joint.

arthroscopy examination of a joint interior using an arthroscope.

bone marrow biopsy removal of bone marrow from sternum, iliac crest, vertebral column, or tibia for detection of leukemias, anemias, multiple myelomas, or any diseases affecting bone marrow. Red or white blood cells are evaluated for appearance, number, development, and infection (also called *bone marrow aspiration*).

bone scan radioactive material is injected into a vein. As seen by x-ray, concentration of this material in any specific area reveals an abnormal condition of bone, particularly metastatic bone cancer.

bone x-ray radiographic examination of bone for presence of disease or fractures.

computerized tomography (CT) imaging device using x-rays at multiple angles through specific sections of the body, analyzed by computer to provide a total picture of the part being examined (also called *computerized axial tomography—CAT*).

discogram x-ray of vertebral disk for diagnostic purposes.

dual energy radiography (DER) a low-level radiation method of measuring bone mass to diagnose osteoporosis (also called *dual energy x-ray absorptiometry—DEXA*).

endoscopy use of an endoscope to examine the interior of a joint, particularly the knee, for presence of torn cartilage.

hydroxyproline urine test to detect bone diseases.

long bone x-ray to determine growth patterns, joint deterioration, and growth of bone spurs.

lumbar puncture needle aspiration of spinal canal fluid in lumbar area, to diagnose traumatic head, neck, or back injury.

magnetic resonance imaging (MRI) noninvasive method of scanning the body by use of an electromagnetic field and radio waves, which provides visual images on a computer screen and magnetic tape recordings (also called *nuclear magnetic resonance* or *NMR*). Used to examine tendons, ligaments, and bone marrow.

nuclear magnetic resonance (NMR) see *magnetic resonance imaging.*

rheumatoid factor blood test to detect rheumatoid arthritis.

skull x-ray examination of bones and sinuses of the skull to detect pathologic conditions.

spinal x-ray for detection of diverse abnormalities.

synovial fluid tests of blood and synovial fluid to diagnose infections, inflammations, and other conditions.

▲ EXERCISES   THE SKELETAL SYSTEM THE FRAMEWORK OF THE BODY

Exercise 6.1   *Complete the following:*

1. The hard outer shell of bone is called ___Compact bone___ .
2. The inner latticelike, spongy structure of bone is called ___Cancellated or cancellous___ bone.
3. The shaft of long bone is called the ___diaphysis___ .
4. The developing ends of long bones are called ___epiphyses___ .
5. The names of the anatomic classifications of the skeleton are ___appendicular___ and ___axial___ .

Exercise 6.2   *Classify the following bones according to shape.*

1. humerus ___long___
2. wrist ___short___
3. anklebone ___short___
4. sternum ___flat___
5. scapula ___flat___

Exercise 6.3   *Multiple choice*

1. Which of the following bones is the only movable one in the skull?
   a. frontal
   b. mandible
   c. ear ossicles
   d. maxillary

2. In which of the following bones are the mastoid sinuses located?
   a. frontal
   b. parietal
   c. temporal
   d. sphenoid

3. Which is the butterfly-shaped bone of the skull?
   a. ethmoid
   b. sphenoid
   c. occipital
   d. frontal

4. Which bones form the posterior portion of the hard palate?
   a. turbinates
   b. palatines
   c. lacrimals
   d. zygomatics

5. What does the sagittal suture separate?
   a. the eye sockets
   b. the parietals
   c. frontal sinuses
   d. the temporals

Exercise 6.4   *Matching*

B	1. periosteum	A. seam
H	2. red bone marrow	B. tough fibrous membrane covering
D	3. osteoblast	C. phagocytic cell
C	4. osteoclast	D. immature bone cell
F	5. fossa	E. small, smooth area
J	6. sulcus	F. basinlike depression
E	7. facet	G. high ridge
G	8. crista	H. hematopoietic tissue
A	9. suture	I. opening or hole
I	10. foramen	J. open, ditchlike groove

Exercise 6.5   *Using the list of terms below, identify each bone in Figures 6.8 and 6.9 by writing its name in the corresponding blank. (Some of these terms may be shown more than once.)*

Acromion	Carpals	Cervical vertebrae
Clavicle	Ischium	Lesser trochanter
Lumbar vertebrae	Mandible	Maxilla
Metacarpals	Metatarsals	Occipital bone
Coccyx	Costal cartilage	Cranium
Femur	Fibula	Orbit
Parietal bone	Olecranon process of ulna	Patella
Phalanges	Pubis	Radius
Sacrum	Greater trochanter	Humerus
Ilium	Innominate bone	Scapula
Sternum	Tarsals	Thoracic vertebrae
Tibia	Ulna	Vertebral column
Xiphoid process		

1. Cranium
2. orbit
3. maxilla
4. mandible
5. Clavicle
6. Sternum
7. humerus
8. Xiphoid process
9. Costal Cartilage
10. vertebral column
11. innominate bone
12. ilium
13. pubis
14. ischium
15. lesser trochanter
16. ulna

17. radius
18. Sacrum
19. greater trochanter
20. carpals
21. metacarpals
22. phalanges
23. femur
24. patella
25. tibia
26. fibula
27. tarsals
28. metatarsals
29. Phalanges
30. acromion
31. Scapula
32. humerus

33. olecranon process of ulna
34. radius
35. ulna
36. femur
37. fibula
38. tibia
39. parietal bone
40. occipital bone
41. cervical vertebrae
42. thoracic vertebrae
43. lumbar vertebrae
44. ilium
45. Sacrum
46. coccyx
47. ischium

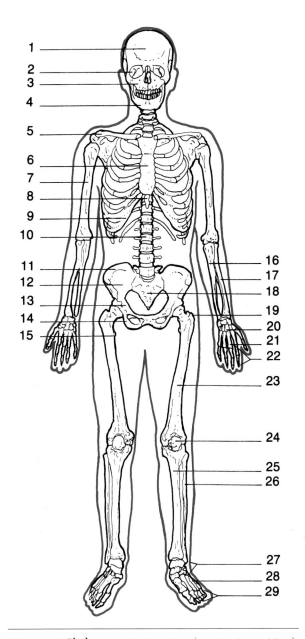

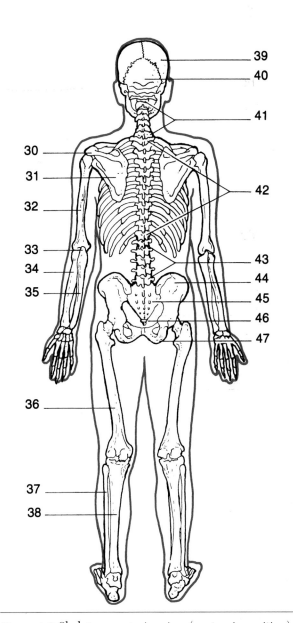

Figure 6.8 Skeleton, anterior view (anatomic position).

Figure 6.9 Skeleton, posterior view (anatomic position).

Exercise 6.6   *Matching*

H   1. sacrum
E   2. clavicle
I   3. femur
S   4. humerus
L   5. sternum
T   6. zygomatic (or malar)
J   7. patella
A   8. coccyx
G   9. scapula
F   10. vomer
D   11. tibia
B   12. mandible
C   13. fibula
Q   14. pubis
N   15. ischium
R   16. carpals
O   17. ilium
P   18. tarsals
M   19. radius
K   20. ulna

A. extreme tip of vertebral column
B. jawbone
C. smaller bone of lower leg
D. large weight-bearing bone of lower leg
E. collar bone
F. a nasal bone
G. shoulder blade
H. next to last vertebral bone
I. thighbone
J. kneecap
K. medial long bone of the forearm
L. breastbone
M. lateral long bone of forearm
N. small, lower, strongest portion of pelvic bone
O. broad upper portion of pelvic girdle
P. anklebones
Q. most anterior part of pelvic girdle
R. wrist bones
S. upper arm bone
T. a cheekbone

Exercise 6.7   *Using the list of terms below, identify each bone in Figure 6.10 by writing its name in the corresponding blank.*

Capitate bone
Trapezoid bone
Hamate bone
Olecranon process
Trapezium bone
Head

Navicular bone
Radial tuberosity
Phalanges
Ulna
Coronoid process

Lunate bone
Radius
Pisiform bone
Triquetrum bone
Metacarpal bones

1. Radial tuberosity
2. radius
3. Navicular bone
4. Capitate bone
5. trapezium bone
6. trapezoid bone
7. olecranon process
8. coronoid process
9. ulna
10. lunate bone
11. pisiform bone
12. triquetrum bone
13. hamate bone
14. metacarpal bones
15. Phalanges
16. head

Exercise 6.8 *Using the list of terms below, identify each bone in Figure 6.11 by writing its name in the corresponding blank.*

Cuboid bone

Fibula

Proximal phalanx

Medial cuneiform

Navicular bone

Middle phalanx

Metatarsal bones

Lateral cuneiform

Tibia

Talus

Intermediate cuneiform

Distal phalanx

Calcaneus

1. _fibula_
2. _Calcaneus_
3. _cuboid bone_
4. _Lateral cuneiform_
5. _distal phalanx_

6. _tibia_
7. _talus_
8. _navicular bone_
9. _intermediate cuneiform_

10. _medial cuneiform_
11. _metatarsal bones_
12. _proximal phalanx_
13. _middle phalanx_

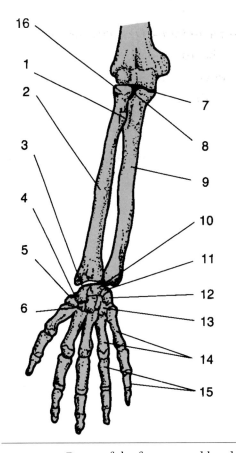

Figure 6.10 Bones of the forearm and hand.

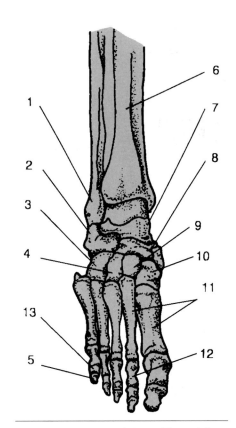

Figure 6.11 Bones of the ankle and foot.

Exercise 6.9   *Using the list of terms below, identify each part in Figure 6.12 by writing its name in the corresponding blank.*

Coronal suture

Maxilla

Zygomatic bone

Parietal bone

Squamous suture

External auditory meatus

Lacrimal bone

Sphenoid bone

Nasal bone

Occipital bone

Mastoid process

Zygomatic arch

Temporal bone

Lambdoidal suture

Frontal bone

Styloid process

Ethmoid bone

Mandible

1. Coronal suture

2. parietal bone

3. temporal bone

4. Squamous suture

5. lambdoidal suture

6. occipital bone

7. external auditory meatus

8. Mastoid process

9. Styloid process

10. frontal bone

11. sphenoid bone

12. ethmoid bone

13. lacrimal bone

14. nasal bone

15. zygomatic or malar bone

16. zygomatic arch

17. maxilla

18. mandible

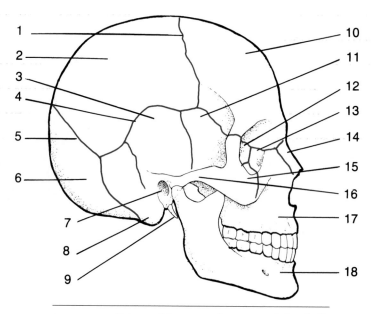

Figure 6.12 Principal bones and sutures of the skull.

Exercise 6.10   *Complete the following:*

1. Freely movable joints are classified as ___diarthroses___ .
2. Slightly movable joints are classified as ___amphiarthroses___ .
3. Immovable joints are classified as ___synarthroses___ .
4. The bones that enter into the formation of the foot articulating with the tarsals and the phalanges are called ___metatarsals___ .
5. A ___ball-and-socket___ joint permits movement in different directions.
6. A ___gliding___ joint is one in which the adjacent bone surfaces glide upon each other to permit movement.
7. Joints are described according to tissue structure as three types: ___synovial___ , ___fibrous___ , and ___cartilaginous___ .
8. The cartilages attaching the first seven pairs of ribs to the sternum are ___costal___ cartilages.
9. When movement is permitted in only one direction, the joint is called a ___hinge___ joint.
10. The sacs that contain synovial fluid, relieving pressure on moving parts, are called ___bursae___ .

Exercise 6.11   *Define each of the following different types of motion.*

1. Flexion ___bending of joint___
2. Extension ___straightening or unbending (a joint)___
3. Abduction ___drawing of a body part away from the midline___
4. Adduction ___drawing of a displaced body part toward midline___
5. Rotation ___turning of a body part on its own axis___
6. Pronation ___turning down or downward___
7. Supination ___turning upward___
8. Circumduction ___movement describing a circle___
9. Eversion ___turning outward___
10. Inversion ___turning inward___

Exercise 6.12   *Give the meaning of the components of the following words and then define the word as a whole. Suffixes meaning* pertaining to *or* state or condition, *shown following a slash mark (/), are not to be defined separately. Before reaching for your medical dictionary, check the Related Terms list in the chapter.*

1. Carpometacarpal: _forming palm of hand_
   carpo _____ wrist _____
   metacarp/al _____ between wrist _____
   _____ and fingers _____

2. Costosternal:
   costo _____ ribs _____
   stern/al _____ sternum _____
   _____ junction of ribs w/ sternum _____

3. Interphalangeal: _articulation between_ _phalanges_
   inter _____ between _____
   phalange/al _____ fingers or toes _____

4. Radiocarpal:
   radio _____ radius _____
   carp/al _____ wrist _____
   _____ forearm bone _____

5. Talonavicular:
   talo _____ ankle bone _____
   navicul/ar _____ navicular bone _____
   _____ articulation between ankle and _____
   _____ navicular bone _____

6. Temporomandibular:
   temporo _____ temporal _____
   mandibul/ar _____ mandible _____
   _____ jawbone _____

7. Sacroiliac:
   sacro _____ sacrum _____
   iliac _____ ilium _____
   _____ joint between sacrum + ilium _____

8. Cuneocuboid:
   cuneo _____ cuneiform _____
   cuboid _____ cuboid _____
   _____ junction between cuneiform and _____
   _____ cuboid bones _____

9. Osteomyelitis: _inflammation of bone_
   osteo _____ bone _____
   myel _____ marrow _____
   itis _____ inflammation _____

10. Spondylarthritis: _inflammation of vertebrae_
    spondyl _____ spine _____
    arthr _____ joint _____
    itis _____ inflammation _____

11. Amelia:
    a _____ no, not _____
    mel/ia _____ limbs _____
    _____ absence of a limb/limbs _____

12. Anencephalia: _____
    an _____ no _____
    encephal/ia _____ brain _____
    _____ absence of cranial vault _____

13. Osteoarthritis: _inflammation of bone joint_
    osteo _____ bone _____
    arthr _____ joint _____
    itis _____ inflammation _____

14. Osteodystrophy: _defective bone formation_
    osteo _____ bone _____
    dys _____ bad _____
    troph/y _____ nutrition _____

15. Osteolysis:
    osteo _____ bone _____
    lysis _____ dissolution _____
    _____ dissolution of bone _____

CROSSWORD PUZZLE

CHAPTER 6

ACROSS

6. Fluid-filled sacs
7. Shoulder blades
8. Upper arm bone
9. U-shaped bone in neck
10. Hip socket
12. Hollow within skull or face bones
15. Chest vertebrae
17. Membrane covering bone
18. Long, lateral bone of lower leg
20. Referring to backbone
22. An opening or hole in bone
25. One of two forearm bones
26. Crescent-shaped carpal bone
27. Kneecap
28. Lower back vertebrae

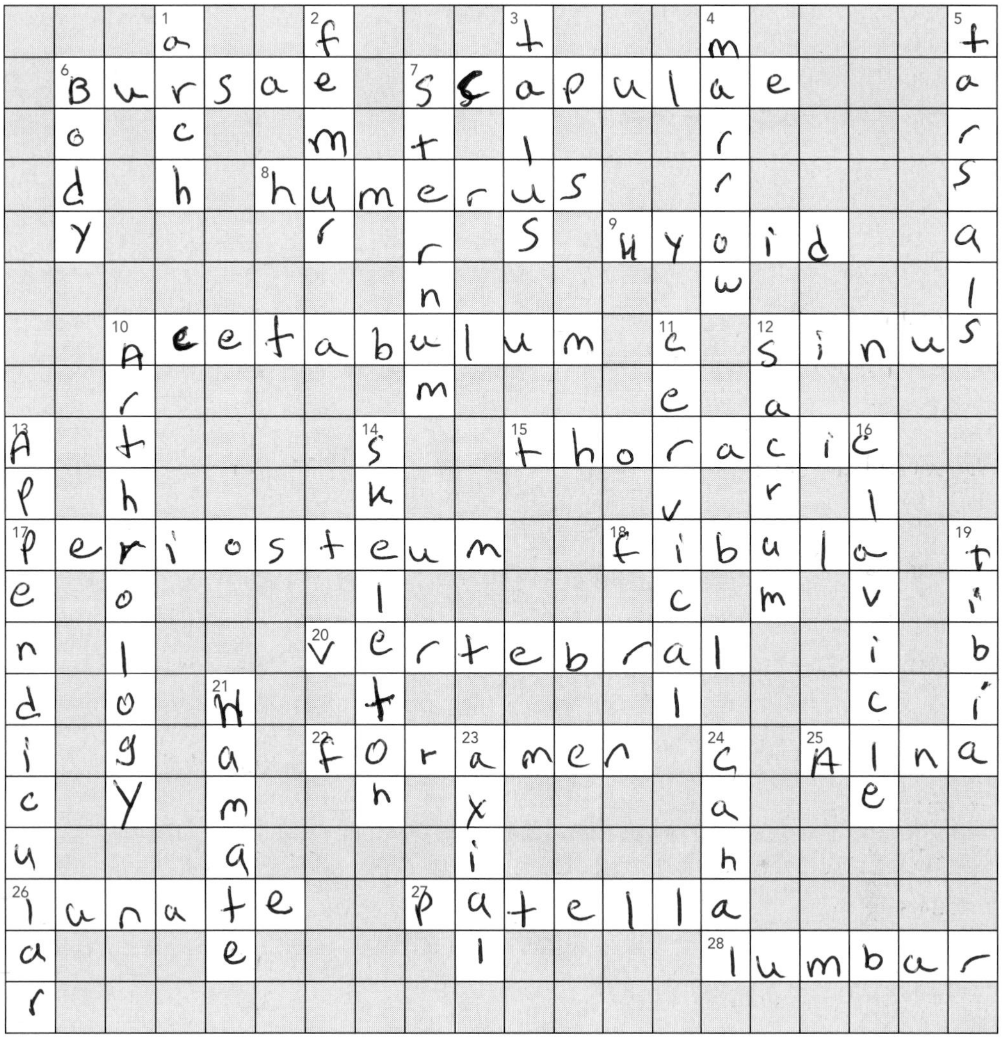

The completed crossword grid (handwritten answers):

- 6 Across: BURSAE
- 7 Across: SCAPULAE
- 8 Across: HUMERUS
- 9 Across: HYOID
- 10 Across: ACETABULUM
- 12 Across: SINUS
- 15 Across: THORACIC
- 17 Across: PERIOSTEUM
- 18 Across: FIBULA
- 20 Across: VERTEBRAL
- 22 Across: FORAMEN
- 25 Across: ULNA
- 26 Across: LUNATE
- 27 Across: PATELLA
- 28 Across: LUMBAR
- 1 Down: ARCH
- 2 Down: FEMUR
- 3 Down: TALUS
- 4 Down: MARROW
- 5 Down: TARSALS
- 6 Down: BODY
- 7 Down: STERNUM
- 10 Down: ARTHROLOGY
- 11 Down: CERVICAL
- 12 Down: SACRUM
- 13 Down: APPENDICULAR
- 14 Down: SKULL
- 16 Down: CLAVICLE
- 19 Down: TIBIA
- 21 Down: HAMATE
- 23 Down: AXIAL
- 24 Down: CANAL

DOWN

1. Posterior portion of a vertebra
2. Thighbone
3. One of the seven tarsal bones
4. Contained in medullary cavities
5. Anklebones
6. Anterior portion of a vertebra
7. Breastbone
10. Study of joints
11. Neck vertebrae
12. Triangular bone of spine
13. One main part of skeleton
14. 206 bones
16. Collarbone
19. Shinbone
21. Hooklike carpal bone
23. Other main part of skeleton
24. Tunnel

HIDDEN WORDS PUZZLE

```
S  L  L  A  R  O  Z  S  R  O  X  P  H  A  C  B  N  B  E  O
D  I  A  P  H  Y  S  I  S  B  R  V  O  W  V  M  T  F  F  Q
Y  B  S  G  V  M  S  T  E  R  N  U  M  E  U  K  C  Y  C  D
N  I  P  X  M  M  N  C  C  L  L  O  U  S  K  T  U  Z  O  R  B
I  Y  G  Z  M  M  Y  J  X  T  P  B  F  A  K  F  K  J  A  Y  B
E  O  H  Q  U  O  X  H  T  P  B  F  A  K  K  E  W  H  Q  V  W
V  M  E  D  U  L  L  A  R  Y  U  L  O  K  K  E  W  L  A  R  Y
Q  E  P  I  P  H  Y  S  E  S  R  M  A  X  I  L  L  A  R  Y  P
F  P  R  P  J  O  E  R  M  E  S  A  F  S  J  Y  E  G  H  P
M  R  T  T  E  O  R  L  I  R  A  K  X  K  T  S  T  T  Y  W
H  M  O  R  E  R  U  R  T  P  E  L  V  I  S  S  C  Q  O  S
R  V  C  N  I  B  I  E  I  W  Y  V  V  K  A  Y  L  A  I  N
D  J  F  H  T  P  R  O  E  W  R  P  K  V  Z  L  K  U  D  J
I  T  X  U  E  A  N  A  S  T  O  M  O  S  E  S  F  Y  V  M
X  C  W  T  N  R  L  L  E  T  T  S  C  A  P  U  L  A  L  P
W  Q  B  P  I  I  X  H  E  Q  T  K  T  D  G  I  Z  Q  V
H  O  K  H  C  E  N  V  J  Z  I  U  Y  E  O  T  E  I  G  V  B
X  F  G  E  E  T  C  A  B  F  D  S  M  M  O  K  E  W  N  B
N  D  W  Z  R  A  C  F  Y  M  T  V  V  H  D  L  T  L  V  R  R
U  H  Q  R  Z  L  S  P  E  N  K  V  R  I  X  S  O  B  S  R  R
D  F  J  X  G  O  L  I  E  O  G  N  C  M  R  Z  Q  G  G  J  L
F  K  X  T  C  U  B  R  N  D  P  Y  J  V  T  J  N  J  Y  L
```

Can you find the 20 words hidden in this puzzle? All hidden word puzzles have words running from top to bottom, left to right, and diagonally downward.

ANASTOMOSES	OSTEOLOGY	AXIAL
PERIOSTEUM	FONTRAL	CANCELLOUS
MEDULLARY	PELVIS	MAXILLARY
SKELETON	OSTEOBLASTS	PARIETAL
BURSAE	EPIPHYSES	STERNUM
EXTREMITIES	VERTEBRAE	HYOID
DIAPHYSIS	SCAPULA	

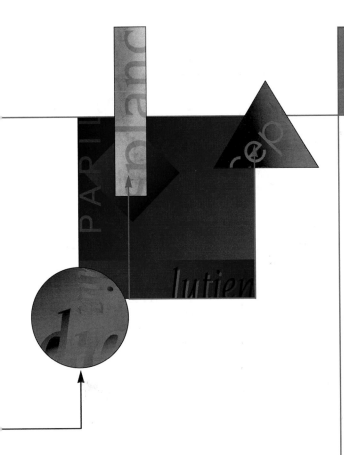

The Muscular System

the moving force

This chapter presents the different muscles of the body and their composition, classification, and relationship to other structures that aid in movement.

MUSCLES

The study of muscles is called *myology* (*myo*—muscle; *logy*—study of). All human activity is carried on by muscles in conjunction with the skeleton to achieve movement. Although the skeleton provides attachment points and support for the muscles, it is the muscle tissue and its ability to extend and contract that effects movement.

There are more than 600 muscles in the human body. Muscles constitute the major part of the fleshy portions of the body and one half of its weight, varying in proportion to the size of the individual. The form of the body is largely determined by the muscles covering the bones.

In addition to movement, the muscles have other roles, such as supporting and maintaining posture and producing body heat. They help form many of the internal organs (heart, uterus, lungs, and intestines). There is never a time when all the muscles are in a quiescent state, because the muscles of the heart, intestines, arteries, and stomach are at work, even though we are not aware of it.

It's a FACT

Contrary to popular belief, the muscles that lose strength first in the average person are the back and head muscles.

97

ALLIED MUSCULAR STRUCTURES AND TERMS

Tendons

Tendons are the strong, fibrous, white bands that attach muscles to bones, enabling the movement of a part located some distance from the contracting muscle. For example, the muscles of the calf of the leg, by means of their tendons, control the movement of the ankles and toes. If the ankle's movement depended on its own muscles, it would need to be many times its present size. Similarly, the wrists and fingers are controlled by the muscles of the upper forearm by means of their tendons. One type of tendon, called an *aponeurosis,* is flat and ribbonlike.

Fascia

Fascia is a sheet of fibrous membrane that encloses muscles and separates them into groups.

Ligaments

Ligaments are strong bands of fibrous tissue connecting bones or cartilage that aid or restrict movement and support organs.

Origin

The origin is the bone attached to a muscle, which remains relatively immovable when that particular muscle is contracted.

Insertion

The insertion is the bone attached to a muscle, which moves when that particular muscle is contracted.

Motor Nerve

A motor nerve causes a muscle to move by stimulating a definite group of muscle fibers. The combination of the nerve cell and its group of muscle cells is called a *motor,* or *neuromotor,* unit.

Tone

The tone of a muscle is the state of tension that is present when one is awake.

REVIEW 7.A

Complete the following:

1. The study of muscles is called _my ology_ .

2. Movement is produced by the ability of muscle to ___extend___ and ___contract___ .

3. The relatively immovable bone to which a muscle is attached is known as its _____ _origin_ .

4. The movable bone to which a muscle is attached is known as its _insertion_ .

5. The state of tension present in a muscle while one is awake is known as _tone_ .

COMPOSITION OF MUSCLE

Like other tissues of the body, muscle tissue is composed of cells. Muscle cells are long and slender and, because of their shape, are called *fibers.* These fibers vary greatly in size, depending on their function, but they are always gigantic when compared to other body cells. The plasma membrane of a muscle cell is called a *sarcolemma,* and its cytoplasm is called *sarcoplasm.* The muscle fibers are held together by connective tissue and enclosed in *fascia* (fibrous membrane sheath). The fibers are able to contract, producing movement of the body or its organs. The speed of muscle contraction varies with individual muscles and the size of the structure to be moved. The smaller the structure to be moved, the more rapid is the muscle action. For example, the muscles that move the eyeball contract much more rapidly than those that move a large muscle such as the gluteus maximus of the hip.

Many movements of the body are carried out by several muscles or muscle groups acting together. The muscles have a rich vascular (blood) supply. Exercise increases muscle fiber thickness but does not produce new fibers.

CLASSIFICATION OF MUSCLES

Muscles are divided into three types according to their function, shape, and structure. These three types are *skeletal, visceral,* and *cardiac* (see Figure 5.4).

Skeletal (Voluntary, Striated) Muscle

Skeletal muscles, which are attached to the skeleton, are called voluntary because they are controlled at will. They are called striated because, under a microscope, they have a cross-striated (striped) appearance. Other voluntary muscles, not attached to the skeleton, are those that move the eyeballs, tongue, pharynx, and some portions of the skin.

A typical voluntary muscle is made up of a fleshy mass of elongated muscle fibers held together in a casing of white fibrous tissue and supplied with a nerve that makes the muscle contract and extend. When muscles contract, the fibers become shorter and thicker. An example of the contraction of a voluntary muscle is flexing the forearm and squeezing it tightly so that the biceps muscle becomes thick and hard. Skeletal muscle is supplied by both the central and peripheral nervous systems (Chapter 15).

Visceral (Involuntary, Nonstriated, or Smooth) Muscle

Visceral muscles, which are found in parts of the body such as the stomach, intestines, blood vessels, and iris of the eye, are made up of nonstriated or smooth, spindle-shaped fibers. These muscles are involuntary (not controllable at will) and are supplied by the autonomic nervous system (Chapter 15).

Cardiac (Involuntary, Striated) Muscle

The cardiac (heart) muscle, although involuntary, shows fine transverse striations under the microscope. Its appearance is an exception to other involuntary muscle tissue. The cardiac muscle is controlled by the autonomic nervous system (Chapters 9 and 15).

ATTACHMENT OF MUSCLES

The attachment of muscles to tendons, which extend to the fingers and toes, results in graceful movement and reduction of bulk that would be necessary for muscles to extend to the digits. Voluntary muscles usually attach to bone; but an exception is the larynx and thorax, where muscle is attached to cartilage. Usually, muscle is attached to the capsule of joints over which its tendon passes; other muscles may be attached to the skin, as in the cheeks, or to mucous membrane, as in the tongue. Muscles may also be attached to fascia of other muscles, like the flat muscles of the abdomen, or to body structures, like the eyeball.

MOVEMENT OF MUSCLES

A muscle does not act alone, but is dependent upon other muscles to assist in executing a desired movement. For this reason, muscles are referred to as *prime movers, antagonists,* and *synergists* (*syn-* means together; *-erg-* refers to work).

The *prime movers* are those that actively produce a movement.

The *antagonists* are those in opposition to the prime movers, relaxing as the prime movers contract.

The *synergists* contract simultaneously with the prime mover to help execute a movement or steady a part.

The muscles, in conjunction with the skeleton, move the body. The different types of movements have been listed and described in Chapter 6.

REVIEW 7.B

Complete the following:

1. Muscle cells are ___long___ and ___slender___.

2. ___Sarcolema___ is the plasma membrane of a muscle cell.

3. ___Sarcoplasm___ is the cytoplasm of a muscle cell.

4. Three types of muscle tissue are _____ ___Skeletal___, ___Visceral___, and ___Cardiac___.

5. Muscles are classified according to how they produce movement and are called ___prime movers___, ___antagonists___, and ___synergists___.

HOW MUSCLES ARE NAMED

Muscle names are based on six points of identification:

1. Muscles may be named for their *action.* Example—ulnar flexor muscle of wrist (flexes wrist).

2. Muscles may be named for their *origin* and *insertion.*

Example—occipitofrontal (between occipital and frontal skull bones).
3. Muscles may be named for their *location*. Example—external oblique muscle of abdomen (abdomen).
4. Muscles may be named for their *shape* or *use*. Examples—pyramidal (shaped like a pyramid); buccinator (cheek muscle used in blowing a trumpet).
5. Muscles may be named for the *direction* of their fibers. Example—orbicular muscle of eye (around eye).
6. Muscles may be named according to the *number* of sections. Example—biceps (*bi-* means two, *-cep* means head).

ADJECTIVES FOR MUSCLES

The following are some important adjectives that aid in the description of muscles:

azygous—not paired.
bi-, tri-, and *quadri*—two, three, and four.
externus—external, or outer.
gracilis—slender.
latissimus—wide.
longissimus—long.
longus—long.
medius—intermediate.
orbicularis—surrounding.
quadratus—square.
rectus—straight.
rhomboideus—diamond or kite shaped.
scalenus—unequally triangular.
serratus—saw-toothed.
teres—round or cylindric.
transversus—crosswise.
vastus—great.

REVIEW 7.C

Complete the following:

1. There are six points of identification in naming muscles: _action_ , _orryin + insertion_ , _location_ , _shape or use_ , _fiber direction_ , and _# of sections/divisions_ .

2. Orbicularis, in relation to muscle, means _Surronding_ .
3. Quadratus, in relation to muscle, means _Square_ .
4. Rhomboideus, in relation to muscle, means _diamond or kite shaped_ .
5. Teres, in relation to muscle, means _round_ .

MUSCLE GROUPS

The following paragraphs name and describe various muscles and their actions, according to their location in the body. Only a few muscles will be covered to provide the student with a basic understanding of this system. However, a more complete listing of the muscles and their related anatomic terms can be found in the Related Terms list in this chapter.

Muscles of the Scalp

There are no muscles over the top of the skull, only skin covering a broad, flat tendon called the *galea aponeurotica* (Figure 7.1, *A*). This tendon connects to three muscle groups:

Occipitofrontal group: the *occipitalis* muscle pulls the scalp backward. The *frontalis* muscle raises the eyebrows, creates horizontal wrinkles on the forehead, and pulls the scalp forward;
Temporoparietal group: tightens scalp and moves ears upward;
Auricular group: three muscles (anterior, superior, posterior) that move the ear forward, upward, and backward.

Facial Muscles

There are many facial muscles that produce a variety of movements (Figure 7.1, *B*). Some of these are:

Orbicularis oculi (*ocul-* eye): muscle that moves the eyelids;
Orbicularis oris (*or-* mouth): muscle that draws the lips into a pucker;
Buccinator: muscle that compresses the cheek for smiling and blowing (also called *trumpeter* muscle);

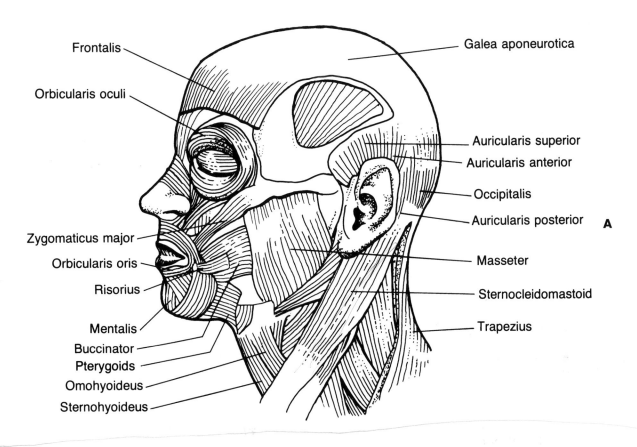

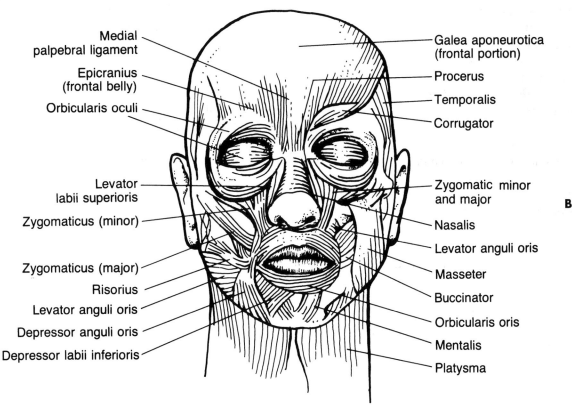

Figure 7.1 **A,** Lateral view of facial and cranial muscles and several muscles of mastication. **B,** Anterior view of muscles of face and cranium.

Platysma: muscle (origin is in fascia of chest wall) that pulls down the corners of the mouth;

Risorius: muscle that draws out the angle of the mouth;

Masseters: muscles of mastication (chewing), which raise the mandible (and close the jaw);

Pterygoids: muscles that raise and move the mandible from side to side (open and close mouth).

Muscles of the Neck and Shoulder

Although there are a number of muscles in the neck, one of the most important is:

The *sternocleidomastoid:* muscle that tilts the head forward, or to one side, and rotates it. This muscle is named for its origin in the sternum and clavicle and its insertion in the mastoid process of the temporal bone (Figures 7.2 and 7.3).

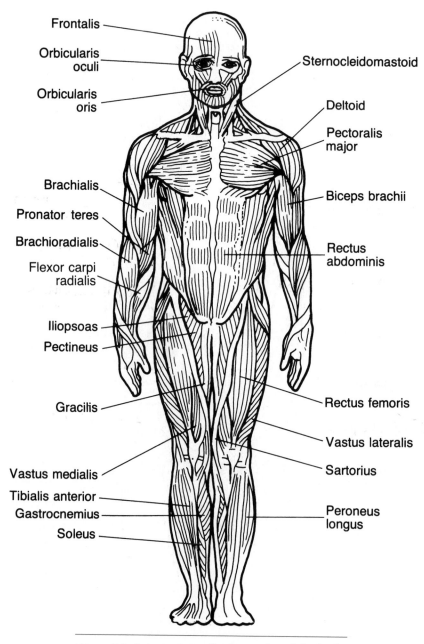

Figure 7.2 Anterior superficial muscles of the body.

Other muscles in the neck and upper thorax assist in rotation of the head, flexing the head upon the neck, and breathing.

The **trapezius** muscle: superficial (surface) muscle of the back of the neck and upper trunk. Broad and flat, it raises, lowers, and shrugs the shoulder;

The **pectoralis major** muscle: adducts and flexes the upper arm, drawing the arms across the chest;

The **latissimus dorsi** muscle: the broadest muscle in the back, extends and adducts the upper arm;

The **teres major** muscle: extends and adducts the upper arm and rotates it medially;

The **deltoid** muscle: abducts, flexes, and extends the upper arm.

Muscles of the Arms and Hands

In addition to the action of the muscles of the shoulder, back, and upper thorax, the muscles of the arms

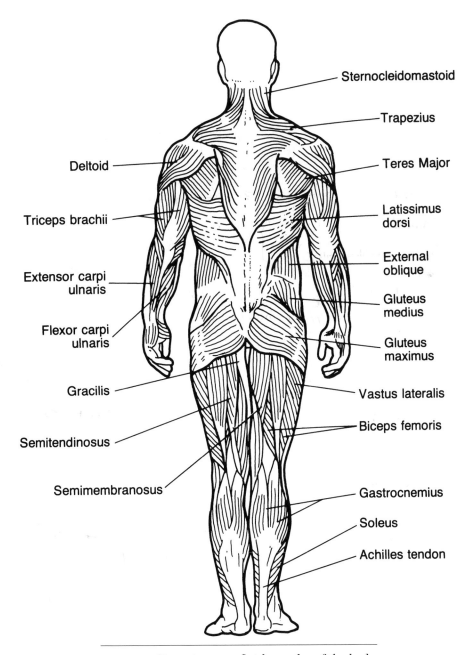

Figure 7.3 Posterior superficial muscles of the body.

also contribute to the movement of the arms (see Figures 7.2 and 7.3).

> The *triceps brachii:* extends the lower arm;
> The *brachialis:* flexes the lower arm;
> The *biceps brachii:* flexes the lower arm and supinates the lower arm and hand;
> The *pronator teres:* flexes and pronates the lower arm.

A group of *flexor* and *extensor* muscles, in conjunction with other muscles of the radius, ulna, and phalanges, control the movements of the wrists, hands, and fingers. Each of the fingers has long flexor and extensor tendons leading from the forearm muscles. The flexors bend the fingers and aid in flexing the wrist and other finger joints. The extensors abduct and adduct the wrist and extend the wrist and fingers. The thumb also has abductors, adductors, extensors, and flexors.

Muscles of the Back

Some of the major muscles in the upper part of the back have already been discussed under shoulder movements. Small muscles deep in the back control the joints between the vertebrae, steadying the vertebral column so that it can be used as a lever by long muscles. Specific muscles steady the vertebral column, maintain posture, abduct and rotate the trunk, and aid in movement of the head (see Figures 7.2 and 7.3).

Muscles of the Thorax

The muscles of the thorax are:

> The *external intercostals;*
> The *internal intercostals;*
> The *diaphragm.*

During respiration, the external intercostals lift the ribs, the internal intercostals lower the ribs, and the diaphragm contracts and flattens out, causing the thorax to enlarge, and creating more room for the lungs to expand.

Abdominal Muscles

The abdominal muscles (see Figures 7.2 and 7.3) are:

> The *external oblique;*
> The *internal oblique;*
> The *rectus abdominis;*
> The *transversus abdominis.*

These muscles keep the viscera in place, support and compress the abdomen, help to maintain posture, and contract during childbirth, defecation, coughing, and sneezing. Additionally, they assist in flexing and rotating the vertebral column.

Muscles of the Pelvic Floor

The chief muscles of the pelvic floor (Figure 7.4, *A* and *B*) are:

> The *perineum:* region between anus and vagina in the female, and anus and scrotum in the male; forms part of the supporting pelvic floor;
> The *coccygeus* muscle and the *levator ani* muscle: two muscles that are important in supporting the pelvic organs, and take part in defecation and childbirth;
> The *sphincter ani:* keeps the anus closed.

Muscles of the Thigh and Leg

The muscles of the thigh and leg (see Figures 7.2 and 7.3) have several functions in movement. The most important of these muscles are:

> The *obturator internus:* laterally rotates the thigh;
> The *obturator externus:* laterally rotates the thigh;
> The *gemellus superior:* laterally rotates the thigh;
> The *gemellus inferior:* laterally rotates the thigh;
> The *piriformis:* laterally rotates, abducts, and extends the thigh;
> The *quadratus femoris:* flexes and extends the leg and laterally rotates the thigh.

> The *gluteal* group includes:
> The *gluteus minimus:* abducts and rotates the thigh;
> The *gluteus medius:* abducts and rotates the thigh;
> The *gluteus maximus:* extends and rotates the thigh.

> The *tensor fasciae latae:* abducts the thigh.
> The *iliopsoas:* flexes the thigh and trunk.

> The *adductor* group includes:
> The *longus, brevis,* and *magnus:* powerful adductors;
> The *gracilis:* flexes the leg and adducts leg and thigh.

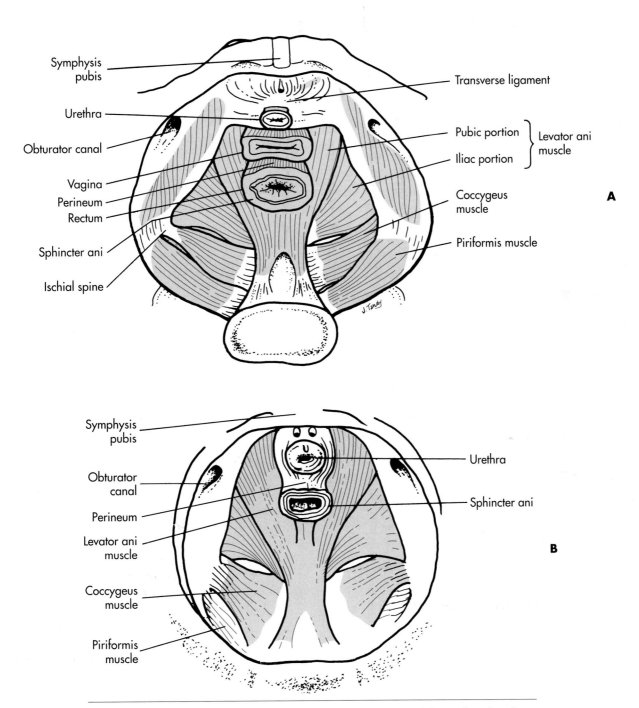

Symphysis pubis

Urethra

Obturator canal

Vagina

Perineum

Rectum

Sphincter ani

Ischial spine

Transverse ligament

Pubic portion ⎫
Iliac portion ⎬ Levator ani muscle

Coccygeus muscle

Piriformis muscle

A

Symphysis pubis

Obturator canal

Perineum

Levator ani muscle

Coccygeus muscle

Piriformis muscle

Urethra

Sphincter ani

B

Figure 7.4 **A**, Muscles of the female pelvic floor. **B**, Muscles of the male pelvic floor.

The *quadriceps femoris* group includes:
The *rectus femoris:* flexes the thigh and extends the leg;
The *vastus lateralis:* extends the leg;
The *vastus medialis:* extends the leg;
The *vastus intermedius:* extends the leg.

The *sartorius:* flexes and adducts the leg.

The *hamstring* group of muscles descend in the back of the thigh, their tendons forming the *hamstrings.* They include:
The *semimembranosus:* extends the thigh;
The *semitendinosus:* extends the thigh;
The *biceps femoris:* extends the thigh and flexes the leg.

The *gastrocnemius:* flexes the leg and extends the foot. This muscle, and the soleus (see Muscles of the Foot following) are commonly called the calf muscles, and their tendon is the *Achilles* tendon.

Muscles of the Foot

The chief muscles of the foot (see Figures 7.2 and 7.3) include:
The *soleus:* extends the foot;
The *tibialis anterior:* turns the foot in and flexes it;
The *tibialis posterior:* turns the foot in and extends it;
The *peroneus longus:* turns the foot outward and extends it;
The *peroneus brevis:* turns the foot outward and flexes it;
The *peroneus tertius:* turns the foot outward and flexes it.

Like the muscles in the fingers, those of the toes have flexor, abductor, adductor, and extensor tendons. In the foot the tendons move the phalangeal joints, keep the foot and toes firmly on the ground, and aid in walking, dancing, running, jumping, dorsiflexion of the ankle, and eversion and inversion of the foot.

REVIEW 7.D

Complete the following:

1. The broad, flat tendon over the top of the skull is called the ___galea aponeurotica___

2. The auricular group of muscles move the ___ear___.

3. The buccinator muscle is also called the ___trumpeter___.

4. The ___sternocleido mastoid___ muscle is named for its origin in the sternum and clavicle and its insertion in the mastoid process.

5. The diaphragm is a muscle of respiration located in the ___thorax___.

6. ___abdominal___ muscles contract when an individual coughs or sneezes.

7. The gluteal group of muscles is divided into ___3___ sections.

8. The muscle that pulls down the corner of the mouth is the ___platysma___.

9. A broad, flat, superficial muscle of the back of the neck and trunk is the ___trapezius___.

10. Muscles for chewing are the ___masseters___

ANATOMY

Muscles

abduction (ab-duk′shun) movement that draws a body part away from the midline of the body.

abductor muscles muscles that abduct.

Achilles tendon (ah-kil′ez) a powerful tendon of the gastrocnemius and soleus at the back of the heel (also called *calcaneal tendon*), named for a Greek hero whose only vulnerable spot was his heel.

adduction (ad-duk′shun) movement that draws a body part toward the midline of the body.

adductor muscles muscles that adduct.

adductor longus, magnus, and **brevis** a group of adductor muscles of the thigh that also assist in flexion, extension, and rotation.

antagonist a muscle acting in opposition to another.

aponeurosis (ap″o-nu-ro′sis) a flattened, ribbonlike, white tendon that connects a muscle to the part it moves (plural—*aponeuroses*).

auriculares (aw″rik-u-la′rez) group of muscles of the ear; *anterior, posterior,* and *superior.*

biceps (bi′seps) indicates two origins (or heads) of a muscle.

brachialis (bra-ke-a′lis) arm muscle that flexes the forearm.

brachioradialis lower arm muscle that flexes the forearm.

buccinator (buk′si-na″tor) a cheek muscle (also called *trumpeter*).

cardiac muscle of the heart.

coccygeus (kok-sij′e-us) muscle supporting and raising the coccyx.

constrictor pharyngis muscle group that constricts the pharynx; *inferior, medius,* and *superior.*

deltoid (del′toid) muscle that abducts, flexes, and extends upper arm.

diaphragm (di′ah-fram) musculomembranous wall between abdominal and thoracic cavities.

erector spinae deep muscle of the back that aids in maintaining balance (also called *sacrospinalis*).

extensors muscles that extend a part.

fascia (fash′e-ah) sheet of fibrous membrane that encloses muscles and separates them into groups (plural—*fasciae*).

fascia lata femoris broad external fascia enveloping muscles of the thigh.

fasciculus (fah-sik′u-lus) a small bundle or cluster (referring to muscle, tendon, or nerve fibers; plural—*fasiculi*).

fibromuscular composed of muscular and fibrous tissue.

fixator muscles muscles that steady a part while other muscles execute movement.

flexor muscle that flexes or bends a joint.

galea aponeurotica (ga′le-ah) the broad, flat tendon over the top of the skull.

gastrocnemius (gas″trok-ne′me-us) muscle of the lower leg (calf), resembling the shape of the stomach, that flexes the leg and extends the foot.

gemellus (je-mel′us) twin thigh muscles, inferior and superior, that aid in lateral rotation of the thigh (plural—*gemelli*).

gluteal (gloo′te-al) referring to the buttock, a group of muscles, *gluteus maximus, medius,* and *minimus,* which abduct, rotate, and extend the thigh.

gracilis (gras′i-lis) flexes leg and adducts leg and thigh.

hamstring group three large muscles that descend in the back of the thigh, their tendons forming the "hamstrings," are the *semimembranosus* and the *semitendinosus,* which extend the thigh, and the *biceps femoris,* which extends the thigh and flexes the leg.

iliacus (il-i′ah-kus) muscle that flexes thigh and trunk.

iliocostalis muscle group including the *iliocostalis dorsi,* which keeps the thoracic spine erect; the *iliocostalis lumborum,* which extends the lumbar spine; and the *iliocostalis cervicis,* which extends the cervical spine.

iliopsoas (il″e-o-so′as) *iliacus* and *psoas major* muscles combined and referred to as one muscle, which flexes the thigh and trunk.

infrahyoid muscles small, flat, ribbonlike muscles of the neck, including the *sternothyroid, sternohyoid, thyrohyoid,* and *omohyoid* muscles, which hold the hyoid bone to the sternum, scapula, and clavicle.

infraspinatus (in″frah-spi-na′tus) muscle that rotates the humerus laterally.

inspiratory muscles muscles that aid in inspiration, such as the *diaphragm* and the *intercostals.*

intercostals respiratory muscles, situated between the ribs.

interossei (in″ter-os′e-i) muscles of the hand and foot that flex, abduct, and adduct fingers and toes.

interspinales (in″ter-spi-nal′ez) muscle group that extends the vertebral column in the cervical, thoracic, and lumbar regions.

involuntary muscle muscle that cannot be moved at will.

latissimus dorsi (lah-tis′i-mus dor′si) the broadest muscle of the back, which extends and adducts the upper arm.

levator ani (le-va′tor) muscle of the pelvic floor.

levator scapulae muscle that raises the scapula.

ligaments strong bands of fibrous tissue connecting bones or cartilage, which aid or restrict movement and support organs.

longissimus muscles (lon-jis′i-mus) group of muscles, including the *capitas,* which draws the head backward and rotates it; the *cervicis,* which extends the cervical vertebrae; and the *thoracis,* which extends the thoracic vertebrae.

lumbricales (lum′bri-ka′les) phalangeal muscles of the foot and hand.

masseter (mas-se′ter) chewing muscle.

multifidus spinae (mul-tif′i-dus) muscles that extend and rotate the vertebral column.

oblique external abdominal muscle that compresses and supports the abdominal viscera.

oblique internal abdominal muscle that compresses and supports the abdominal viscera.

obturator externus and internus (ob′tu-ra″tor) muscles that rotate the thigh laterally.

occipitofrontal (ok-sip″i-to-fron-t′al) a group of flat muscles of the forehead and scalp.

orbicularis oculi (or-bik″u-la′ris) muscle that moves the eyelids.

orbicularis oris muscle that draws lips into a pucker.

orbitalis muscle that makes eye protrude.

palatoglossus (pal″ah-to-glos′us) muscle for elevating the tongue and constricting the passage from mouth to throat.

palatopharyngeus aids in swallowing.

pectineus muscle that flexes and adducts the thigh.

pectoralis major and minor (pek″to-ra′lis) muscles that adduct and flex upper arms *(major)* and draw shoulder forward and down *(minor).*

peroneus longus, brevis, and tertius (per″o-ne′us) lower leg muscles aiding in movement of the feet.

piriformis (pir″i-for′mis) pear-shaped muscle that laterally rotates, abducts, and extends the thigh.

platysma (plah-tiz′mah) facial muscle of expression that pulls down the corners of the mouth.

popliteal (pop″li-te′al) muscle that flexes and rotates the leg medially.

pronator teres and quadratus muscles that flex and pronate the lower arm.

psoas major and minor (so′as) muscles that flex the trunk and thigh, medially rotating the thigh.

pyramidal (pi-ram″id′al) muscle that tenses the abdominal wall.

quadratus femoris (kwod-ra′tus) thigh muscle for adduction and lateral rotation.

quadratus lumborum muscle that laterally flexes the trunk.

quadriceps femoris (kwod′ri-seps) muscle (four-headed) that extends the leg.

rectus abdominis (rek′tus ab′dom′i-nis) muscle supporting abdomen and flexing lumbar vertebrae.

rectus capitis muscles of head, anterior, lateral, and posterior major and minor muscles that support, flex, and extend the head.

rectus femoris muscle that extends the leg and flexes the thigh.

rhomboideus major and minor (rom-boi′de-us) rhomboid muscles (kite shaped) that elevate, adduct, and retract the scapulae.

risorius (ri-so′re-us) facial muscle that draws out the angle of the mouth.

sarcolemma plasma membrane of muscle cells.

sarcoplasm the cytoplasm of muscle cells.

sartorius (sar-to′re-us) muscle of the thigh, deriving its name from its ability to flex and adduct the leg to that position assumed by a tailor sitting cross-legged at work *(sartorius* means tailor).

scalenus group of muscles that raise the first and second ribs.

semimembranosus muscle that extends the thigh.

semispinalis (sem″e-spi-na′lis) group of muscles for movement of the vertebral column and head.

semitendinosus (sem″e-ten″di-no′sus) muscle that extends the thigh.

serratus (ser-ra′tus) muscle group *(anterior, posterior superior,* and *posterior inferior)* that rotates scapula, raises shoulder, abducts arm, and raises and lowers ribs during respiration.

soleus (so′le-us) muscle that extends the foot.

sphincters (sfingk'ters) circular muscles that constrict an orifice, such as the anus, urethra, and pyloris.

splenius (sple'ne-us) muscle group (*capitis* and *cervicis*) that extends and rotates the head and neck.

sternocleidomastoid (ster"no-kli"do-mas'toid) muscle that tilts the head forward, or to one side, and rotates it.

subclavius (sub-kla've-us) muscle that moves the clavicle.

subcostals muscles that raise the ribs in inspiration.

subscapularis (sub"skap-u-la'ris) muscle that rotates the arm medially.

supinator (su"pi-na'tor) muscle that turns the forearm upward.

supraspinatus (su"prah-spi-na'tus) muscle that abducts the arm.

synergists (sin'er-jists) muscles that work together.

tensor fasciae latae muscle that abducts the thigh.

teres major and **minor (te'rez)** muscles that extend and adduct the upper arm and rotate it medially.

tibialis anterior and **posterior (tib"e-a'lis)** muscles that extend, flex, and turn the foot in.

tone state of tension, present to a degree in muscles when one is awake.

transversus abdominis the transverse abdominal muscles that compress and support the viscera of the abdomen.

trapezius (trah-pe'ze-us) a trapezoid-shaped muscle of the back of the neck and upper trunk that controls shoulder movements.

triceps brachii (tri'seps) muscle that extends the forearm.

vastus intermedius, lateralis, and **medialis (vas'tus)** muscle group that extends the leg.

voluntary muscle muscle that can be moved at will.

PATHOLOGIC CONDITIONS

Inflammations and Infections

dermatomyositis (der"mah-to-mi"o-si'tis) connective tissue disease characterized by inflammation of the skin, underlying tissues, and muscles, with necrosis of muscle fibers.

fasciitis (fas"e-i'tis) inflammation of the fascia (also called *fascitis*).

myocellulitis (mi"o-sel"u-li'tis) myositis with cellulitis (inflammation of cellular tissue).

myochorditis (mi"o-kor-di'tis) inflammation of the muscles of the vocal cords.

myofascitis (mi"o-fas-i'tis) inflammation of a muscle and its fascia.

myositis (mi"o-si'tis) inflammation of voluntary muscle.

myositis ossificans (o-sif'i-kans) a myositis characterized by bony deposits in muscle tissue.

myotenositis (mi"o-ten"o-si'tis) inflammation of a muscle and its tendon.

polymyalgia rheumatica (pol'i-mi-al'je-ah) pain caused by inflammation in more than one muscle group.

shin splints swelling and pain caused by strain of pretibial muscle following overexertion.

tenositis inflammation of a tendon (also called *tendinitis, tenontitis,* and *tenonitis*).

tenostosis (ten"os-to'sis) conversion of tendon tissue into bone or bony substance.

tenosynovitis (ten"o-sin"o-vi'tis) inflammation of a tendon sheath (also called *tenovaginitis* or *tendovaginitis*).

torticollis (tor"ti-kol'is) an acute myositis of the cervical muscles (also called *wryneck*).

trichiniasis or **trichinosis (trik"i-ni'ah-sis; trik"i-no'sis)** disease caused by eating undercooked, parasite-infected meat with symptoms of nausea, diarrhea, colic, and fever, followed by stiffness, pain, and swelling of muscles.

Degenerative and Innervative Disorders

amyotrophy or **amyotrophia** atrophy of muscles.

Dupuytren's contracture (du-pwe'trahnz) disease affecting the palmar fascia of the hand, causing the ring and little finger to contract toward the palm (named for its discoverer).

muscular atrophy wasting away of muscle tissue (types and causes are multiple).

myasthenia gravis (mi"as-the'ne-ah) debilitating, muscular disease, with progressive paralysis of the muscles, especially affecting muscles of the face, lips, tongue, throat, and neck.

myofibrosis (mi"o-fi-bro'sis) overgrowth of fibrous tissue, replacing muscle tissue.

myoparalysis paralysis of a muscle or muscles.

myotonia (mi"o-to'ne-ah) increased muscular irritability and contractility (tonic spasm), with delayed relaxation.

myotonia acquisita myotonia caused by injury or disease.

spastic paralysis paralysis marked by spasticity of muscles of the affected part and heightened tendon reflexes.

Volkmann's contracture (folk'mahnz) contracture of the fingers and sometimes the wrists (named for its discoverer), with loss of muscle power, caused by vascular (blood flow) blockage (also called *ischemic muscular atrophy*).

Hereditary, Congenital, and Developmental Disorders

congenital amyotonia (ah'mi"o-to'ne-ah) term used to describe several rare congenital diseases of infants and children, characterized by lack of muscular development (also called *atonic pseudoparalysis*, *amyotonia congenita*, and *Oppenheim's disease*).

muscular dystrophy a group of hereditary diseases characterized by progressive weakness and atrophy of muscles without nervous system involvement (also called *idiopathic muscular atrophy* and *myodystrophia*).

myotonia congenita hereditary, congenital disease, characterized by spasm and rigidity of muscles when moved after rest or when mechanically stimulated, with stiffness disappearing as muscles are used (also called *paramyotonia congenita*, *myotonia hereditaria*, *Eulenburg's disease*, and *Thomsen's disease*).

pseudohypertrophic muscular dystrophy progressive dystrophy of the muscles of the shoulder and pelvic girdles, beginning in childhood, with hypertrophy progressing to atrophy of the muscles (also called *Duchenne's muscular dystrophy*, *Erb's paralysis*, and *pseudohypertrophic muscular atrophy*).

Werdnig-Hoffman disease hereditary, progressive, muscular atrophy, beginning in infancy and followed by early death (also called *familial spinal muscular atrophy* and *progressive spinal muscular atrophy of infants*).

Oncology

desmoid tumor very hard fibroma, most frequently in abdominal muscles, especially in women who have borne children.

leiomyoma (li"o-mi-o'mah) benign tumor of smooth muscle, usually found in the uterus (commonly known as *fibroid tumor*).

leiomyosarcoma* (li"o-mi"o-sar-ko"mah) malignant tumor of smooth muscle usually found in uterus or retroperitoneal region.

myoblastoma (mi"o-blas-to'mah) a benign lesion of soft tissue (also called *myoblastomyoma*).

myofibroma tumor with muscular and fibrous elements.

myoma (mi-o'mah) tumor composed of muscle tissue.

myosarcoma* malignant tumor of muscular tissue.

rhabdomyoma benign tumor arising from striated muscle.

rhabdomyochondroma (rab"do-mi"o-kon-dro'mah) benign tumor composed of two or more types of cells (also called *rhabdomyomyxoma*).

rhabdomyosarcoma* (rab"do-mi"o-sar-ko'mah) very malignant tumor of striated muscle (also called *rhabdomyoblastoma*).

SURGICAL PROCEDURES

fasciectomy (fas"e-ek'to-me) excision of fascia.

fasciodesis (fas"e-od'e-sis) suturing of fascia to tendon or other fascia.

fascioplasty (fash'e-o-plas"te) plastic repair of fascia.

fasciorrhaphy (fash"e-or'ah-fe) repair of torn fascia.

fasciotomy (fash"e-to'o-me) incision of fascia.

myectomy (mi-ek'to-me) excision of a part of a muscle.

myoplasty (mi'o-plas"te) plastic repair of muscle.

myorrhaphy (mi-or'ah-fe) repair of a divided muscle (also called *myosuture*).

myotenotomy (mi"o-ten-ot'o-me) cutting of muscle and tendon (also called *tenomyotomy* and *tenontomyotomy*).

myotomy incision or dissection of a muscle.

tenodesis (ten-od'e-sis) suturing of a tendon to a bone.

tenoplasty (ten'o-plast"te) plastic repair of a tendon.

tenorrhaphy (ten-or'ah-fe) suturing of a divided tendon (also called *tenosuture*).

tenosynovectomy (ten"o-sin"o-vek'to-me) excision of the sheath of a tendon.

tenotomy cutting of a tendon.

---

*Indicates a malignant condition.

DESCRIPTIVE AND DIAGNOSTIC TERMS

myalgia (mi-al′je-ah) pain in a muscle (also called *myodynia*).

myoclonus (mi-ok′lo-nus) spasm of a muscle or muscles.

myodiastasis (mi″o-di-as′tah-sis) muscle separation.

myodystonia (mi″o-dis-to′ne-ah) muscle tone disorder.

myoedema (mi″o-e-de′mah) fluid accumulation in muscle.

myogelosis (mi″o-je-lo′sis) hardening of muscle in a specific area, especially in the gluteal region.

myokinesis (mi″o-ki-ne′sis) movement of a muscle or its fibers, especially during a surgical procedure.

myology study of muscles.

myolysis disintegration of muscle tissue.

myomalacia (mi″o-mah-la′she-ah) softening of a muscle.

myomelanosis (mi″o-mel″ah-no′sis) area of black pigment in a muscle.

myonecrosis (mi″o-ne-kro′sis) death of muscle fibers.

myopathy (mi-op′ah-the) any disease of the muscles.

myosclerosis (mi″o-skle-ro′sis) hardening of muscle tissue.

myospasm (mi′o-spazm) spasm of a muscle.

myotasis (mi-ot′ah-sis) stretching of a muscle.

tenodynia (ten″o-din′e-ah) pain in a tendon (also called *tenalgia*).

tetany paroxysmal spasms.

tic twitch or spasm of a muscle.

LABORATORY TESTS

biopsy removal of tissue for microscopic examination.

computerized tomography (CT) imaging device using x-rays at multiple angles through specific sections of the body, analyzed by computer to provide a total picture of the part being examined to detect tumors in muscle tissue (also called *computerized axial tomography—CAT*).

creatine phosphokinase blood serum test to detect enzyme elevations found in patients with muscular dystrophy and other muscle conditions.

electromyography electrical recording of the changes in skeletal muscle resulting from electrical stimulation.

inulin clearance a urine test to evaluate the rate at which inulin is excreted, to diagnose muscle diseases.

magnetic resonance imaging (MRI) noninvasive method of scanning the body by use of an electromagnetic field and radio waves, which provides visual images on a computer screen, and magnetic tape recordings, to detect muscle disease (also called *nuclear magnetic resonance—NMR*).

3-methoxy-4-hydroxymandelic acid a urine test in which elevated levels of adrenaline and noradrenaline indicate muscle conditions such as muscular dystrophy and myasthenia gravis.

myoglobin test for protein found in normal muscle tissue, which, when present in urine, indicates extensive muscle destruction.

myokinesimeter testing device to measure muscular contractions by stimulation with electrical current.

nuclear magnetic resonance (NMR) see *magnetic resonance imaging.*

trichina agglutinin test of blood serum that reveals the presence of trichinosis.

EXERCISES   THE MUSCULAR SYSTEM THE MOVING FORCE

Exercise 7.1   *Complete the following:*

1. The strong fibrous white bands that attach muscles to bones are called ___tendons___ .
2. The strong bands of tissue that hold bones together and support organs are called ___ligaments___ .
3. A particular type of tendon that is flat and ribbonlike is called a(n) ___aponeurosis___ .
4. The immovable attachment of a muscle, or the point at which it is anchored by a tendon to a bone, is called its ___origin___ .
5. The nerve that causes a muscle to move is called a(n) ___motor nerve___ .

Exercise 7.2   *Matching*

___D___   1. skeletal
___F___   2. visceral muscle
___H___   3. cardiac muscle
___B___   4. prime mover
___G___   5. antagonist
___J___   6. sarcolemma
___A___   7. synergist
___I___   8. insertion
___C___   9. striated
___E___   10. nonstriated

A. muscles that work together
B. muscle that actively produces a movement
C. striped
D. muscle that can be moved voluntarily
E. smooth
F. muscle that cannot be moved at will
G. muscle acting in opposition to another
H. heart muscle
I. movable bone attached to muscle
J. plasma membrane of a muscle cell

Exercise 7.3   *Multiple choice*

1. Unpaired muscles are described as:
   a. azygous
   b. gracilis
   c. serratus

2. Long muscles are referred to as:
   a. longissimus
   b. latissimus
   c. medius

3. Muscles surrounding a part are described as:
   a. orbicularis
   b. externus
   c. transversus

4. Muscles that have four insertions may include the term:
   a. *bi-*
   b. *tri-*
   c. *quadri-*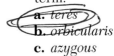

5. A round or cylindrical muscle may include the term:
   a. *teres*
   b. *orbicularis*
   c. *azygous*

Exercise 7.4   *Muscles may be named in six ways. Study the statements below carefully and identify the manner in which the following muscles are named by placing the correct letter in the space provided.*

A. Action: has a verb-based root with a suffix, followed by the name of the structure affected.

B. Joining the names of the points of origin and attachment, with an adjective suffix.

C. Location: usually includes an adjective, followed by the location of the muscle.

D. For their shape or for the way the muscle is used.

E. According to the direction of the muscle fibers.

F. According to the number of sections or divisions forming them.

B	1. brachioradialis
D	2. buccinator
A	3. extensor carpi
C	4. external oblique abdominal
F	5. biceps brachii
E	6. orbicularis
D	7. platysma
A	8. levator scapulae
A	9. flexor carpi radialis
C	10. tibialis anterior

Exercise 7.5   *Using the list of terms below, identify each muscle in Figure 7.5 by writing its name in the corresponding blank.*

Frontalis   Rectus femoris   Tibialis anterior   Brachioradialis

Sternocleidomastoid   Sartorius   Iliopsoas   Soleus

Biceps brachii   Orbicularis oculi   Vastus lateralis   Vastus medialis

Flexor carpi radialis   Deltoid   Pronator teres   Rectus abdominis

Gastrocnemius   Brachialis   Orbicularis oris   Pectineus

Gracilis   Peroneus longus   Pectoralis major

1. Frontalis
2. orbicularis oculi
3. orbicularis oris
4. brachialis
5. pronator teres
6. brachioradialis
7. Flexor carpi radialis
8. iliopsoas
9. pectineus
10. gracilis
11. vastus medialis
12. gastrocnemius
13. tibialis anterior
14. soleus
15. sternocleidomastoid
16. deltoid
17. pectoralis major
18. biceps brachii
19. rectus abdominis
20. rectus femoris
21. vastus lateralis
22. sartorius
23. peroneus longus

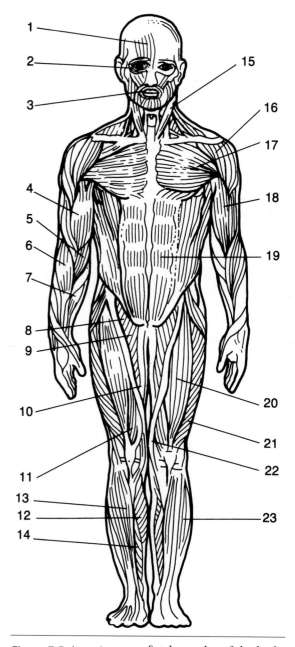

Figure 7.5 Anterior superficial muscles of the body.

Exercise 7.6   *Using the list of terms below, identify each muscle or tendon in Figure 7.6 by writing its name in the corresponding blank.*

Sternocleidomastoid   Semitendinosus   Gluteus medius   Flexor carpi ulnaris

Triceps brachii   Achilles tendon   Biceps femoris   Gluteus maximus

Extensor carpi ulnaris   Trapezius   Gastrocnemius   Semimembranosus

External oblique   Teres major   Deltoid   Soleus

Vastus lateralis   Gracilis   Latissimus dorsi

1. _deltoid_
2. _triceps_
3. _extensor carpi ulnaris_
4. _flexor carpi ulnaris_
5. _gracilis_
6. _semitendinosus_
7. _sternocleidomastoid_
8. _trapezius_
9. _teres major_
10. _latissimus dorsi_
11. _external oblique_
12. _gluteus medius_
13. _gluteus maximus_
14. _vastus lateralis_
15. _biceps femoris_
16. _semimembranosus_
17. _gastrocnemius_
18. _soleus_
19. _achilles tendon_

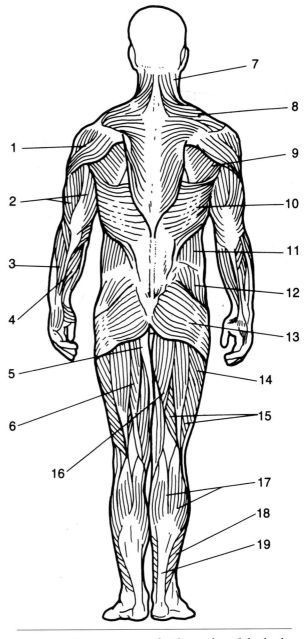

Figure • 7.6 Posterior superficial muscles of the body.

Exercise 7.7   *Matching*

_B___ **1.** orbicularis oculi

_K___ **2.** masseters

_D___ **3.** sternocleidomastoid

_C___ **4.** trapezius

_G___ **5.** buccinator

_F___ **6.** pronator teres

_I___ **7.** serratus

_H___ **8.** gluteus maximus

_J___ **9.** latissimus dorsi

_E___ **10.** rectus abdominis

_A___ **11.** orbicularis oris

A. surrounding the mouth

B. surrounding eyes

C. back of neck and upper trunk controlling shoulder movements

D. sternum and clavicle to mastoid process

E. frontal abdominal muscle

F. flexes and pronates lower arm

G. cheek muscle

H. hip muscle

I. sawtooth muscle

J. broad muscle of back

K. facial muscle for chewing

Exercise 7.8   *Give the meaning of the components of the following words and then define the word as a whole. Suffixes meaning pertaining to or state or condition, shown following a slash mark (/), are not to be defined separately. Before reaching for your medical dictionary, check the Related Terms list in this chapter.*

1. Amyotrophia:

   a ___no___

   myo ___muscle___

   troph/ia ___nourishment___

   ___atrophy of muscle___

2. Myofibrosis:

   myo ___muscle___

   fibr/osis ___fibrous tissue___

   ___muscle tissue replaced by fibrous tissue___

3. Fasciodesis:

   fascio ___fascia___

   desis ___binding___

   ___suturing of fascia to skeletal___

4. Myotenotomy:

   myo ___muscle___

   teno ___tendon___

   tomy ___surgical incision of tendon of a muscle___

5. Myalgia:

   my ___muscle___

   algia ___pain___

   ___painful muscle___

6. Myoedema:

   myo ___muscle___

   edema ___swelling___

   ___swelling of muscle___

7. Tenostosis:

   ten ___tendon___

   ost/osis ___bone___

   ___ossification of tendon___

8. Myoma:

   my ___muscle___

   oma ___tumor___

   ___tumor of muscle___

9. Myorrhaphy:

   myo ___muscle___

   rrhaphy ___suturing___

   ___suturing of muscle___

10. Myosclerosis:

    myo ___muscle___

    scler/osis ___hardening___

    ___hardening of muscle___

11. Tenosynovectomy:

    teno ___tendon___

    synov ___synovial sheath___

    ectomy ___excision___

    ___surgical excision of tendon sheath___

12. Myomelanosis:

    myo ___muscle___

    melan/osis ___melanin pigment___

    ___area of black pigment in a muscle___

CROSSWORD PUZZLE

CHAPTER 7

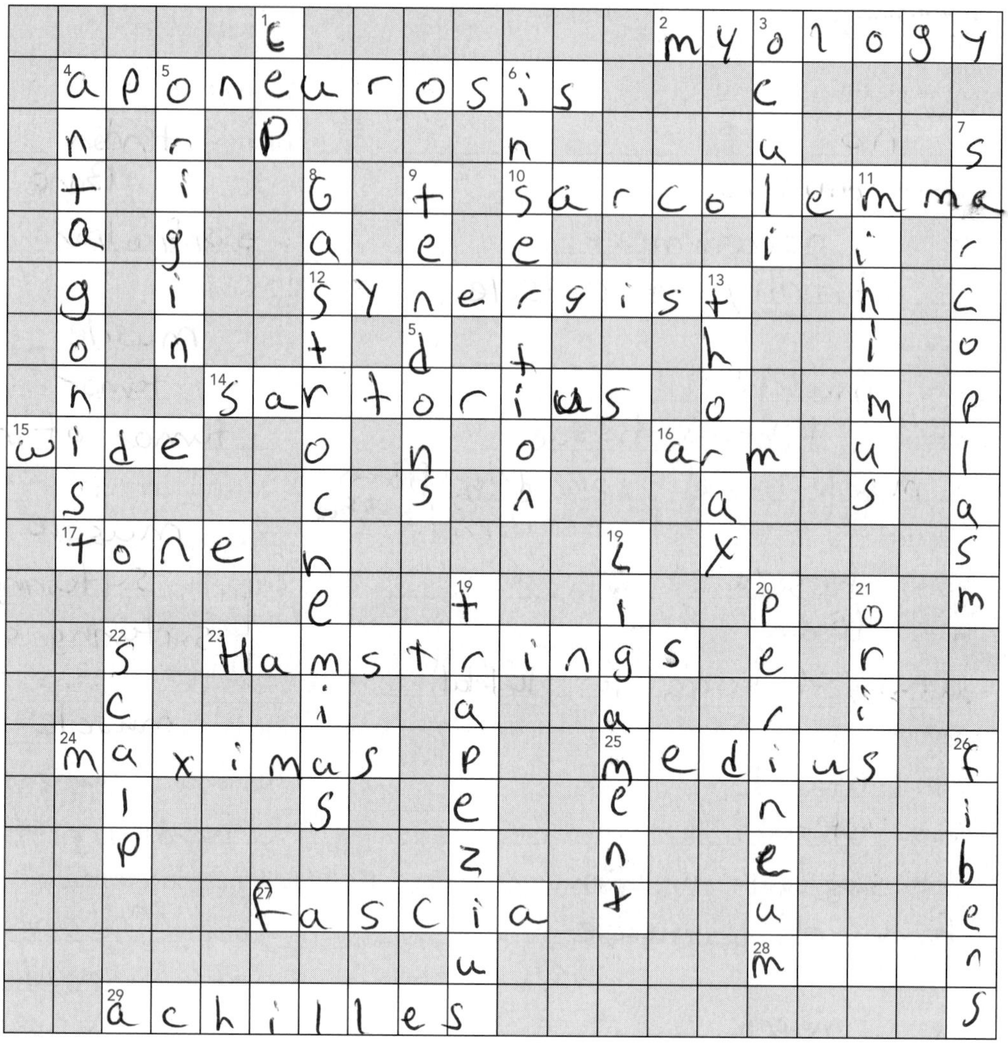

ACROSS

2. The study of muscles
4. Flat, ribbonlike type of tendon
10. Plasma membrane of a muscle cell
12. Contracts with a prime mover to move or steady a part
14. Name this "tailor" muscle
15. The meaning of latissimus
16. Location of the brachialis
17. Waking state muscle tension
23. Muscle group and tendons descending back of thigh
24. One of three gluteal muscles
25. Second of three gluteal muscles
27. Fibrous membrane sheet
28. Nerve type causing muscle to move
29. Tendon of calf muscles

DOWN

1. Root meaning "head"
3. Orbicularis of eyelid
4. Muscle that opposes prime mover
5. Immovable attachment of muscle
6. Movable attachment of muscle
7. Muscle cell cytoplasm
8. One of two calf muscles
9. Bands attaching muscles to bones
11. Third of gluteal muscle group
13. Diaphragm location
18. Supporting and connecting band
19. Muscle of neck and upper back
20. Supports part of pelvic floor
21. Orbicularis of the lips
22. Three groups moving forehead and ears
26. Term for muscle cells

HIDDEN WORDS PUZZLE   CHAPTER 7

Can you find the 20 words hidden in this puzzle? All hidden words puzzles have words running from top to bottom, left to right, and diagonally downward.

CLASSIFICATION

SYNERGISTS

LIGAMENT

CARDIAC

MUSCLE

ANTAGONISTS

INSERTION

SKELETAL

FASCIA

ORIGIN

APONEUROSIS

VOLUNTARY

STRIATED

FIBERS

SMOOTH

INVOLUNTARY

EXTENSOR

VISCERAL

FLEXOR

TENDON

```
E C F G Q S A B B S R D L P X C W S Q X U V
T P V L T O H I S K E L E T A L Y F N Q N U
F H V M E O J N Y C H Q B T J H Q R V M H G
B R S Y N X U S N L K E J M G W S O T E N E
D F W B D O O E E F T X B U J Y N A W K S L
U E A E O R G R R K Q T T L B J C E V C X X
C F E S N I V T G S J E T T U M G D U S C D
M Z S M C G C I I J O N M L R H S Y X L N S
M R N O W I L O S V I S C E R A L O S T L F
F E P O M N A N T A G O N I S T S L A P U O
V I S T O U S P S Z B R L D G R Q P A E A K
H O B H R T S L O J W S G C F C G P V C T T
E V L E H V I C I N V O L U N T A R Y K X U
M C F U R N F W L G E K C H L N R R Y I M C
I X U Y N S I G N E A U E R X J J F D K Y L
O Q O H P T C G W D S M R C G T B S R I M W
I P S J Q R A M Q G M W E O D D D Q B S A F
P Q U X F I T R E Q D L B N S O D I U C K C
I T R Q B A I P Y N E H J V T I N L Q F E T
B A S J X T O R D C F P I V T M S E D U D I
R M H Q R E N Y S U V Q R F Y M O U W U Q R
F G K N T D W U J B U C W Z R I M B V A E J
```

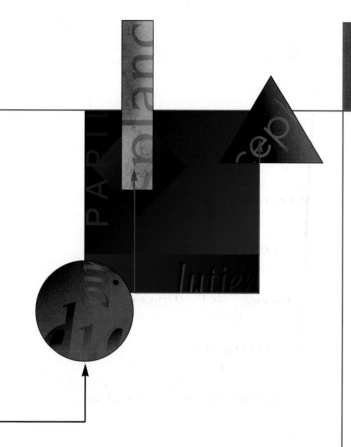

The Integumentary System

the skin and its

accessory structures

This chapter describes the skin, the largest and one of the most remarkable organs of the body, and its accessory organs—hair, sweat glands, sebaceous glands, and nails—which form the integumentary system.

SKIN

The study of skin is called *dermatology* (*derm*—skin; *logy*—study of). The skin, which covers the body, has a variety of functions necessary to survival. It acts as a barrier against the invasion of microorganisms, protects underlying structures from injury, helps to maintain and regulate body temperature, and acts as a receptor for the sensations of touch, heat, cold, pressure, and pain. Along with the kidneys, intestines, and lungs, the skin plays a crucial role in disposing of waste products.

Under normal conditions the temperature of the body is maintained through a heat-regulating mechanism that keeps a balance between heat production and heat loss. The body produces heat by metabolism of the food ingested, and the amount of heat produced is directly connected to the amount of work done by the muscles.

Its a FACT

The average adult changes his or her outer skin about every 27 days, making a rough total of 1000 skins in a 70-year period.

Most body heat loss occurs through the skin by:

1. transfer from the skin to a cooler surface without direct contact—called *radiation;*
2. transfer from the skin to objects in direct contact—called *conduction;*
3. transfer from the skin by movement of fluid or air—called *convection;*
4. perspiration—called *evaporation.*

The remainder of heat loss occurs through the mucous membranes of the respiratory, digestive, and urinary tracts.

R E V I E W 8 . A

Complete the following:

1. The accessory organs of the skin are the ___hair___, ___Sweat Glands___, ___sebaceous glands___ and ___nails___.
2. The study of skin is called ___dermatology___.
3. The body produces heat by ___metabolism___ of food taken in.
4. Heat loss due to perspiration is called ___evaporation___.
5. Transfer of heat from skin to a cooler surface without direct contact is called ___radiation___.

Composition of the Skin

The skin is composed of two principal layers, the *epidermis,* the outer, thinner layer visible to the naked eye, and the *dermis* (or *corium*), the inner, thicker layer (Figure 8.1).

Epidermis. The epidermis is made up of stratified squamous epithelial tissue. The layers of the epidermis, from the dermis outward, are:

The *stratum germinativum* (basal layer)—the cells in this innermost layer multiply continuously to compensate for the constant loss of cells from the surface of the epidermis. These new cells push upward into each succeeding layer, eventually die, and are sloughed off. The process is continuous.

The *stratum granulosum* (granular layer)—so-called because it contains granules visible in the cytoplasm of the cells, which begin to die in this layer. The stratum granulosum may not be present in some areas of thin skin.

The *stratum lucidum* (clear layer)—so-called because of its closely packed, clear cells, and found only in the thicker skin of the soles of the feet and the palms of the hands.

The *stratum corneum* (horny layer)—composed of flat, lifeless, *keratinized* (*kerat-* means horny tissue) cells, which appear as overlapping dry scales making up the outer skin layer. If these scales are unbroken, they can prevent the entrance of microorganisms. Dead cells are continuously sloughed off this layer and replaced by new ones from the stratum germinativum.

Skin color is determined by the amount of *melanin* (skin pigment) in the stratum germinativum layer of the epidermis. Melanin serves as protection by screening ultraviolet rays from harming the underlying tissue. Heredity is the chief factor influencing the lightness or darkness of a person's skin color, in conjunction with sunlight and some hormones.

Dermis. The dermis (corium) is made up of a dense, fibrous connective tissue containing blood vessels and nerves. A subcutaneous layer under the dermis consists of *areolar* (loose, ordinary) and *adipose* (fatty) tissue. In the dermis are the hair shafts, with small bundles of involuntary muscle called the *arrector pili* attached to the hair follicles. When one is frightened, or exposed to cold, these muscles contract, the hair "stands up," and the skin forms what is known as "gooseflesh." *Sebaceous* (oil-producing, to lubricate the hair) glands, sweat glands, and receptors for the sensations of touch, heat, cold, and pain are also found in the dermis.

Structure of the Skin

The structure of the skin differs throughout the body. It is tough and stretchable and varies in thickness. It is thick on the palms of the hands and soles of the feet and thin on the eyelids. There are differences in moistness, roughness, dryness, and smoothness, according to the presence of sebaceous and sweat glands. The skin is firm and elastic in youth, but with age it becomes wrinkled, dry, loose, and saggy, particularly in the regions of the neck, hands, and around the eyes and mouth.

The structure of the skin over the palms of the hands and soles of the feet is different from that of the

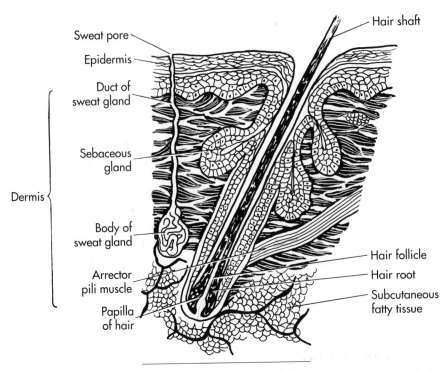

Figure 8.1 Composition of skin.

rest of the body. It has ridges, unique to each individual, particularly on the fingers and toes, that do not change throughout life. Each individual pattern differs from all others, providing a basis for the use of fingerprints as a means of positive identification.

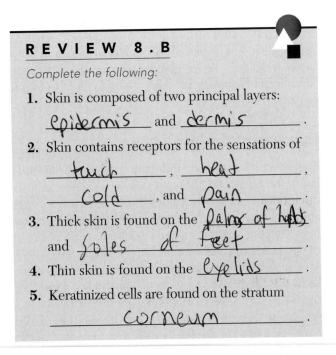

REVIEW 8.B

Complete the following:

1. Skin is composed of two principal layers: __epidermis__ and __dermis__ .

2. Skin contains receptors for the sensations of __touch__ , __heat__ , __cold__ , and __pain__ .

3. Thick skin is found on the __palms of hands__ and __soles of feet__ .

4. Thin skin is found on the __eyelids__ .

5. Keratinized cells are found on the stratum __corneum__ .

Hair. Almost all parts of the body are covered by hair, although in many areas it is so fine that it is scarcely discernible. There is no hair on the palms of the hands, the soles of the feet, and the palmar and plantar surfaces of the fingers and toes. Hair first appears on the fetus. At puberty, there is an added growth of body hair, especially in the areas of the pubes and axillae in both sexes, with males developing facial hair.

Hair develops from a structure in the dermis called the *hair papilla,* located at the base of a tube, the *hair follicle,* extending to the outside of the epidermis. The growing cells in the *hair root* at the base of the follicle increase, push upward, and keratinize, forming the visible *hair shaft* at the surface.

The texture, amount, distribution, and color of hair vary, with hereditary factors playing a major role. Hair loses pigment and "grays" with increasing age, and hair loss is associated with root cell death.

There seems to be no known function for body hair. Head and facial hair affords some protection against cold and sunlight. The *cilia* (eyelashes), *supercilia* (eyebrows), and the hair in the ears and nose provide some protection against entry by insects and dust, and the eyelashes and brows also provide shade.

Sweat glands. The *sudoriferous* (sweat) glands are excretory organs of the skin and serve a function in the cooling of the body. They are the most numerous of the skin glands, and there are more on the palms, soles, forehead, and axillae. An *eccrine* (ordinary) sweat gland is a coiled, tubular structure, in the form of a ball, embedded in the dermis, with its duct emerging on the skin surface as a sweat pore (see Figure 8.1).

Perspiration is constantly secreted and usually evaporates as fast as it is formed, except during muscular exercise or exposure to heat, when it increases more rapidly than it can evaporate. *Apocrine* glands, located in the axillae, around the anus, and in the genital area, are larger sweat glands, with a strong smelling secretion stimulated by excitement and emotion.

Sebaceous glands. The sebaceous glands are saclike structures, secreting a substance called *sebum,* which lubricates the skin and hair. Sebaceous glands are far more numerous on the scalp, forehead, face, and chin than in other parts of the body and are mainly associated with hair follicles. However, some open on the surface independently of hairs, on the eyelids, labia minora (vaginal lips), prepuce (sheath of the clitoris or penis), and areola (area around the nipple). When sebaceous gland ducts become blocked with sebum, a pimple or blackhead may develop.

Ceruminous glands. Ceruminous glands are classified as modified sweat glands, located in the external ear canal, secreting a yellowish, waxy substance called *cerumen* (earwax).

Nails. The nails are a modified form of epidermis that grows from epithelial cells located at the base of each nail under the *lunula* (half-moon shaped white portion). The nails are keratinized, flat, translucent, resilient plates that derive their pink appearance from the underlying blood vessels.

REVIEW 8.C

Complete the following:

1. Cells at the base of the ___hair follicle___ increase, push upward, keratinize, and form the visible hair shaft.
2. The word ___supercilia___ means eyebrows.
3. Another word for sweat gland is ___sudoriferous___
4. Sebaceous glands secrete ___sebum___.
5. The yellowish, waxy secretion in the ears is called ___cerumen___

■ RELATED TERMS   THE INTEGUMENTARY SYSTEM THE SKIN AND ITS ACCESSORY STRUCTURES

ANATOMY

apocrine glands (ap′o-krin) sweat glands, larger than the eccrines, with a strong-smelling secretion, located in the regions of the axillae, anus, and genitalia.

areola (ah-re′o-lah) a circular, pigmented area, surrounding another area of a different color (as around the nipple).

arrector pili (pe′le) small muscle of the skin that raises the skin surface, creating gooseflesh.

cilia (sil′e-ah) eyelashes (singular—*cilium*).

corium (ko′re-um) another term for dermis.

derma (der′mah) skin.

dermis inner, thicker layer of skin.

duct (dukt) tubelike passage, especially for excretions or secretions (also called *ductus*).

ductule (dukt′ule) tiny duct.

eccrine glands (ek′rin) ordinary sweat glands (also called *exocrine glands*).

epidermis (ep″i-der′mis) outer layer of skin.

exocrine glands (ek-so′krin) duct glands that empty secretions on skin surface (e.g., sweat glands).

hair bulb the expansion at the proximal (root) end of the hair.

hair follicle (fol′i-kl) the tube in which the hair grows.

hair papilla nipple-shaped cluster of cells at the base of the follicle where hair growth begins.

hair root invisible growing part of the hair within the follicle.

hair shaft the portion extending beyond the surface of the skin.

keratin (ker′ah-tin) hard, protein constituent of hair, nails, epidermis, horny tissues, and tooth enamel.

lunula (lu′nu-lah) whitish, half-moon shaped, base of the nail.

melanin (mel′ah-nin) dark pigment of skin, hair, and other areas of the body.

sebaceous gland (se-ba′shus) secretes sebum that lubricates skin and hair.

sebum (se′bum) oily secretion of the sebaceous glands.

stratum corneum outer (horny) layer of the epidermis.

stratum germinativum (jer″mi-na″-te′vum) innermost layer of epidermis (also called *basal layer*).

stratum granulosum grainy layer of epidermis above the basal layer, which may not be present in thin skin (also called *granular layer*).

stratum lucidum (lu′sid-sum) translucent layer of epidermis found only on the palms and soles (also called *clear layer*), above the granular layer.

subcutaneous located under the skin.

sudoriferous glands (su″dor-if′er-us) sweat glands.

supercilia (su″per-sil′e-ah) eyebrows (singular—*supercilium*).

supernumerary (su″per-nu′mer-ar″e) occurring in more than the usual number.

DESCRIPTIVE TERMS

anhidrosis (an″hi-dro′sis) abnormal reduction of sweating.

bulla (bul′ah) a large lesion filled with fluid (also called a *blister, bleb,* or *vesicle*).

cicatrix (sik-a′triks) scar (plural—*cicatrices*).

cyanosis (si″ah-no′sis) bluish skin color due to an excess of oxygen-starved hemoglobin in the blood.

dyskeratosis an abnormal alteration in keratinization.

ecchymosis (ek′i-mo′sis) minute, flat, circumscribed, reddish-purple spot caused by intradermal or submucous hemorrhages (also called *petechia*).

erythema term referring to redness of the skin, caused by congestion of the capillaries, usually followed by name of specific condition or cause.

exanthema (ek-san′the′mah) any rash caused by fever or disease (also called *exanthem*).

exfoliation shedding or desquamation of the horny layer of the epidermis.

fissure crack or groove.

hirsutism (her′sut-izm) abnormal hairiness.

hyperhidrosis excessive sweating.

hyperkeratosis overgrowth of the horny layer of the epidermis (also called *acanthokeratodermia*).

keloid (ke′loid) scar tissue.

macula (mak′u-lah) small, discolored spot on skin that can be seen but not felt.

nodule (nod′ul) a small, visible knot protruding above the skin.

pallor paleness of skin.

papule (pap′ul) small, rounded, solid elevation of the skin.

purpura (pur′pu-rah) group of conditions with purplered or brown-red discolorations on the epidermis, caused by hemorrhage into the tissues (small ones are *petechiae*, large ones are *ecchymoses*).

pustule (pus′tul) pus collected in a hair follicle or pore.

scale horny epithelial cells on epidermis, or shed from it.

spongiosis (spon″je-o-sis) edematous swelling within the cells of the epidermis.

PATHOLOGIC CONDITIONS

Many eruptive skin diseases are symptoms of specific, multiple-system diseases (see Chapter 18).

Inflammations and Allergies

acne inflammation of the skin, caused by plugging of sebaceous glands, with development of papules and pustules.

actinic dermatitis inflammation of the skin produced by exposure to ultraviolet and other radiation.

allergic dermatitis (der″mah-tit′is) skin inflammation caused by allergy.

angioneurotic edema condition in which there is sudden onset of swollen (edematous) areas of skin, mucous membranes, or other tissues caused by allergy or unknown causes (also called *giant urticaria*).

aphthous stomatitis (af'thus sto-mah-ti'tis) inflammation of mucous membranes of the mouth, characterized by small, white, ulcerlike lesions (also called *canker sores*).

chilblain localized, painful erythema, caused by frostbite, with itching and swelling of ears, fingers, and toes (also called *erythema pernio*).

contact dermatitis caused by contact with various allergy-producing substances (also called *dermatitis venenata*).

decubitus ulcer skin surface lesion caused by pressure on affected areas resulting in defective circulation (also called *bedsore*).

dermatitis (der"mah-ti'tis) inflammation of the skin.

dermatitis herpetiformis (her-pet"i-form'is) chronic, recurrent, inflammatory dermatitis with grouped skin eruptions and severe itching and burning (also called *Duhring's disease* and *dermatitis multiformis*).

dermatitis medicamentosa (med"i-kah-men-to'sah) caused by sensitivity to drugs.

dermatocellulitis (der"mah-to-sel"u-li'tis) inflammation of the skin and underlying connective tissue.

dermatoconiosis (der"mah-to-ko"ne-o'sis) dermatitis caused by dust.

dermatographia (der"mah-to-graf'e-ah) a type of urticaria in which wheals or welts appear with very slight pressure or scratching.

dermatosis (der"mah-to'sis) any skin disease, especially those not usually associated with inflammation.

discoid lupus erythematosus (DLE) a limited form of lupus (see Chapter 18), a systemic disease, with cutaneous lesions of the face appearing as erythema, overgrowth of horny tissue, plugging of follicles, and usual butterfly pattern over nose and cheeks.

eczema (ek'ze-mah) general term for acute or chronic dermatitis.

exfoliative dermatitis dermatitis, with scaling, itching, loss of hair, and redness of skin, resulting from any of several abnormal skin conditions.

frostbite tissue damage caused by exposure to extreme cold, or by contact with chemicals that have a rapid freezing action.

occupational dermatitis produced by exposure to materials in the workplace (also called *industrial dermatitis*).

parakeratosis scaly dermatosis caused by overabundance of keratinocyte nuclei in the horny layer of the epidermis.

rosacea (row-zay'-shuh) reddening of the nose and adjoining areas produced by dilation of inflamed surface blood vessels, accompanied by an acne condition caused by plugged oil glands (also called *acne rosacea*).

seborrheic dermatitis (seb"o-re'ik) chronic, inflammatory dermatitis with yellowish, greasy scaling of the skin, especially the scalp, face, ears, and forehead, accompanied by pruritus (itching).

urticaria (ur"ti-ka're-ah) skin reaction, usually allergic, with wheals appearing on skin, accompanied by pruritus (also called *hives*).

wheal (wheel) round, smooth, slightly elevated lesion on the skin, whiter or redder than surrounding area, that itches severely and is usually evidence of an allergy.

Bacterial, Fungal, Viral, and Parasitic Infections

carbuncle (kar'bung-kl) infection of the skin and underlying tissues in the form of *furuncles* (boils), usually caused by *Staphylococcus aureus*.

cellulitis inflammation, usually bacterial, possibly purulent, involving loose subcutaneous tissue.

chiggers infestation by larvae of mites, causing severe itching and dermatitis.

dermatophytosis (der"mah-to-fi-to'sis) fungal infection of the skin, especially the feet (also called *dermomycosis* and *epidermomycosis*).

ecthyma (ek-thi'mah) form of impetigo or skin infection with shallow lesions and crusting, caused by streptococci and staphylococci.

erysipelas (er"i-sep'e-las) acute, contagious infections of the skin and subcutaneous tissue with swelling and redness of affected regions, caused by hemolytic streptococci.

erythema infectiosum childhood illness caused by parvovirus B19 (not related to dog parvovirus). The contagious stage is a 4- to 14-day incubation period preceding the breakout of a facial rash signaling the end of the contagious stage (also called *fifth disease*).

felon abscess of distal end of finger, usually around the nail.

furunculosis (fu-rung"ku-lo'sis) persistent, consecutive occurrence of boils over a period of time.

herpes (her'pez) recurrent, infectious, inflammatory disease of the skin or other epithelial tissue, characterized by clusters of small vesicles, caused by herpesvirus (usually followed by a modifying term to identify the particular condition).

herpes febrilis herpes simplex (type 1) virus–produced condition (also called cold sore or fever blister).

herpes genitalis herpes simplex (type 2) virus–produced condition of the genital areas of both sexes.

impetigo streptococcal-caused skin infection, with groups of minute vesicles that rupture and spread (also called *impetigo contagiosa*).

onychomycosis (on"i-ko-mi-ko'sis) a disease of the nails in which they become opaque, white, thickened, brittle, and easily crumbled (also called *ringworm* of the nails).

paronychia (par"o-nik'e-ah) bacterial or viral inflammation of the skin around the fingernail.

pediculosis infestation by head, body, or pubic lice, causing intense itching.

scabies contagious skin disease caused by invasive mites, producing intense itching and eczema.

tinea (tin'e-ah) general name for a variety of superficial fungal skin infections (ringworm), with a modifier to identify the type (e.g., *tinea pedis*—of foot (athlete's foot), *tinea capitis*—of scalp, *tinea cruris*—jock itch, etc.).

toxic epidermal necrolysis (TEN) staphylococcus infection, usually affecting children younger than 10 years, causing outer layers of skin to split, separate, and peel, resembling skin after scalding (also called *scalded skin syndrome*).

wart virus-caused, benign, small, tumorlike epidermal growth (also called *verruca*).

Hereditary, Congenital, and Developmental Disorders

albinism congenital defect in melanin development, causing lack of pigment in skin, hair, and eyes.

cutis hyperelastica (hy'per-e-las'ti-kah) hereditary disorder marked by hyperextensibility of the joints with fragile and hyperelastic skin (also called *Ehlers-Danlos syndrome*).

ectodermal dysplasia genetic condition with poorly functioning or no sweat glands, sparse hair follicles, missing or abnormal fingernails or toenails, and a rash-prone skin, in addition to other systemic abnormalities.

epidermolysis bullosa (EB) (ep"i-der-mol'i-sis bul-lo-sah) a group of grave, inherited, noncontagious skin disorders characterized by soft, peeling epidermis, with formation of bullae and vesicles at sites exposed to trauma.

ichthyosis congenita (ik"the-o'sis kon-jen'i-tah) rare hereditary condition in which infant is covered with a "fish-scale" membrane, which peels off within 24 hours of birth, followed by healing or recurrence of the condition.

keratosis follicularis (fo-lik"u-lah'ris) rare, hereditary skin disorder marked by areas of crusting, itching, and rough papules on the scalp, face, neck, and trunk (also called *Darier's disease*).

pachyonychia congenita (pak"e-o-nik'ee-ah) rare inherited condition with thickening of nails, thickening of skin on soles of feet and palms of hands, and leukoplakia of mouth mucous membranes (also called *Jadassohn-Lewandowsky syndrome*).

psoriasis hereditary, chronic dermatosis, with bright red macules covered by scales, most commonly involving the scalp, elbows, knees, and shins.

xeroderma pigmentosum (ze"ro-der'mah pig-men-to'sum) rare, inherited, frequently fatal disease in which skin and eyes are unusually sensitive to light; the condition can progress to malignancy.

Other Skin Conditions

alopecia (al-o-pe'shi-ah) hair loss.

Beau's lines horizontal depressions across nail plate, possibly caused by illness or malnutrition.

calcinosis cutis (kal"si-no'sis) condition characterized by calcium salts being deposited in the skin.

callosities (kah-los'i-tez) localized overgrowths of the outer (horny) layer of the epidermis.

koilonychia (koy-lo-nik'ee-ah) nail plates become depressed and spoon-like, possibly due to thyroid disease or anemia (also called *spoon nails*).

necrobiosis lipoidica (nek"ro-bi-o'sis li-poi'di-kah) skin condition marked by degeneration of the connective and elastic tissues especially in the upper dermis, with lesions usually occurring on the shins; commonly found in diabetic individuals (also known as *necrobiosis lipoidica diabeticorum*).

pemphigus formerly fatal, debilitating skin and mucous membrane disease, cause unknown; characterized by weeping bullae (blisters) that rupture and leave raw spots, leading to possible infection; treated with corticosteroids and other immunosuppressive medications.

skin tag small outgrowth of skin, most commonly on the neck (also called *cutaneous papilloma, acrochordon,* or *soft fibroma*).

vitiligo (vit-i-li'go) loss of pigment-producing cells, resulting in irregularly shaped, lighter or white patches on the surface of the skin. Authorities theorize it may be hereditary, acquired, or possibly an autoimmune disease.

xanthoma (zan-tho'mah) lipid deposits in the skin forming yellow papules or nodules.

yellow nail syndrome nails become thick and yellow; related to chronic respiratory disease, as well as lymph and thyroid diseases.

Oncology

ABCD a visual grading system for differential diagnosis of pigmented skin tumors; *A* refers to asymmetry of the lesion, *B* refers to unevenness and lumpiness around the *borders,* *C* refers to variations in *color,* and *D* refers to size in *diameter.*

actinic keratosis* flat or raised, reddish or skin-colored growth affecting middle-aged or elderly people, caused by exposure to the sun's rays; it may develop into squamous cell carcinoma.

angiolipoma a lipoma containing many small blood vessels (may be painful).

basal cell carcinoma* malignant tumor of the epithelium that seldom metastasizes or spreads (also called *hair-matrix carcinoma*).

carcinoma cutaneum* malignant tumor of the epithelium.

dermatofibroma (der"mah-to-fi-bro'mah) fibrous tumor of the skin.

epithelial carcinoma* malignant epithelioma.

epithelioma tumor of epithelial tissue.

hidradenoma (hi"drad-e-no'mah) benign skin tumor composed of epithelial elements of sweat glands (also called *syringocystadenoma*).

intraepidermal carcinoma* confined to the epidermis, without penetration of basal layer.

intraepidermal epithelioma* (ep"i-the"le-o'mah) precancerous tumor of the epidermis.

leiomyoma cutis (li"o-mi-o'mah) benign smooth muscle tumor of arrector pili muscles.

lenticular carcinoma* skin cancer with flattened nodules and papules running together into surface masses.

lipoma common benign fatty tissue tumor.

melanocytic nevus pigmented nevus (see *nevus*).

melanoma* malignant, pigmented, skin tumor that can develop from a melanocytic nevus.

nevus circular overgrowth on skin (also called *mole*).

sebaceous cyst cyst of a sebaceous gland plugged with sebum.

seborrheic keratosis benign tumor of the epidermis with many yellow or brown raised lesions on the skin (also called *seborrheic wart*).

squamous cell carcinoma* type of carcinoma from squamous epithelium (also called *epidermoid carcinoma*).

syringocystadenoma see *hidradenoma.*

tuberous carcinoma* skin cancer with nodular projections.

verrucous carcinoma* epidermoid cancer usually in mucosa of cheek, but can affect other soft tissues such as larynx and genitals.

SURGICAL PROCEDURES

dermabrasion surgical removal of epidermis and some dermis as needed to remove scar tissue, tattoos, moles, and other skin irregularities (also called *planing*).

excisional biopsy surgical incision to remove tissue of all or part of a lesion and surrounding normal-appearing tissue.

Mohs' micrographic surgery a specialized technique for removal of successive layers of a skin cancer for microscopic examination, until no more cancer cells are detected.

punch biopsy sample of tissue obtained by use of a punch.

skin graft surgical procedure to replace nonregenerative skin.

   accordion graft graft skin with multiple slits to permit stretching over large area.

° Indicates a malignant condition.

° Indicates a malignant condition.

artificial skin graft graft derived from laboratory-grown epidermis sheets started from a postage stamp–size sample of skin taken from individual for autograft or other donor sources; appears to minimize rejection.

autodermic graft skin graft taken from patient's own body.

cutis graft grafting of skin after removal of epidermis and subcutaneous fat to replace fascia in plastic procedures.

delayed graft original graft shifted to new area.

heterodermic graft skin graft from donor of another species (also called *dermatoheteroplasty*).

LABORATORY TESTS

biopsy removal of tissue for microscopic examination.

buccal smear scraping of cells from inner surface of cheek for detection of hereditary abnormalities.

computerized tomography (CT) imaging device using x-rays at multiple angles through specific sec-

tions of the body, analyzed by computer to provide a total picture of the part being examined (also called *computerized axial tomography—CAT*). Used to detect tumors in epithelial tissue.

intradermal tests several tests using injection of substances subcutaneously to observe reaction.

PPD (purified protein derivative) test for tuberculosis (also called *Mantoux test*).

Schick test for diphtheria.

Dick test for scarlet fever.

patch test skin test for sensitivity to particular allergens, by placing small amount of substance in solution on skin and covering for several days to note skin allergic response.

scratch test a test for allergy by inserting suspected substances into scratches on skin surface to observe allergic reaction.

tissue culture epithelial cells, taken from body, grown in a medium for diagnostic or research purposes.

EXERCISES **THE INTEGUMENTARY SYSTEM** THE SKIN AND ITS ACCESSORY STRUCTURES

Exercise 8.1   *Complete the following:*

1. The epidermis is composed of four layers of cells. They are:

   a. _Stratum germinativum or basal layer_   c. _Stratum lucidum or clear layer_

   b. _Stratum granulosum or granular layer_   d. _Stratum corneus or horny layer_

2. Body heat is lost through the skin by _radiation_, _Conduction_, _Convection_, and _evaporation_.

3. Hair covers almost all parts of the body except the _palms_ of the hands and the _soles_ of the feet.

4. The _Cilia (eye lashes)_ and _Super-cilia (eyebrows)_ serve as a protection to shade the eyes and keep out harmful objects and dust.

5. Another term for dermis is _Corium_.

Exercise 8.2   *Using the list of terms below, identify each part in Figure 8.2 by placing its name in the corresponding blank.*

Hair shaft

Subcutaneous fatty tissue

Sebaceous gland

Hair follicle

Epidermis

Papilla of hair

Body of sweat gland

Sweat pore

Dermis

Duct of sweat gland

Arrector pili muscle

Hair root

1. _Sweat pore_
2. _dermis_
3. _epidermis_
4. _duct of sweat gland_
5. _sebaceous gland_
6. _body of sweat gland_

7. _arrector pili muscle_
8. _papilla of hair_
9. _hair shaft_
10. _hair follicle_
11. _hair root_
12. _subcutaneous fatty tissue_

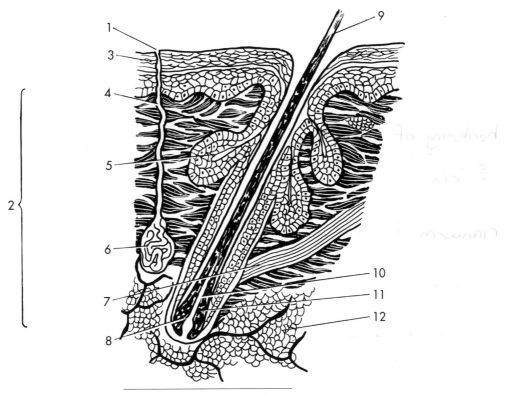

Figure 8.2 Composition of skin.

Exercise 8.3   *Matching*

_____ B _____ **1.** sebaceous glands
_____ C _____ **2.** apocrine glands
_____ I _____ **3.** ceruminous glands
_____ F _____ **4.** dermis
_____ H _____ **5.** lunula
_____ J _____ **6.** arrector pili
_____ G _____ **7.** areola
_____ D _____ **8.** melanin pigment
_____ E _____ **9.** sebum
_____ A _____ **10.** skin

A. barrier, receptor, waste disposal
B. glands with ducts opening around hair follicles
C. large sweat glands with strong-smelling secretion
D. pigment of skin or hair
E. secretions of sebaceous glands
F. dense, fibrous connective tissue
G. area around the nipple
H. crescent-shaped portion at nail base
I. modified sweat glands located in the external ear canal
J. small muscles of the skin that produce "gooseflesh"

Exercise 8.4   *Give the meaning of the components in the following words and then define the word as a whole. Suffixes meaning pertaining to or state or condition, shown following a slash mark (/), are not to be defined separately. Before reaching for your medical dictionary, check the Related Terms list in this chapter.*

1. Dermatosclerosis:
derm/ato _Skin_
scler/osis _hardening_
hardening of the Skin

2. Tinea barbae:
tinea _ring worm_
barb/ae _beard_
ringworm of bearded area of face

3. Cutis hyperelastica:
cutis _Skin_
hyper _increase_
elastic/a _elastic tissue_
hyper elasticity of Skin

4. Ichthyosis congenita:
ichthy/osis _fish (scales)_
congenita _congenital_
Skin resembling fish scales

5. Anhidrosis:
an _no Sweat_
hidr/osis _Condition_
inability to sweat

6. Neurofibroma:
neuro _nerve_
fibr _fibrous_
oma _tumor_
tumor of nervous and fibrous elements

7. Dyskeratosis:
dys _disordered_
kerat/osis _Keratin_
faulty development of epidermis

8. Purpura:
purpura _purple Petechiae_
Cluster of petechiae w/ purple appearance

9. Exfoliative dermatitis:
exfolia/tive _Shedding_
derm/at/itis _Skin_
Scaling or redness of Skin

10. Actinic dermatitis:
actin/ic _ultraviolet light_
derm/at/itis _Skin_
inflamation of Skin caused by ultraviolet light

CROSSWORD PUZZLE

ACROSS

1. Term for sweat gland
4. Study of the skin
6. One of four epidermal layers
8. Form fingerprints
9. An accessory organ gland
10. Number of principal skin layers
11. One of the skin layers
15. Heat loss by direct contact
17. A type of sweat gland
20. One of four epidermal layers
21. One of four epidermal layers
23. Skin pigment
24. A skin accessory organ
25. Skin color is due to
   _____

DOWN

2. Heat loss by perspiration
3. Heat loss by fluid/air movement
5. Heat loss without direct contact
7. Sebaceous gland secretion
12. A type of sweat gland
13. Outer layer of skin
14. Largest organ of body
16. Another word for inner skin layer
18. Yellow ear secretion
19. Tube from which hair grows
22. Half-moon portion of nail

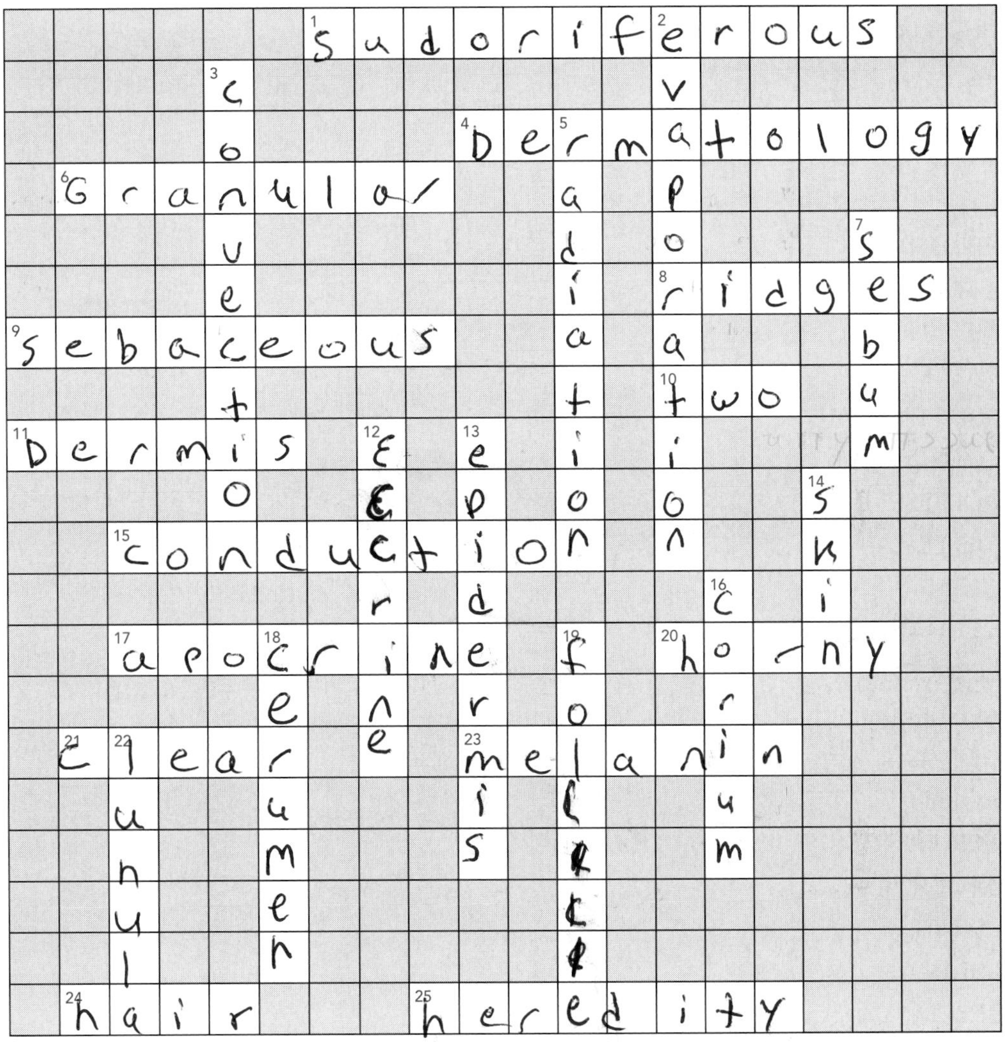

Completed puzzle answers (handwritten):
- 1 Across: sudoriferous
- 4 Across: dermatology
- 6 Across: granular
- 8 Across: ridges
- 9 Across: sebaceous
- 10 Across: two
- 11 Across: dermis
- 15 Across: conduction
- 17 Across: apocrine
- 20 Across: horny
- 21 Across: clear
- 23 Across: melanin
- 24 Across: hair
- 25 Across: heredity

HIDDEN WORDS PUZZLE

Can you find the 20 words hidden in this puzzle? All hidden words puzzles have words running from top to bottom, left to right, and diagonally downward.

INTEGUMENTARY

EPIDERMIS

GRANULAR

MELANIN

BASAL

SUDORIFEROUS

FOLLICLES

ADIPOSE

PAPILLA

CLEAR

DERMATOLOGY

SEBACEOUS

AREOLAR

DERMIS

HORNY

CERUMINOUS

APOCRINE

KERATIN

LUNULA

SEBUM

```
L U N U L A R G S U F W H Y P H O W V A E Y J
B K M Y D E R M I S U C T F Y E F F E E J L T
A P O C R I N E T R E M V F O I G O I X V P T
S C D M O Q M P O X O B T A I V U I B T C U Y
A G K E R A T I N L X K U V R R G I Q V X F H
L I P L A Q I D W R A J A M F Q V U N B D R W
H Q U A U T R E N K A R X M J S B M M P E B N
R I Q N X H O R N Y D I N A A E M W S S W I T
U N U I D P U M M B I Y H L G B O L K F F D X
H O M N N L H I D O P Q X M U A K R L O L W H
D T A T G X Z S N A O P M V V C E U H Y X N B
T H E H X H E U U C S G G W F E U Y C M D Q E
D S Q F J D C H U D E R M A T O L O G Y Y L K
O S M Q G U L C K G O R K D W U L Y D B C S Z
I R U L K U E W C R R U H K S T L M U O I R
S I Y H P P A P I L L A I M W U N Y I X N T Y
Y P L R U G R F M M G J N F I P H N T C D C G
K B Y A A R A M G I H B T U E N L F K W L S L
W F X P B T I J D R F F E Q L R O K S T T E Y
J B L N E H F F N O R W G C E A O U E T A Y S
G P M U D S F U V T P D U V H U R U S N U Y G
B U M J V M R K G U M W M H S V S H S J E F S
J L W K I O R W U T J Z E G M J U K F Q V Y X
W J D N X Z B O P S W K N N X L H K W C B K I
R R Y H E P R I T P L Z T E P B H I L U O A R
L Y H A K J G T I J I Q A P Z K U K Y L A Z Y
L F Y J J J E C M I M T R B G C B B Z Z J H W
P T S X T A C S X B Q I Y P P H V E B W K P P
```

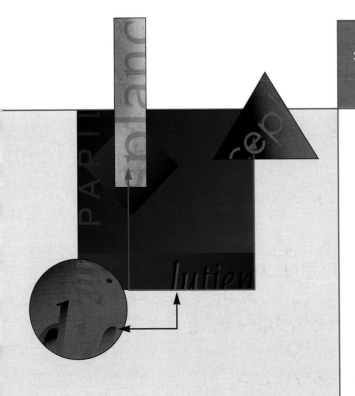

The Internal Mechanisms of the Body

This is the third of the five sections of *Learning Medical Terminology*. This section contains five chapters that describe the internal workings of the body.

Chapter 9 presents the cardiovascular system and its relation to the production and circulation of blood throughout the body.

Chapter 10 discusses the respiratory system and its importance in providing the body with oxygen and eliminating waste gases from cell metabolism.

Chapter 11 describes how the gastrointestinal system functions, from digestion of food through the elimination of solid wastes.

Chapter 12 presents the urinary system and its role in eliminating liquid waste.

Chapter 13 describes the reproductive system and its functions in both sexes.

As in the previous section, there are drawings within the chapters illustrating the principal parts of the anatomy in that particular chapter. In addition, please refer to the color plates at the front of the text that provide more vivid detail.

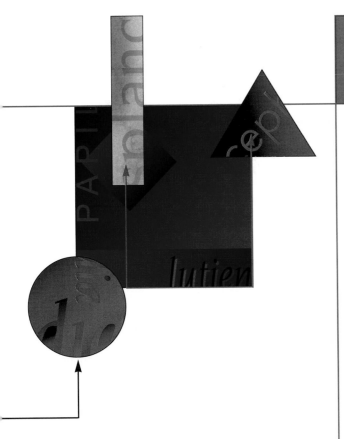

The Cardiovascular System

the transports of the body

This chapter explains the structures and functions of the heart, the various types of blood vessels, the characteristics of blood, and the mechanism of circulation. The cardiovascular system includes the heart, blood vessels, blood, and its circulation.

THE HEART

The *cardiac muscle* (heart) is a hollow muscular organ, divided into four chambers and about the size and shape of a large clenched fist (Figures 9.1 and 9.2). It lies between the lungs, in the middle of the chest, behind the sternum, with about two thirds to the left and one third to the right. The *base*, or upper border, of the heart is just below the second rib, and the *apex*, or lower border, of the heart points downward and to the left, separated from the anterior chest wall by the lungs and pleura. The heart is a pump that circulates the blood in the body, to nourish and to remove waste products from the tissues.

It's a **FACT**

The blood in the average adult body travels 168 million miles every 24 hours.

135

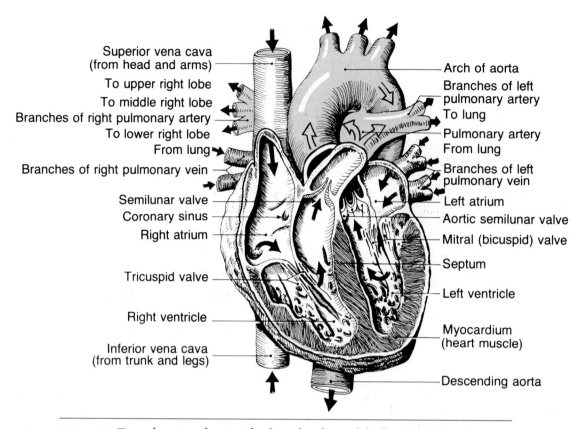

Superior vena cava (from head and arms)

To upper right lobe

To middle right lobe

Branches of right pulmonary artery

To lower right lobe

From lung

Branches of right pulmonary vein

Semilunar valve

Coronary sinus

Right atrium

Tricuspid valve

Right ventricle

Inferior vena cava (from trunk and legs)

Arch of aorta

Branches of left pulmonary artery

To lung

Pulmonary artery

From lung

Branches of left pulmonary vein

Left atrium

Aortic semilunar valve

Mitral (bicuspid) valve

Septum

Left ventricle

Myocardium (heart muscle)

Descending aorta

Figure 9.1 Frontal section showing the four chambers of the heart and the valves, openings, and major blood vessels. Arrows indicate direction of the blood flow. (The branches of the right pulmonary vein continue from the right lung, behind the heart, to enter the left atrium.)

Structure of the Heart

The heart is covered by a saclike membrane, which has three layers:

The *pericardium*—tough, fibrous external layer and two internal serous layers;

The *parietal* layer—lining the pericardium; and

The *visceral* layer *(epicardium)*—covering the surface of the heart.

There is a space between the two layers of serous membrane called the *pericardial space,* which contains several drops of pericardial fluid.

The heart wall is composed of three layers. The outer layer is the *epicardium* (visceral layer) described above. The middle layer, the *myocardium,* is the *cardiac* (heart) muscle itself; and the innermost layer, the *endocardium,* lines the chambers of the heart and covers its valves.

Chambers of the heart. The hollow of the heart is divided into four chambers. Each of the upper two chambers is called an *atrium* (plural—*atria*) and each of the lower two chambers is called a *ventricle.* A wall

called the *interatrial septum* divides the atria into right and left sides, and a similar wall, the *interventricular septum,* divides the ventricles into right and left sides. The two sides do not communicate (see Figure 9.1).

The atria have thin walls and are the receiving chambers. The ventricles, which do the pumping, have thick walls. The right side of the heart receives blood from the body tissues and sends it to the lungs to be oxygenated. The left side of the heart receives blood from the lungs and sends it to the tissues. The walls of the left ventricle are thicker than the walls of the right ventricle because the left ventricle pumps blood to all the blood vessels of the body; the right ventricle pumps blood only to the lungs.

Valves. Between the atria and ventricles are valves that close to ensure that blood flows in one direction, preventing blood backflow into the atria. The left atrium and the left ventricle are separated by the *mitral* or *bicuspid* (two flaps) *valve.* The right atrium and the right ventricle are separated by the *tricuspid* (three flaps) *valve.* The *semilunar* (half-moon shaped)

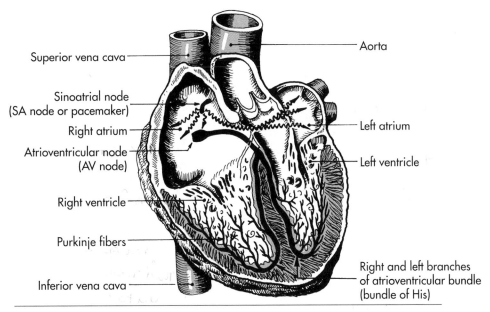

Superior vena cava

Sinoatrial node
(SA node or pacemaker)

Right atrium

Atrioventricular node
(AV node)

Right ventricle

Purkinje fibers

Inferior vena cava

Aorta

Left atrium

Left ventricle

Right and left branches
of atrioventricular bundle
(bundle of His)

Figure 9.2 The conduction system of the heart. The sinoatrial node (pacemaker) located in the wall of the right atrium sets the basic heart rhythm.

valves, located at the bases of the *pulmonary artery* and the *aorta,* prevent a backflow of blood from the arteries into the ventricles (see Figure 9.1).

Conduction System

The heart begins pumping in utero and is dependent on a conduction system that includes:

The *sinoatrial node (SA node)*—also called the *pacemaker,* consists of cells in which electrical impulses originate, producing atrial contractions, and forcing blood into the ventricles;

The *atrioventricular node (AV node)*—consists of conductile cells through which the electrical impulses continue down to

The *atrioventricular bundle* (or *bundle of His*)— and on to

The *Purkinje fibers*—that move the impulses on to stimulate the contraction of the ventricles.

After a brief rest period, the entire process repeats itself (see Figure 9.2).

Nerve Function in Heart Action

The *autonomic* nervous system has two divisions with opposite actions on the heart:

The *parasympathetic* division, mainly supplying the sinoatrial (SA) and atrioventricular (AV) nodes, slows the heart rate, reduces impulse conduction, and dilates the coronary arteries;

The *sympathetic* division, through the cardiac nerves, also acts on the sinoatrial and atrioventricular nodes to increase the heart rate and impulse conduction, and both constricts and dilates the coronary arteries (see Chapter 15).

Cardiac Cycle

The cardiac cycle includes the *systole* (contraction) and *diastole* (relaxation) of the atria and the ventricles. The heart chambers do not contract all at one time. The two atria contract in unison; as the atria relax, the two ventricles contract. Similarly, as the ventricles relax, the atria contract, and the cycle is repeated.

When the atria contract, the blood is forced into the ventricles through the bicuspid and tricuspid valves, which open to allow the blood to pass from the atria to the ventricles, while the semilunar valves close to prevent blood from entering the aorta or the pulmonary artery.

When the atria relax, blood enters the atrial chambers from the pulmonary veins and venae cavae, and the ventricles contract. When the ventricles contract, the bicuspid and tricuspid valves close to prevent backflow to the atria, and the semilunar valves open to permit the blood to flow from the ventricles into the aorta and pulmonary artery.

When the ventricles relax, the semilunar valves close, the bicuspid and tricuspid valves open, the atria contract, and blood from the atria again starts to fill the ventricles, repeating the cycle.

TYPES OF BLOOD VESSELS

The human body has three major types of blood vessels: *arteries*, *capillaries*, and *veins*.

Arteries

Oxygenated blood is carried from the heart to all structures of the body by the arteries, which are elastic tubes with thick walls composed of three layers:

The *tunica intima* (also called *intimal layer* or *tunica interna*)—a lining of endothelium;

The *tunica media* (or *medial layer*)—a muscle layer;

The *tunica adventitia* (or *tunica externa*)—a fibrous outer coat.

Arterioles, Capillaries, and Venules

Arteries become smaller and smaller, branching and re-branching throughout the body, finally becoming *arterioles* (small arteries). The arterioles feed the blood into *capillaries*, which are billions of minute, very thin-walled vessels that communicate with other capillaries. The capillaries distribute the blood to the tissues. Other capillaries pick up the blood from the tissues and return it to *venules* (small veins), which pass the blood to the veins. The veins return the blood to the heart.

Veins

The veins are hollow tubes, similar to the arteries, that have thinner and less elastic walls and transport blood back to the heart. The venules (smallest veins) collect blood from the capillaries, connect to larger veins, and finally join the *venae cavae* (singular—*vena cava*) to return the blood to the heart. Within the venous channels are valves that help to prevent backflow of blood and allow it to be propelled forward, with some assistance from alternate contraction and relaxation of the muscles of the limbs.

REVIEW 9.A

Complete the following:

1. The cardiovascular system includes the
   ___heart___ , ___blood vessel___ ,
   ___blood___ , and ___circulation___ .

---

2. The heart is called the ___cardiac___ muscle.

3. The hollow of the heart is divided into
   ___four___ chambers.

4. The external layer of the saclike membrane covering the heart is called the
   ___pericardium___ .

5. The valves of the heart prevent a _____
   ___back flow___ of blood into the atria.

6. The conduction system of the heart consists of the ___pace maker___ , ___atrio ventricular___
   ___atrioventricular bundle___ , and ___purkinje fibers___ .

7. The ___autonomic___ nervous system has two divisions with opposite actions on the heart.

8. The cardiac cycle includes the systole or
   ___contraction___ and the diastole or
   ___relaxation___ of the atria and ventricles.

9. The three major types of blood vessels are
   ___arteries___ , ___capillaries___ ,
   and ___veins___ .

10. Arteries carry ___oxygenated___
    blood from the heart throughout the body,
    and ___veins___
    transport it back to the heart.

BLOOD

The average adult body contains about 6 quarts of blood, which may vary with the size and health of the individual. Blood is made up of about 55% *plasma* (liquid), and 45% formed elements, which consist of *erythrocytes* (red blood cells), *leukocytes* (white blood cells), and *platelets (thrombocytes)*.

1. Blood transports oxygen from the lungs to the body tissues, collects carbon dioxide waste from the tissues, and brings the waste back to the lungs to be expelled.

2. Blood distributes nutrients throughout the body.
3. Blood collects waste products of metabolism (urea, uric acid, creatinine, etc.) and delivers them to the excretory organs for disposal.
4. Blood carries hormones of the different ductless glands (such as the thyroid and parathyroid glands) to the cells.
5. Blood maintains the fluid content of the tissues.
6. Blood serves as a temperature regulator for the body.

Among the nutrients carried by the blood are *lipids* (fats and oils) such as *cholesterol* and *triglycerides,* which are needed for energy and for manufacturing important hormones and salts. The lipids combine with proteins to form molecules that circulate in the blood as *lipoproteins.* Two of the major lipoproteins are *low-density lipoprotein (LDL)* and *high-density lipoprotein (HDL).* Low-density lipoprotein is commonly called "the bad cholesterol" because it is responsible for the deposit of cholesterol into the walls of the arteries, resulting in *atherosclerosis* (see Terms list). High-density lipoprotein is commonly called "the good cholesterol" because it has a role in metabolizing and eliminating excess cholesterol. Triglycerides function to provide energy for the tissues.

Plasma

The clear, straw-colored, liquid portion of blood, approximately 90% water and 10% solutes, with protein making up the major portion of solutes, is called *plasma.* Other solutes present in plasma, in much smaller amounts, include nutrients (lipids, glucose, and amino acids), end products of metabolism (urea, creatinine, uric and lactic acids), gases (oxygen and carbon dioxide), hormones, enzymes, and antibodies.

Blood Cells

All blood cells have their origin in undifferentiated *stem cells,* the *hemocytoblasts,* which develop in the embryo. In children, blood cells are produced in almost all bone marrow, whereas in the adult, blood cells are produced in red bone marrow only.

Proerythroblasts produce *erythrocytes;*
Myeloblasts produce *granulocytes;*
Lymphoblasts produce *lymphocytes;*
Monoblasts produce *monocytes;*
Megakaryoblasts produce *platelets.*

The logical progression through which the immature cells mature is given in Figure 9.3.

Erythrocytes. At maturity, *erythrocytes* are extremely small, nonnucleated, biconcave (indented on both sides) disks (see Figures 9.3 and 9.4). They contain *hemoglobin (heme*—iron; *globin*—protein), an iron-containing pigment that, in combination with oxygen, gives the blood its red color. Hemoglobin combines with oxygen in the lungs and distributes it to body cells; there the hemoglobin combines with carbon dioxide, which it carries to the lungs for disposal. The average life span of erythrocytes is estimated to be about 120 days. If iron is lacking in erythrocytes, there is a reduction of hemoglobin and the number of red cells, resulting in an anemia.

Leukocytes. Much less numerous than erythrocytes, *leukocytes* are colorless and have nuclei (see Figures 9.3 and 9.4).

Although leukocytes are considered constituents of blood, they are also included in the lymphatic and immune systems (Chapter 17). They are divided into two groups:

granulocytes—originating in bone marrow, have lobed nuclei, cytoplasm that contains fine granules, and are classified according to staining characteristics:

neutrophils—the most numerous, make up about 70% of all leukocytes, have red and blue staining granules, and mainly function in *phagocytosis* (digesting invading microorganisms).

eosinophils—make up about 2% to 5% of all leukocytes, have orange or yellow acid dye staining granules, and function to detoxify foreign proteins from allergens or parasitic infections.

basophils—make up about 1% of all leukocytes, have blue and purple, basic dye staining granules, and function in allergies and blood coagulation.

agranulocytes—originating in lymphatic organs, with clear, nongranular cytoplasm and either a round, or horseshoe-shaped, single nucleus:

lymphocytes—make up about 20% to 25% of all leukocytes, have a rounded nucleus, and function in phagocytosis and in antibody formation.

monocytes—make up about 3% to 8% of all leukocytes, have a horseshoe-shaped nucleus, and mainly function in phagocytosis.

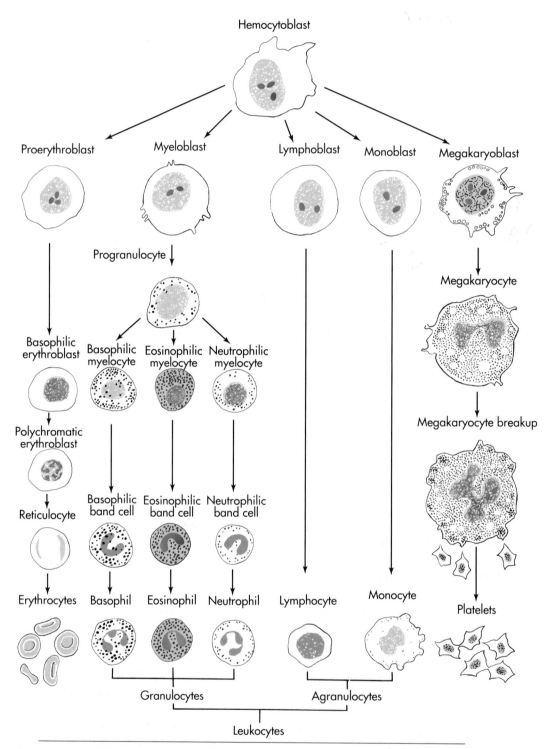

Figure 9.3 Hematopoiesis. All cells are derived from a single progenitor cell, the hemocytoblast, which gives rise to the progenitors of each cell type. (From Seeley RR, Stephens TD, Tate P: *Anatomy and physiology*, New York, 1989, McGraw-Hill.)

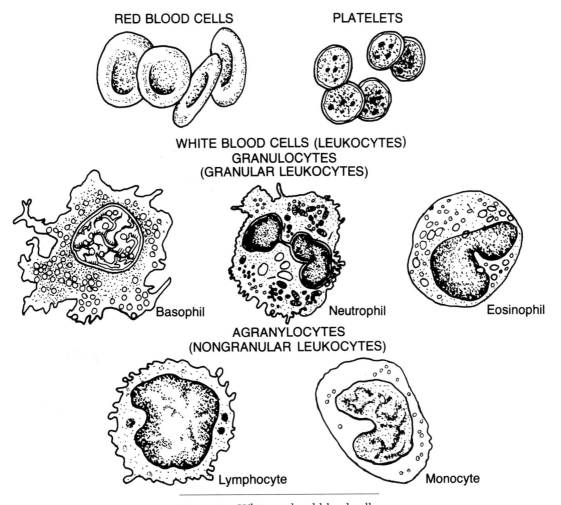

Figure 9.4 White and red blood cells.

Platelets (thrombocytes) and clotting mechanism. *Platelets (thrombocytes)* originate in red bone marrow from *megakaryocyte* cells (see Figure 9.3). Small pieces of the cell break off and become platelets, which function in the clotting mechanism.

Clotting is the result of a chemical reaction. The thrombocytes attach to the injured blood vessel and begin to release several substances that constrict blood vessels and hasten clotting. *Prothrombin* and *fibrinogen* are proteins, made in the liver and present in blood plasma, that are necessary for clotting. Prothrombin is converted to *thrombin,* and thrombin changes fibrinogen to *fibrin,* which enmeshes the red blood cells, platelets, and plasma to form a clot and close the wound.

ABO Blood Group

Blood for transfusion, under normal conditions, is carefully matched to the recipient. Blood is grouped into four types or groups, named for the *antigens* (substances that stimulate the immune system to form antibodies) found on the membranes of red blood cells. For a fuller discussion of antigens and antibodies, see Chapter 17.

The four blood types are:
A: antigen A and anti-B antibodies are present—can only receive types A or O blood in transfusion;
B: antigen B and anti-A antibodies are present—can only receive types B or O blood in transfusion;
AB: both A and B antigens present with no antibodies—generally referred to as *universal recipient,* who in extreme emergency, can receive any blood type in transfusion;
O: neither A nor B antigens, with both anti-A and anti-B antibodies present—can receive only type O blood in transfusion, but is generally referred to as *universal donor,* and in an emergency can give a transfusion to any other blood type.

Rh Factor

In addition to blood being typed in the ABO blood group, blood is classified according to the presence of one or more of a number of **Rh** antigens. Blood is identified as either Rh positive or Rh negative, depending on whether or not an Rh antigen is present on the membranes of the red blood cells.

BLOOD PRESSURE

Blood pressure is the force exerted by the heart in pumping blood through the vessels of the body. **Systolic pressure** is produced by the blood pressing against the walls of the arteries during contraction of the ventricles of the heart. **Diastolic pressure** is produced by the blood pressing against the walls of the arteries during relaxation of the ventricles. Normal blood pressure in the average adult is about 120 (systolic) over 80 (diastolic). The difference between the systolic and diastolic pressures is called **pulse pressure**. Diastolic pressure is considered more important medically because it shows the least amount of pressure to which the arterial walls are subjected. The condition in which the blood pressure is elevated is called **hypertension,** and low blood pressure is called **hypotension.**

THE PULSE

The **pulse** is produced by the blood pumping out of the heart and into the aorta. This action rhythmically increases and decreases the pressure on the walls of the aorta, which, because of their elasticity, expand as the blood enters and relax as it leaves. This rhythm is then transmitted from the aorta to surface arteries, where the rhythm is felt as the pulse.

R E V I E W   9 . B

Complete the following:

1. There are about _____ 6 _____ quarts of blood in the average adult.

2. The clear, straw-colored, liquid portion of blood is called _____ Plasma _____.

3. Erythrocytes contain an iron-containing pigment called _____ hemaglobin _____.

4. A lack of iron in erythrocytes results in _____ anemia _____.

5. Small, nonnucleated, biconcave, disklike blood cells are called _____ red blood cells _____

6. Leukocytes are divided into two groups, _____ granulocytes _____ and a _____ granulocytes _____

7. _____ Platelets _____ originate in red bone marrow and function in the clotting mechanism.

8. The four blood types are _____ A _____, _____ B _____, _____ AB _____, and _____ O _____.

9. The difference between systolic and diastolic pressure is called _____ pulse pressure _____

10. The pumping of blood from the heart into the aorta produces the _____ pulse _____.

CIRCULATION OF THE BLOOD

The blood circulates throughout the body in a closed vascular system. One circuit of the blood, taking it through most of the body, is known as **systemic circulation,** which includes a segment called **hepatic portal circulation.** A second circuit, **pulmonary circulation,** takes the blood through the lungs.

Systemic Circulation

Blood circulates from the left ventricle to the aorta, arteries, arterioles, capillaries, venules, and veins of the body and returns to the right atrium. This **systemic circulation** includes a circuit through the abdominal digestive organs known as **hepatic portal circulation.**

Hepatic Portal Circulation

Blood from veins in the visceral walls and organs (gallbladder, pancreas, spleen, stomach, and intestines) is carried to the liver by the hepatic portal vein. From the liver, the hepatic veins carry the blood to the inferior vena cava, which drains into the right atrium, where pulmonary circulation begins.

Pulmonary Circulation

Blood passes from the right atrium into the right ventricle, which contracts, forcing blood into the pulmonary artery, which has two branches, one going to each lung. In the lung the blood discharges carbon dioxide, is oxygenated, and then drains into the pulmonary veins, which empty into the left atrium, and finally into the left ventricle, where another systemic circuit begins.

Pulmonary veins are the only veins that carry oxygenated blood, which is a bright crimson color. All other veins carry waste products in the blood, making it a darker red color.

Tracing the Circulation

It takes about 1 minute for the blood to make a complete circuit of the body and return, always following the same pattern:

Left ventricle → arteries → arterioles → capillaries of body tissues → venules → veins → right atrium → right ventricle → pulmonary artery → arterioles of lung → lung capillaries → lung venules → pulmonary veins → left atrium → left ventricle (Figure 9.5).

THE MAJOR BLOOD VESSELS

The Arteries

The *aorta,* the largest artery in the body, originating from the left ventricle of the heart, arches up around

the left lung and passes down along the spinal column through the diaphragm. It branches into other arteries that supply the head, neck, arms, chest, and abdomen (abdominal aorta), finally dividing into arteries that supply the lower extremities (Figure 9.6).

The branches from the *aorta* include the:
ascending aorta—branches into the two arteries:
right coronary } arteries that supply the right
and } and
left coronary } left sides of the myocardial
muscle
aortic arch—branches into three large arteries:
the **brachiocephalic (innominate)** divides into
the **right subclavian,** supplying the right arm, and
the **right common carotid,** supplying the right side of the head, branches into
the **right internal carotid,** supplying the cranial cavity, and
the **right external carotid,** supplying the neck and head outside the cranial cavity.
the **left common carotid,** the second large artery, supplying the left side of the head, branches into
internal and **external** divisions, which function similar to those of the right common carotid.
the **left subclavian,** the third large artery, supplying the left arm with blood.

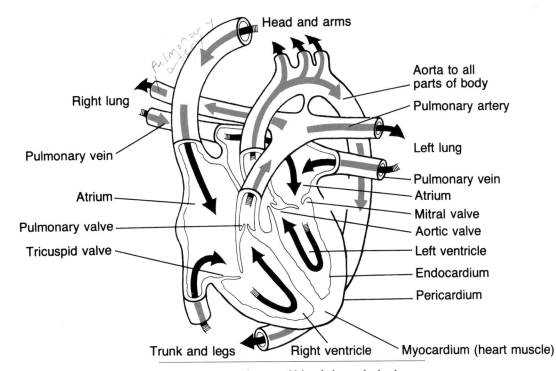

Figure 9.5 Circulation of blood through the heart.

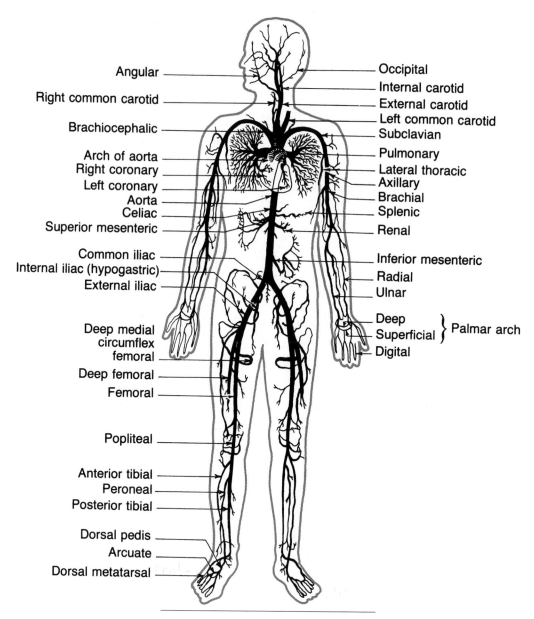

Angular
Right common carotid
Brachiocephalic
Arch of aorta
Right coronary
Left coronary
Aorta
Celiac
Superior mesenteric
Common iliac
Internal iliac (hypogastric)
External iliac
Deep medial circumflex femoral
Deep femoral
Femoral
Popliteal
Anterior tibial
Peroneal
Posterior tibial
Dorsal pedis
Arcuate
Dorsal metatarsal

Occipital
Internal carotid
External carotid
Left common carotid
Subclavian
Pulmonary
Lateral thoracic
Axillary
Brachial
Splenic
Renal
Inferior mesenteric
Radial
Ulnar
Deep
Superficial } Palmar arch
Digital

Figure 9.6 Principal arteries of the body.

The right and left subclavian arteries branch into:

the *vertebral*—supplying the neck and brain, and

the *axillary*—the largest artery of the arm, passing from the armpit down the inner side of the arm, continuing into

the *brachial*—in the upper arm, branching at the elbow into

the *radial* and *ulnar* (named for lower arm bones)—branching into smaller arteries supplying the hands. (The radial artery can be felt at the wrist where the pulse is taken).

descending aorta—which divides into two segments:

descending thoracic aorta—divides into branches:

the *visceral*—supplying pericardium, bronchi, mediastinum, and esophagus;

the *parietal*—supplying diaphragm, mammaries, and chest muscles.

descending abdominal aorta—has four branches:

the *visceral* and the *parietal* } supplying abdominal and pelvic organs

the *right common iliac* the *left common iliac* } divides into

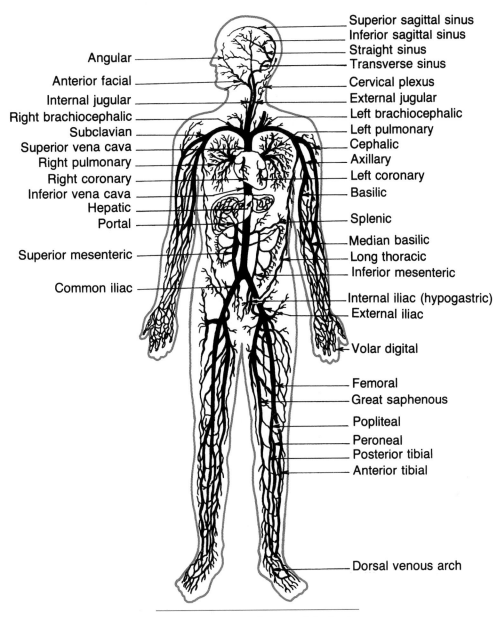

Angular
Anterior facial
Internal jugular
Right brachiocephalic
Subclavian
Superior vena cava
Right pulmonary
Right coronary
Inferior vena cava
Hepatic
Portal
Superior mesenteric
Common iliac

Superior sagittal sinus
Inferior sagittal sinus
Straight sinus
Transverse sinus
Cervical plexus
External jugular
Left brachiocephalic
Left pulmonary
Cephalic
Axillary
Left coronary
Basilic
Splenic
Median basilic
Long thoracic
Inferior mesenteric
Internal iliac (hypogastric)
External iliac
Volar digital
Femoral
Great saphenous
Popliteal
Peroneal
Posterior tibial
Anterior tibial
Dorsal venous arch

Figure 9.7 Principal veins of the body.

right and *left internal iliacs,* supplying the
pelvic wall and viscera, and the
right and *left external iliacs,* supplying the
legs and continuing into the *femoral,*
popliteal, and *anterior* and *posterior tib-*
ials into the toes.

The Veins

The previous section traced the blood from the heart,
through the arteries, to the extremities. This section
will describe the return of the blood, through the
veins, to the heart (see Figures 9.1 and 9.7).

The *pulmonary* veins are four veins that return the
blood from the lungs to the *left atrium* of the heart

and are the only veins that carry freshly oxygenated
blood.

Veins lying deep within the tissues are called *deep*
veins; those close to the surface, and sometimes visible
through the skin, are called *superficial* veins. The large
veins of the cranium are called *sinuses* but bear no relation to the sinuses of bony tissue (see Figure 9.7).

The *internal jugular* veins are deep veins draining
the skull and brain. The superficial *external*
jugular veins drain the scalp, face, and neck.
Both jugulars empty into the *subclavian* veins.
The *axillary, scapular,* and *thoracic* deep veins
and the *cephalic* and *basilic* superficial veins also
empty into the *subclavian* veins.

The *subclavian* veins empty into the *brachio-cephalic* (also called *innominate*) veins. The *brachiocephalic* veins empty into the *superior vena cava* to the *right atrium*.

The veins draining the lower extremities are both superficial and deep. The veins of the feet and lower legs drain into two superficial veins, the *small saphenous* and the *great saphenous*.

The *small saphenous* veins drain into the *popliteals*, deep veins draining into the *femorals*.

The *great saphenous* veins drain into the *femorals*.

The *femorals* are deep veins of the thigh that drain into the *external iliacs*.

The *external iliacs* are deep veins of the groin that join

The *internal iliacs* (or *hypogastrics*), deep veins draining the pelvic viscera. The *external* and *internal iliacs* join to form the *common iliacs*.

The *common iliacs* join to become the *inferior vena cava*.

The *inferior vena cava* empties into the *right atrium*.

Specific veins drain the blood from the stomach, intestines, spleen, pancreas, gallbladder, and liver and empty into the *inferior vena cava* for return to the *right atrium*, as described in *hepatic portal circulation*.

The veins of the stomach are the *right* and *left gastroepiploic*, the *pyloric*, and the *gastric* (also called *coronary*).

The veins of the intestines are the *superior* and *inferior mesenteric*, *right* and *left colic*, *ileocolic*, and *sigmoid*.

The veins of the spleen are the *splenic*.

The veins of the pancreas are the *pancreatic*.

The veins of the gallbladder are the *cystic*.

All these veins connect with, and drain into, the *hepatic portal vein*, which enters the liver. From there the blood leaves through the *hepatic vein*, which drains into the *inferior vena cava*, finally emptying into the *right atrium*.

REVIEW 9.C

Complete the following:

1. Blood circulation consists of two circuits: _Systemic_ circulation, which includes a segment called _portal_ circulation; and a second circuit called _pulmonary_ circulation.

2. _Pulmonary_ veins are the only veins carrying oxygenated blood.

3. The blood makes a complete circuit of the body in about _1_ minute(s).

4. The _aorta_ is the largest artery in the body.

5. The _coronary_ arteries supply the myocardial muscle.

6. The pulse of the _radial_ artery can be felt at the wrist.

7. The three branches of the aorta are the _ascending aorta_, _aortic arch_, and _descending aorta_.

8. Veins lying close to the surface are called _superficial_ veins, and those within the tissues are called _deep_ veins.

9. The internal and external _jugular_ veins drain regions of the head and neck.

10. The _inferior vena cava_ drains into the right atrium.

ANATOMY

Heart

aortic valve semilunar valve that prevents backflow of blood from the aorta to the heart.

apex (a′peks) rounded tip of heart, pointing left and downward.

atrial appendage ear-shaped continuation of the left and right upper part of the atria.

atrioventricular node located in the right atrium near the lower portion of the interatrial septum, and composed of a small mass of atypical cardiac muscle tissue (also called *AV node, Aschoff's node,* and *Tawara's node*).

atrioventricular valves valves between atria and ventricles of the heart (the left valve is the *bicuspid,* or *mitral,* and the right valve is the *tricuspid*).

atrium (a′tre-um) left or right upper chamber of the heart.

bundle of His a band of specialized cardiac muscle fibers that arise in the atrioventricular node and branch down on both sides of the interventricular septum, transmitting the atrial contraction rhythm to the ventricles (also called *atrioventricular bundle*).

chordae tendineae (kor′de ten″din′e-ay) tendinous strings resembling cords that extend from the cusps of the atrioventricular valves to the papillary muscles of the heart, which prevent valve inversion.

conus arteriosus (ko′nus ar-te″re-o′sus) upper, anterior angle of the right ventricle where the pulmonary artery begins (also called *infundibulum of the heart*).

cor another name for the heart.

coronary arteries and veins blood vessels of the heart.

cusp leafletlike segment of the cardiac valve.

diastole (di-as′to-le) relaxation stage of the heart action.

ductus arteriosus blood vessel in fetal circulation connecting pulmonary artery to descending aorta.

endocardium endothelial membrane lining the chambers of the heart.

epicardium outermost serous layer covering the heart.

foramen ovale cordis (fo-ra′men o″vah′le) opening between the atria in the fetal heart, normally closed after birth.

interventricular between ventricles.

myocardium thick middle muscle layer of the heart wall.

pacemaker sinoatrial node, which initiates the heartbeat and regulates its rate.

pericardium external layer of the membrane covering the heart.

pulmonary valve valve at the base of the pulmonary artery (also called *semilunar valve*).

Purkinje fibers specialized cardiac muscle fibers that are involved in the impulse-conducting system of the heart.

semilunar valves refers to the half-moon shape of the valves at the base of the pulmonary artery and aorta.

sinoatrial node see *pacemaker.*

systole (sis′to-le) contraction stage of heart action.

valves membranous structures in passages that close to prevent the reflux of contents.

Blood and Blood Vessels

basophil (ba′so-fil) granular leukocyte cell that stains with basic dyes.

capillary small blood vessel that connects arterioles with venules, forming a vast network throughout the body.

eosinophil (e″o-sin′o-fil) granular leukocyte cell that stains readily with orange or yellow acid eosin dyes.

erythrocyte (e-rith′ro-site) red blood cell.

erythropoiesis (e-rith″ro-poi-e′sis) red blood cell production.

granulocyte (gran′u-lo-site) cell containing granules (leukocytes with cytoplasmic granules of neutrophils, basophils, or eosinophils).

granulocytopoiesis (gran″u-lo-si″to-poi-e′sis) production of granulocytes.

hematopoiesis (hem″ah-to-poi-e′sis) production of red blood cells (also called *hemopoiesis*).

heme insoluble, nonprotein, iron-containing portion of hemoglobin.

hemoglobin iron-containing red pigment (heme) that combines with a protein substance (globin), giving blood its red color.

heparin (hep′ah-rin) anticoagulant substance.

leukocyte (lu″ko-site) white blood cell.

leukocytopoiesis leukocyte production (also called *leukopoiesis*).

lymphocyte (lim″fo-site) clear, nongranular leukocyte with single, round nucleus that functions in phagocytosis and antibody formation.

lymphopoiesis (lim″fo-poi-e″sis) production of lymphocytes.

macrocyte (mak′ro-site) abnormally large erythrocyte.

megakaryocyte (meg″ah-kar′e-o-site) giant cell of bone marrow that produces mature blood platelets.

megalocyte (meg′ah-lo-sit) large nonnucleated erythrocyte.

monocyte phagocytic, mononuclear white blood cell (leukocyte).

monocytopoiesis (mon″o-si″to-poi-e′sis) formation of monocytes.

neutrophil (nu′tro-fil) neutral dye staining granular leukocyte containing lobed nucleus (also called *polymorphonuclear leukocyte*).

phagocytosis (fag″o-si-to′sis) the ingestion and destruction of microorganisms, cells, and foreign matter.

plasma liquid portion of blood.

plasmocyte plasma cell.

platelet disklike, nonnucleated element in the blood, originating in the red bone marrow and necessary for coagulation of blood (also called *thrombocyte*).

prothrombin factor in the blood plasma that converts to thrombin and is part of the blood clotting mechanism.

reticulocyte (re-tik′u-lo-site) immature red blood cell, which shows basophilic reticulum (network) under vital staining.

sinusoid (si′nus-oid) large, variable, anastomosing, terminal blood vessel, with reticuloendothelium lining, found in organs such as liver, suprarenals, and heart (also called *sinusoidal capillary*).

thrombin enzyme of prothrombin, that changes fibrinogen to fibrin.

thrombocyte blood platelet.

thromboplastin (throm″bo-plas′tin) substance in blood and body tissue that aids in converting prothrombin to thrombin.

tunica term for a coat or covering of a blood vessel, organ, or body part.

tunica adventitia or **tunica externa vasorum** the fibrous elastic outer covering of blood vessels.

tunica intima vasorum inner coat of blood vessel.

tunica media vasorum middle coat of blood vessel.

vas vessel.

Arteries. Most of the arteries in this Related Terms list are frequently encountered arteries and their branches, appearing in records of procedures and disorders.

aorta (a-or′tah) largest artery in the body and main trunk of the entire arterial system.

aortic arch continuation of the ascending portion of the aorta.

arteriole (ar-te′re-ohl) tiny arterial branch.

ascending pharyngeal branch of the external carotid artery that distributes to the pharynx, soft palate, ear, and meninges.

auricular posterior (aw-rik′u-lar) branch of the external carotid artery that serves the middle ear, mastoid cells, parotid gland, auricle of the ear, and various muscles.

axillary (ak′si-lar″e) branch of the subclavian artery that distributes to the axilla, chest, shoulder, and upper extremity.

basilar (basi-lar) branch of the vertebral artery distributing to the brainstem, cerebellum, posterior cerebrum, and internal ear.

brachial (bra′ke-al) axillary artery branch distributing to the shoulder, arm, and hand.

brachiocephalic (innominate) (brak″e-o-se-fal′ik) aortic arch branch distributing to the right side of the head, neck, and arm.

carotids (kah-rot′ids) right and left common carotids, originating from the brachiocephalic artery and the aortic arch respectively, distributing to the right and left sides of the head.

celiac trunk branch of the abdominal aorta distributing to the stomach, liver, pancreas, spleen, and duodenum.

cerebellar (ser″e-bel′ar) three cerebellar arteries distributing to the cerebellum and/or medulla, pineal body, and midbrain.

cerebral (ser′e-bral) distributes to cerebrum and its structures.

colic distributes to the colon.

coronary left and right arteries distributing to the left and right sides of the myocardial muscle (atria and ventricles).

cystic distributes to the gallbladder.

deferential distributes to the ureter, ductus deferens, testes, and seminal vesicles.

dorsalis pedis distributes to the foot and toes.

epigastric three arteries serving respectively the abdominal muscles and peritoneum; the abdominal muscles, skin, and diaphragm; and the skin of the abdomen, the inguinal lymph nodes, and superficial fascia.

esophageal thoracic aorta branch that distributes to the esophagus.

femoral branch of the external iliac artery that distributes to the external genitalia, lower leg, and lower abdominal wall.

gastric three arteries distributing to the esophagus and curvatures of the stomach.

gastroduodenal branch of the hepatic artery that distributes to the stomach, duodenum, pancreas, and greater omentum.

gastroepiploic (gas″tro-ep″i-plo′ik) two arteries distributing to the stomach and greater omentum.

gluteal two arteries that distribute to the buttocks and thighs.

hemorrhoidal (hem″o-roi′dal) three arteries distributing to the anal canal and rectum.

hepatic distributes to the stomach, pancreas, duodenum, liver, gallbladder, and greater omentum.

ileal (il′e-al) branch of the superior mesenteric artery that distributes to the ileum.

ileocolic branch of the superior mesenteric artery distributing to the cecum, appendix, ascending colon, and ileum.

iliac (il′e-ak) the common iliac artery and its branches distribute to the pelvis, abdominal wall, lower limbs, external genitalia, pelvic visceral wall, buttocks, reproductive organs, and the midthigh.

iliolumbar branch of the internal iliac artery that distributes to the pelvic bones and muscles, fifth lumbar vertebra, and sacrum.

intercostal thoracic aorta branch distributing to thoracic wall.

internal spermatic branch of the abdominal aorta that distributes to the ureter, epididymis, and testis (also called *testicular artery*).

intestinal branch of the superior mesenteric artery that distributes to the jejunum, ileum, duodenum, and colon.

laryngeal (lah-rin′je-al) inferior and superior branches of the thyroid arteries, which distribute respectively to the larynx (superior), trachea (inferior), and esophagus (both superior and inferior).

lingual branch of the external carotid artery that distributes to the tongue, sublingual glands, tonsils, and epiglottis.

lumbar branch of the abdominal aorta that distributes to the abdominal walls and the renal capsule.

malleolar two arteries distributing to the ankle joint.

mammary distributes to the anterior thoracic wall, diaphragm, and mediastinal structures (also called *internal thoracic artery*).

maxillary two arteries distributing to the jaws, teeth, chewing muscles, ears, nose, nasal sinuses, palate, and meninges.

mesenteric inferior and superior branches of the abdominal aorta distributing respectively to the lower half of the colon and rectum; and the small intestine and proximal half of the colon.

nutrient any artery that supplies blood to the bone marrow (also called *medullary artery*).

obturator branch of the internal iliac artery that distributes to the pelvic muscles and hip joint.

occipital branch of the external carotid artery that distributes to the muscles of the neck, scalp, meninges, and mastoid cells.

ophthalmic branch of the internal carotid artery that distributes to the eyes, orbits, and adjacent facial structures.

ovarian branch of the abdominal aorta that distributes to the ovaries, uterine tubes, and ureters.

pancreaticoduodenal (pan″kre-at″i-ko-du″o-de′nal) two arteries that distribute to the pancreas and duodenum.

peroneal branch of the posterior tibial artery that distributes to the ankle and deep calf muscles.

phrenic two pairs of arteries, inferior and superior, distributing to the diaphragm and suprarenal glands.

popliteal femoral artery branch distributing to the knee and calf.

pudendal external and internal branches of the femoral and internal iliac arteries, respectively, distributing to the external genitalia.

pulmonary the only arteries in the body that carry nonoxygenated blood, which is delivered to the lungs for oxygenation.

radial brachial artery branch distributing to forearm and hand.

renal branch of the abdominal aorta that distributes to the kidneys, suprarenals, and ureters.

sacral two arteries distributing respectively to adjacent structures of the coccyx and sacrum, and to the sacrum, coccyx, and rectum.

sigmoid branch of the inferior mesenteric artery that distributes to the sigmoid colon.

splenic branch of the celiac trunk that distributes to the spleen, stomach, pancreas, and greater omentum.

subclavian two arteries distributing to the neck, upper limbs, thoracic wall, spinal cord, brain, and meninges.

subcostal branch of the thoracic aorta that distributes to the upper posterior abdominal wall.

subscapular branch of the axillary artery that distributes to the shoulder and scapular areas.

temporal three pairs of arteries, *superficial, middle,* and *deep,* distributing to the head.

thoracic three arteries, *lateral, superior,* and *internal,* distributing respectively to the pectoral muscles and mammary glands; the axillary area of the chest wall; and the diaphragm, structures of the mediastinum, and the anterior thoracic wall.

thyrocervical trunk branch of the subclavian artery distributing to the scapular area, deep neck, and thyroid.

thyroid two arteries distributing to the thyroid gland and neighboring structures.

tibial two arteries that distribute to the leg, ankle, and foot.

transverse cervical branch of subclavian artery distributing to the neck and scapular muscles.

ulnar brachial artery branch distributing to forearm and hand.

uterine branch of the internal iliac artery that distributes to the uterus, uterine tubes, vagina, and ovaries.

vertebral subclavian artery branch distributing to the neck, vertebral column, cerebellum, internal cerebrum, and spinal cord.

Veins. Most of the veins in this listing are frequently encountered veins and their branches, appearing in records of procedures and disorders.

auricular two veins that are anterior and posterior to the ear.

axillary basilic and brachial vein continuation to subclavians.

azygos (az′i-gos) three veins of the trunk that empty into the superior vena cava.

basalis veins of the cerebral area.

basilic (bah-sil′ik) veins of the forearm and hand.

brachiocephalic (innominate) (brak″e-o-se-fal′ik) left and right branches unite to form the superior vena cava.

bronchial veins that bring blood back from the lung.

cardiac veins of the heart, including coronary veins (also called *venae cordis*).

cephalic (se-fal′ik) veins of the forearm and arm.

cerebellar veins of the cerebellum.

cerebral numerous veins that drain blood from the brain (also called *venae cerebri*).

cervical deep vein of the neck.

choroid (ko′roid) veins of choroid plexus and other brain areas.

circumflex a group of veins serving femoral and iliac areas.

colic right, medial, and left veins of intestines.

comitans (kom′i-tans) veins accompanying corresponding arteries or nerves.

common iliac large veins draining blood from pelvis and leg, joining to form inferior vena cava.

cutaneous small subcutaneous veins draining into deep veins.

cystic vein of the gallbladder.

digital group of veins serving the palms, fingers, soles, and toes.

dorsal veins of clitoris deep and superficial veins of the clitoris.

dorsal veins of penis deep and superficial veins of the penis.

epigastric comitans veins of the epigastric arteries.

esophageal veins of the esophagus.

facial superficial and deep veins of the facial structures.

femoral comitans veins of the femoral artery of the thigh.

gastric group of veins serving the stomach, including the pyloric vein and the coronary vein of the stomach.

gastroepiploic comitans right and left veins of the stomach and omentum.

gluteal comitans veins of the thighs and buttocks.

hemorrhoidal group of veins of the rectal area.

hepatic veins that drain the liver.

hepatic portal carries blood from the digestive system to the liver.

hypogastric veins of the lower and middle abdomen, joining the external iliac to form the common iliac vein.

ileocolic veins draining the ileum, cecum, appendix, and part of the ascending colon.

iliac external and internal, join with the saphenous to form the common iliac vein.

iliolumbar comitans vein of the iliolumbar artery, serving the iliac and lumbar regions.

intercostal comitans veins that accompany intercostal arteries.

interlobular renal and hepatic veins.

intervertebral numerous comitans veins of spinal nerves.

jejunal and ileal veins draining the jejunum and ileum and joining the superior mesenteric vein.

jugular two pairs of veins, *internal* and *external*, serving the head and neck.

labyrinthine (lab″i-rin′thin) comitans veins of the ear.

laryngeal inferior and superior veins of the larynx.

lateral thoracic veins draining the side of the thoracic wall.

lingual veins serving the tongue, area below the tongue and mandibular glands, and floor of the mouth.

lumbar comitans veins of the lumbar region.

mammary thoracic artery comitans vein (also called *internal thoracic*).

median antebrachial veins of the forearms.

median cubital veins of the elbow and forearm, most commonly used for venipuncture site (also called *intermediate basilic*).

mediastinal veins of the mediastinum.

mesenteric intestinal comitans veins emptying into hepatic portal vein.

nasal vein of the nose.

obturator veins of the hip joint and thigh muscles.

occipital veins of the head.

ophthalmic inferior and superior veins of the orbital area.

ovarian veins of the ovary.

palatine veins of the area of the palate.

pancreatic veins of the pancreas.

pancreaticoduodenal comitans veins of the pancreas and duodenum.

parotid veins of the parotid gland.

pericardiac small veins of the pericardium of the heart.

peroneal comitans veins of the lower leg.

pharyngeal veins of the pharyngeal area.

phrenic veins of the diaphragm.

plexus network of nerves, lymph, or blood vessels.

popliteal veins from the knee area into the femoral vein.

pudendal comitans veins draining perineum and external genitalia.

pulmonary four veins returning oxygenated blood from the lungs to the left atrium of the heart.

renal comitans veins of the kidney.

sacral comitans veins emptying into the iliac veins.

saphenous (sah-fe′nus) *great,* the longest vein in the body running from foot to thigh, and *small,* running from foot to knee.

sigmoid veins of the sigmoid colon.

spermatic veins that drain the testes and epididymis.

spinal veins draining the blood from the spinal cord.

splenic vein draining the spleen (also called *lienal vein*).

subclavian main veins of the upper extremity, joining the internal jugulars to form the two brachiocephalic veins.

supraorbital veins of the anterior scalp.

suprarenals veins of the adrenal glands.

temporal veins draining the temporal region of the head.

thoracoepigastric veins of the trunk.

thyroid veins of the thyroid gland.

tibial comitans veins of the leg emptying into the popliteal.

tracheal veins of the trachea.

ulnar comitans veins of the forearm.

uterine veins of the uterus.

venae cavae two large veins that return blood to the heart, the *superior* from the head, neck, chest, and upper extremities, and the *inferior* from the abdominal viscera, pelvis, and lower extremities.

venae vasorum (va-so'rum) small veins that return blood from the walls of blood vessels.

venules minute veins.

vertebral veins of the vertebrae.

vesical veins of the bladder (usually the urinary bladder).

volar veins of the palm of the hand and sole of the foot.

PATHOLOGIC CONDITIONS

Inflammations and Infections

aortitis inflammation of the aorta.

arteritis (ar"te-ri'tis) inflammation of an artery.

bacteremia bacteria in the blood.

carditis inflammation of the heart.

endarteritis inflammation of the tunica intima of an artery.

endarteritis deformans persistent endarteritis characterized by fatty degeneration of the tissue of the arteries and forming of deposits of lime salts.

endarteritis obliterans endarteritis with narrowing and closure of the arterial lumen (space within a tube).

endocarditis (en"do-kar-di'tis) inflammation of the endocardium (lining) membrane of the heart.

erythrocytosis abnormal increase in red blood cells, usually caused by infection.

leukocytosis temporary increase in number of leukocytes in the blood, caused by inflammation, infection, or hemorrhage.

myocarditis (mi"o-kar-di'tis) inflammation of the heart muscle.

panarteritis inflammatory arterial disease, involving all layers of the arterial wall.

periarteritis inflammation of the adventitia (outer layer) of an artery.

pericarditis (per'i-kar'dit'is) inflammation of the pericardium.

perisplenitis inflammation of the outer covering of the spleen and the surrounding structures.

phlebitis (fle-bi'tis) inflammation of a vein, with formation of a thrombus, accompanied by pain, stiffness, and edema.

polyarteritis inflammatory condition of the arterial system with many destructive lesions.

polyserositis (pol"e-se-ro-si'tis) general inflammatory condition of the serous membranes, accompanied by serous effusion.

pyelophlebitis (pi"e-lo-fle-bi'tis) inflammatory condition of the renal pelvis veins.

septicemia (sep"ta-se'me-ah) general systemic blood infection caused by the presence of pathogenic microorganisms or their toxins (also called *blood poisoning*).

thromboangiitis (throm"bo-an"je-i'tis) thrombi (blood clots) accompanying inflammation of the intima (inner coat) of a blood vessel.

thrombophlebitis inflammation of a vein with clot formation.

Hemorrhages and Related Conditions

disseminated intravascular coagulation (DIC) simultaneous hemorrhage and thrombosis caused by overstimulation of blood clotting mechanisms, as a result of disease or injury.

epistaxis (ep"i-stak'sis) nosebleed.

hemarthrosis (hem"ar-thro'sis) presence of blood in a joint.

hematemesis (hem"at-em'e-sis) vomiting of blood.

hematencephalon (hem"at-en-sef'ah-lon) cerebral hemorrhage.

hematocele (hem'ah-to-sel") blood in a cavity or cyst.

hematocoelia (hem"ah-to-se'le-ah) escape of blood into the peritoneal cavity (*coel* means cavity).

hematocolpos (hem"ah-to-kol'pos) menstrual blood accumulated in the vagina (*colpo* means vagina).

hematoma (hem"ah-to"mah) blood, usually clotted, accumulated in a tissue, organ, or space caused by a blood vessel wall break.

hematometra (hem"ah-to-me'trah) accumulation of blood in the cavity of the uterus.

hematomphalocele (hem"at-om'fal'o-seal) umbilical hernia filled with blood (*cele* means protrusion).

hematomyelia (hem"ah-to-mi-e'le-ah) bleeding into the spinal cord.

hematopericardium (hem"ah-to-per"i-kar"de-um) escape of blood into the pericardium (also called *hemopericardium*).

hematoperitoneum (hem"ah-to-per"it-to-ne'um) escape of blood into the peritoneum.

hematorrhachis (hem-ah-tor'ah-kis) bleeding into the spinal column (*rhachis* means spine).

hematorrhea (hem'ah-to-re'ah) profuse hemorrhage.

hematosalpinx (hem"ah-to-sal'pinks) accumulation of blood in a tube, most frequently a uterine tube (also called *hemosalpinx*).

hematospermatocele (hem"ah-to-sper-mat'o-seal) sperm-filled cyst containing blood.

hematotympanum (hem"ah-to-tim'pah-num) bleeding into the middle ear.

hematuria blood in the urine.

hemophthalmia (he"mof-thal'me-ah) bleeding into the eyeball (also called *hemophthalmos* or *hemophthalmus*).

hemoptysis (he-mop'ti-sis) spitting of blood, or bloody sputum (*ptysis* means spitting).

hemothorax accumulation of blood in the pleural cavity.

melena passing of tarry stools caused by presence of digested blood.

menorrhagia (men"o-ra'je-ah) abnormally heavy menstrual flow.

metrorrhagia (me"tro-ra'je-ah) abnormal uterine bleeding, especially between menstrual periods.

petechial hemorrhages (pe-te'ke-al) small pinpoint hemorrhages in the skin or the mucous membranes.

postpartum hemorrhage hemorrhage following childbirth.

Anemias

anemia reduction in red blood cells.

aplastic anemia anemia resulting from bone marrow disease or destruction.

deficiency anemia anemia caused by lack of necessary nutritional substances.

hemolytic anemia anemia resulting from the destruction of erythrocytes.

hypochromic microcytic anemia iron deficiency anemia.

macrocytic anemia anemia in which erythrocytes are enlarged.

myelophthisic anemia (mi"e-lof'thi-sik) anemia caused by dissolution or crowding out of the blood-forming tissues by lesions (also called *leukoerythroblastosis*).

pernicious anemia megaloblastic anemia resulting from failure of the gastric mucosa to secrete a factor necessary to form erythrocytes and absorb vitamin B_{12}.

Leukemias

This is a limited listing of leukemias. Refer to a medical dictionary for a more detailed listing with definitions.

leukemia (lu-ke'me-ah) malignant, progressive disease, marked by an abnormal increase in the production of leukocytes and a decrease in erythrocytes and platelets, causing an anemia and vulnerability to infection and hemorrhage; classified as: (1) acute or chronic type; (2) cell type involved (myeloid, lymphoid, or monocytic); and (3) increase or nonincrease of abnormal cells.

aleukemic leukemia leukemia in which the peripheral white blood cell count is normal or below normal.

leukemia cutis leukemia with general or localized skin involvement, having nodular lesions with accumulation of leukemic cells in the skin.

monocytic leukemia leukemia in which monocytes are the predominant white blood cells.

myeloblastic leukemia leukemia in which myeloblasts are the predominant white blood cells.

stem cell leukemia leukemia that is difficult to type because the prevailing cells are too immature and may be lymphoblasts, myeloblasts, or monoblasts.

Hereditary, Congenital, and Developmental Disorders

coarctation of aorta (ko"ark-ta'shun) deformity of the aorta causing narrowing of its lumen.

Cooley's anemia one of a group of familial hemolytic anemias occurring in neonates (also called *thalassemia*).

dextrocardia heart is displaced to the right side of the thoracic cavity.

dextroposition of the aorta aorta is displaced to the right (see *tetralogy of Fallot*).

Eisenmenger's complex interventricular septal defect with pulmonary hypertension and hypertrophy of the ventricle on the right side, accompanied by cyanosis.

hemophilia (he"mo-fil'e-ah) hereditary disease in which there is a deficiency in the clotting of blood.

hereditary hemorrhagic telangiectasia (tel-an"je-ek-ta'ze-ah) familial condition marked by many small angiomas of the mucous membranes and skin frequently accompanied by gastrointestinal bleeding or epistaxis.

patent ductus arteriosus duct between the left pulmonary artery and descending aorta in the fetus that normally closes at birth.

pulmonary stenosis narrowing of the passage between the pulmonary artery and the right ventricle.

sickle cell anemia hemolytic anemia caused by a hereditary genetic defect, occurring most frequently in blacks.

tetralogy of Fallot (fal-o′) group of four cardiac anomalies, including pulmonary stenosis, dextroposition of the aorta, interventricular septal defect, and marked hypertrophy of the right ventricle (also called *Fallot's tetrad*).

thalassemia see *Cooley's anemia.*

transposition of aorta and pulmonary artery aorta originates from the right ventricle and the pulmonary artery originates from the left ventricle, causing cyanosis as a result of lack of oxygen in the blood (also called *transposition of great vessels*).

tricuspid atresia absence of a tricuspid valve.

Other Abnormalities

agranulocytosis (ah-gran″u-lo-si-to′sis) disease characterized by a sudden decrease in granulocytes and the appearance of lesions of the mucous membranes, especially in the gastrointestinal tract and on the skin.

altitude alkalosis increased alkalinity in the blood and body tissues caused by high altitude.

aneurysm blood-filled, saclike formation, caused by localized dilation of a blood vessel wall (usually an artery) or the heart.

angialgia pain in a vessel (also called *angiodynia*).

angina refers to any condition with attacks of suffocating, paroxysmal pain.

angina pectoris (an-ji′nah pec′tor-is) an ischemic condition with severe, paroxysmal chest pain, usually radiating from the cardiac area of the chest to the left shoulder and down the left arm (sometimes referred to as a *charley horse of the heart*).

angiomegaly (an″je-o-meg′ah-le) enlargement of a blood vessel.

angionecrosis (an′je-o-ne-kro′sis) necrosis (death) of blood vessel walls.

angioparalysis paralysis affecting a blood vessel.

angiosclerosis sclerosis (hardening) of blood vessel walls.

angiostenosis narrowing of vessels.

aortic insufficiency blood from the aorta flows back to the left ventricle because of malfunctioning of the semilunar valve of the aorta.

arrhythmia (ah-rith′me-ah) abnormal rhythm of the heartbeat.

arteriolonecrosis (ar-te″re-o″lo-ne-kro′sis) necrosis of cells forming arteriole walls.

arteriolosclerosis (ar-te″re-o″lo-skle-ro′sis) thickening and hardening of the walls of arterioles.

arteriomalacia (ar-te″re-o-mah-la′she-ah) softening of arterial coats.

arterionecrosis (ar-te″re-o-ne-kro′sis) necrosis of walls of an artery.

arteriosclerosis (ar-te″re-o-skle-ro′sis) classification of diseases of the arteries, marked by a thickening of the walls of the arteries and loss of their elasticity.

arteriospasm (ar-te′re-o-spazm) spasm of an artery.

arteriostenosis (ar-te″re-o-ste-no′sis) narrowing of the lumen of an artery.

atherosclerosis (ath″er-o″skle-ro′sis) type of arteriosclerosis marked by the formation of plaques containing cholesterol and lipids within the intima of large- and medium-sized arteries.

bradycardia slow heartbeat.

cardiac arrest abrupt stopping of cardiac function and absence of arterial blood pressure.

cardiac edema edema symptomatic of congestive heart failure.

cardiac hypertrophy enlargement of the heart.

cardiac murmur abnormal sound heard between the normal heart sound of lub-dub.

cardialgia pain in the upper anterior chest or abdomen (also called *cardiodynia*).

cardiectasis (kar″de-ek′tah-sis) expansion of the heart.

cardiohepatomegaly (kar″de-o-hep″ah-to-meg′ah-le) swelling of the heart and liver.

cardiomalacia (kar″de-o-mah-la′she-ah) abnormal softening of the heart muscle.

cardiomegaly (kar″de-o-meg′ah-le) enlargement of the heart.

cardiomyoliposis (kar″de-o-mi″o-li-po′sis) fatty deterioration of the muscles of the heart.

cardionecrosis (kar″de-o-ne-kro′sis) death of heart tissue.

cardioptosis (kar″de-o-to′sis) downward displacement of the heart.

carotenemia presence of carotene in the blood, sometimes producing a jaundicelike skin coloring.

congestive heart failure prolonged inability of the heart to pump and maintain the blood flow adequately, resulting in impaired circulation, edema throughout the body, and blood backed up in the veins leading to the heart.

cor pulmonale cardiac condition caused by pulmonary hypertension resulting from disease of the lungs or their blood vessels.

cyanosis bluish skin color caused by reduced amounts of hemoglobin in the blood.

embolism (em′bo-lizm) blocking of a blood vessel by an obstruction, such as a blood clot, air bubble, fat globule, tissue, bacteria clump, or amniotic debris, carried by the flow of blood.

erythremia (er″i-thre′me-ah) chronic polycythemia (excessive formation of red blood cells) with hyperplasia (overgrowth) of bone marrow, and increase of blood volume.

erythrocytosis (e-rith″ro-si-to′sis) increase of red blood cells in circulation.

erythropenia deficiency of erythrocytes (also called *erythrocytopenia*).

fibrillation arrhythmia with uncoordinated, irregular contractions of the heart muscle affecting the atria and/or ventricles.

granulocytopenia (gran′u-lo-si″to-pe′ne-ah) decrease of granulocytes in the blood (also called *granulopenia*).

granulocytosis unusually large number of granulocytes in the blood.

heart block partial or complete interference with the conduction of the cardiac electrical impulses.

hemangiectasis (hem″an-je-ek′tah-sis) dilation of blood vessels (also called *angiectasis*).

hematocytopenia (hem″ah-to-si″to-pe′ne-ah) deficiency in the elements of the blood cells.

hematocytosis increase in the elements of the blood.

hematopenia decrease in blood.

hemoglobinemia (he″mo-glo′bi-ne′me-ah) abnormally large amounts of hemoglobin in blood plasma.

hemolith stone in the wall of a blood vessel.

hypertension high blood pressure.

hypotension low blood pressure.

infarct area of tissue that is damaged or necrotic because of an insufficient blood supply resulting from an obstruction to circulation.

ischemia local, temporary deficiency of blood supply to an area of the body caused by an obstruction in the blood vessel supplying the area (called *charley horse* when affecting calf muscles).

leukopenia reduction in the amount of white blood cells (also called *leukocytopenia*).

lymphocytopenia decrease of lymphocytes in the blood.

lymphocytosis excess of lymphocytes in the blood (also called *lymphocythemia*).

mitral valve prolapse (MVP) protrusion of the mitral valve into the left atrium, causing backflow of blood because of incomplete closure.

Mönckeberg's arteriosclerosis (menk′e-bergz) type of arteriosclerosis affecting the medial arterial coat with calcium deposits, destroying elastic and muscle fibers (also called *medial arteriosclerosis*).

monocytopenia decrease of monocytes in the blood.

monocytosis increase of monocytes in the blood.

myocardial infarction occlusion (blockage) of a coronary artery, resulting in heart muscle damage.

neutropenia decrease of neutrophils in the blood (also called *neutrocytopenia*).

occlusion obstruction of a blood vessel, that may be caused by a thrombus or an embolus.

palpitation rapid action, or tachycardia, of the heart.

paroxysmal tachycardia (par″ok-siz′mal) sudden onset of rapid heartbeat, beginning and ending abruptly.

phlebangioma aneurysm of a vein.

phlebectasia (fleb″ek-ta′ze-ah) swelling of a vein or veins, or a varicosity (also called *phlebectasis*).

phlebemphraxis (phleb″em-frak′sis) obstruction of a vein by a clot or plug (*emphraxis* means stoppage).

phlebolithiasis condition marked by the development of calculi in the veins.

phlebosclerosis hardening of the walls of a vein (also called *venosclerosis*).

phlebostenosis narrowing of the walls of a vein.

polycythemia increase of erythrocytes in the blood.

polycythemia vera (pol″e-si-the′me-ah ver′ah) excess of red blood cells with blood volume increase, along with splenomegaly, leukocytosis, and thrombocythemia.

polyemia excessive amount of blood in the body.

purpura fulminans extremely rare, severe, and often fatal blood disorder, usually occurring after an infectious disease in children, producing clotting and bleeding simultaneously.

Raynaud's disease idiopathic (cause unknown) disorder of arterial circulation, resulting in cyanosis of digits, nose, and/or ears.

Raynaud's phenomenon blanching or cyanosis of digits as a result of arterial spasm, caused by cold or emotion.

restenosis a condition of clogged arteries that may result some time after angioplasty, requiring repetition of the procedure.

reticulocytopenia (re-tik"u-lo-si"to-pe'ne-ah) decrease in the amount of reticulocytes in the blood (also called *reticulopenia*).

Stokes-Adams syndrome sudden loss of consciousness (often with convulsions); may accompany heart block.

superior vena cava syndrome (SVCS) edema of the neck, face, or upper arms caused by excessive venous pressure in the superior vena cava.

tachycardia rapid heartbeat.

thrombocytopenic purpura (throm"bo-si"to-pe'nik pur'pu-rah) progressive, systemic condition, which may be fatal, with hemorrhages of mucous membranes, decrease in platelets, and anemia,

thrombosis development, or presence, of a blood clot or thrombus.

thrombus blood clot obstructing a blood vessel.

transient ischemic attack (TIA) temporary blockage of blood supply to the brain, causing loss of brain function for about 24 hours.

varicose (var'i-kos) lasting, abnormal swelling, as in varicose vein (*varico* means twisted and swollen).

vascular abnormalities abnormal arteries are described as beaded, dilated, obstructed, sclerosed, or tortuous, and abnormal veins are described as dilated, distended, inflamed, varicosed, or thrombosed.

vasoconstriction (vas"o-kon-strik'shun) narrowing of blood vessels.

vasodilation the expansion of blood vessels.

vasospasm blood vessel spasm causing a narrowing in its diameter.

Oncology*

atrial myxoma benign tumor composed of primary connective tissue cells that originate in the interatrial septum.

carotid body tumor benign, encapsulated, spherical mass at the bifurcation (branching) of the common carotid artery.

hemangioma benign tumor caused by a cluster of newly formed blood vessels.

plasmacytoma* plasma cell neoplasm in or outside of bone marrow.

°Indicates a malignant condition.

SURGICAL PROCEDURES

anastomosis (ah-nas"to-mo'sis) creation of a passage between two vessels.

aneurysmectomy (an"u-riz-mek'to-me) completely removing an aneurysm by excising the sac.

aneurysmoplasty (an"u-riz'mo-plas"te) repairing of an aneurysm by plastic surgery.

aneurysmorrhaphy (an"u-riz-mor'ah-fe) suturing of an aneurysm.

aneurysmotomy (an"u-riz-mot'o-me) incision of an aneurysmal sac.

angiectomy (an"je-ek'to-me) excision of a vessel.

angioneurectomy (an"je-o-nu-rek'to-me) excision of vessel and nerve.

angioneurotomy (an"je-o-nu-rot'o-me) cutting of vessels and nerves.

angioplasty (an'je-o-plas"te) repair of a vessel.

angiorrhaphy (an"je-or'ah-fe) suture of a vessel.

angiostomy (an"je-os'to-me) opening of a blood vessel for insertion of a tube.

angiotomy incision of a blood vessel.

aortotomy cutting of the aorta.

arteriectomy excision of a section of an artery.

arterioplasty (ar-te"re-o-plas'te) repair of an artery.

arteriorrhaphy (ar-te"re-or'ah-fe) suture of an artery.

arteriotomy incision of an artery.

artificial cardiac pacemaker device (implanted or external), used in place of a defective sinoatrial node to supply electrical impulses to the heart.

atriotomy incision of the heart atrium.

bone marrow transplantation (BMT) bone marrow is harvested from a compatible donor and transplanted in the recipient for the treatment of anemias, leukemias, and other conditions.

cardiac prosthesis artificial replacement of cardiac tissue, such as plastic or pig valves, and patches or plastic tubular grafts for diseased arteries.

cardiocentesis (kar"de-o-sen-te'sis) surgical puncture or incision of the heart.

cardiotomy (kar"de-ot'o-me) incision of the heart.

coronary artery bypass graft (CABG) a section of a mammary artery or a saphenous vein is sutured to either side of an obstructed coronary artery to improve the flow of blood to the heart muscle.

directional coronary atherectomy (DCA) a method of shaving and removing plaque from clogged arteries in the heart by a motor-driven catheter equipped with a balloon, cutter, and storage chamber.

embolectomy (em″bo-lek′to-me) excision of an embolus.

excimer laser angioplasty a catheter equipped with a laser is guided into a blocked artery having extended plaque segments difficult to treat conventionally (see *percutaneous transluminal coronary angioplasty*). Ultraviolet energy pulses vaporize the plaque into gas that dissolves in the blood.

hemorrhoidectomy (hem″o-roid-ek′to-me) excision of hemorrhoids (varicose veins of the rectal area).

homograft replacement of heart transplant of a healthy human donor heart as a replacement for an irreparably damaged human heart.

open heart surgery surgical procedures requiring prolonged manipulation inside the heart, with the heart detached from systemic circulation and a heart-lung machine replacing its function.

percutaneous transluminal coronary angioplasty (PTCA) commonly called *balloon angioplasty,* because a catheter with a balloon tip is inserted in the coronary artery and inflated, pushing obstructing plaque against the vessel walls to allow free flow of blood.

pericardiectomy excision of the pericardium.

pericardiocentesis puncture of the pericardial cavity (also called *pericardicentesis*).

pericardiotomy incision of the pericardium.

phlebophlebostomy (fleb″o-fle-bos′to-me) anastomosis of two veins.

phleboplasty (fleb′o-plast″te) repair of a vein.

phleborrhaphy (fleb-or′ah-fe) suture of a vein.

sclerolaser therapy use of a laser to obliterate spider veins.

sclerotherapy chemical injections to obliterate spider veins and varicosities.

thrombectomy (throm-bek′to-me) excision of a thrombus from a blood vessel.

thrombolysis dissolving of a blood clot, particularly by injection of chemicals such as streptokinase, urokinase, and tissue plasminogen activator (TPA), which appear to spur the body's own mechanisms.

transmyocardial laser revascularization (TMLR) experimental procedure to increase the blood supply to the heart by using a high-energy laser to puncture tiny holes in the heart muscle.

valvuloplasty (val′vu-lo-plas″te) repair of a valve.

valvulotomy (val″vu-lot′o-me) incision of a valve, like those of the heart (also called *valvotomy*).

venipuncture puncture of a vein, to draw blood or give medication.

ventriculotomy (ven-trik″u-lot′-o-me) incision of a heart ventricle.

Vineberg coronary artery procedure surgical technique to implant a healthy artery into the heart muscle in the area of coronary disease.

LABORATORY TESTS AND PROCEDURES

abdominal aortography x-ray studies of the abdominal aorta and other vessels, using contrast medium.

activated partial thromboplastin time blood test to screen coagulation disorders and clotting factors.

angiocardiogram contrast medium is injected to study the heart and its vessels by use of x-ray examination.

angiogram a contrast medium is injected into the blood vessels and an x-ray film is taken (used to study vessels throughout the body).

apolipoprotein test measures blood content of apolipoprotein, which breaks down cholesterol.

arterial plethysmography noninvasive procedure to rule out occlusion in lower extremities.

aspartate aminotransferase (AST) a blood test to detect myocardial infarction (formerly called *serum glutamic-oxaloacetic transaminase—SGOT*).

ballistocardiogram test that records motion transmitted to the body by the heart pumping.

blood culture sample of blood is incubated in a growth medium to determine the type of organism causing infection.

bone marrow aspiration insertion of a needle into the sternum or iliac crest to obtain samples of bone marrow for analysis, to diagnose disorders involving red and white blood cells, by evaluating them as to appearance, numbers, development, and presence of infection.

capillary fragility test use of a blood pressure cuff to determine the fragility of small blood vessels, which is indicative of various diseases of blood vessels.

cardiac catheterization passage of a small catheter into the heart via a vein in the neck, arm, groin, or leg to inject dye for x-ray examination purposes, to record pressure, and to discover anomalies of the heart.

cholesterol test a test to determine the level of cholesterol, a necessary blood lipid which, if too high, is considered a risk factor in coronary heart disease (also see *lipoprotein tests*).

citrate agar hemoglobin electrophoresis procedure that identifies various forms of hemoglobin, which may indicate various hereditary anemias such as sickle cell.

coagulation tests tests of blood plasma and serum to determine clotting ability.

complete blood count (CBC) tests to determine the number of red blood cells *(RBC)*, white blood cells *(WBC)*, hematocrit *(HCT)*, and hemoglobin *(Hgb)* percent in the blood.

computerized tomography (CT) imaging device using x-rays at multiple angles through specific sections of the body, analyzed by computer to provide a total picture of the part being examined (also called *computerized axial tomography—CAT*).

Coombs' test test to determine the various types of anemia and blood incompatibility in pregnant women and their fetuses.

differential blood count percentages of leukocytes in a blood sample.

echocardiography (cardiac ultrasound examination) use of high-frequency sound waves to visualize the heart for assessment of valvular heart disease, and overall heart function.

electrocardiograph (ECG or EKG) instrument producing a graphic record of the electrical currents of the heart.

erythrocyte sedimentation rate (ESR) measurement of the rate at which red blood cells settle in unclotted blood, as an indication of the presence of inflammatory diseases and infections.

functional magnetic resonance imaging (FMRI) detects blood flow, metabolism, gas and water diffusion and movement in functioning systems (also see *magnetic resonance imaging*).

glucose tolerance test measurement of blood glucose levels at specific intervals following a fasting patient's intake of a quantity of glucose, used to determine effectiveness of metabolism of sugar.

hematocrit (HCT) method to determine erythrocytic volume in whole blood.

hemogram written record of the differential blood count.

hemolysis procedure to separate hemoglobin from red blood cells.

lipoprotein tests evaluates amounts and types of fatty substances in the blood (also see *cholesterol*).

High levels of *high-density lipoproteins (HDLs)* are related to decreased risk of heart disease,

whereas high levels of *low-density lipoproteins (LDLs)* and *triglycerides* are risk factors in heart disease.

magnetic resonance imaging (MRI) noninvasive method of scanning the body by use of an electromagnetic field and radio waves, which provides visual images on a computer screen and magnetic tape recordings (also called *nuclear magnetic resonance—NMR*).

nuclear magnetic resonance (NMR) see *magnetic resonance imaging*.

positron emission tomography (PET) noninvasive method of scanning using computer-analyzed radionuclides to detect abnormalities in heart and blood vessel function (also called *positron emission computerized tomography—PECT*).

prothrombin time test to determine the time necessary for clot formation in plasma, which provides a measure of the activity of various coagulation factors.

radionuclide angiocardiography noninvasive method of imaging the chest as a large volume of a blood-labeling agent (radionuclides like thallium or technetium) circulates through the heart and major blood vessels to assess ventricular function (also called *blood pool imaging*).

reticulocyte count measure of bone marrow activity, which decreases in hemolytic diseases, and elevates after an anemic attack or hemorrhage.

rubacell test blood test to determine immunity to German measles.

serum enzyme tests series of tests measuring enzymes released into the blood after a heart attack.

spatial vectorcardiogram electrocardiogram projected in three planes (three dimensional), showing electrical activity of the heart muscle and its contraction and relaxation.

thallium stress test use of radioactive thallium salts injected in minute amounts to mimic the effect of potassium on heart muscle, used in conjunction with an imaging machine to visualize the action of the heart under resting and stress conditions.

transesophageal echocardiography method of visualizing the heart from behind by passing a probe through the mouth and down the esophagus (also see *echocardiography*).

venography x-ray examination procedure using contrast dye to determine the presence of blood clots.

venous plethysmography noninvasive test to evaluate vein function in the lower extremities.

E X E R C I S E S **THE CARDIOVASCULAR SYSTEM** THE TRANSPORTS OF THE BODY

Exercise 9.1   *Complete the following:*

1. Blood carries ___oxygen___ from the lungs to body tissues and collects ___carbon dioxide waste___ from tissues to take back to the lungs to be expelled.

2. Two components made in the liver that are necessary for clotting blood are ___prothrombin___ and ___fibrinogen___ .

3. Blood is made up of ___plasma___ , ___white blood cells___ ___red blood cells___, and ___platelets___ .

4. The iron-containing pigment in red blood cells is ___hemoglobin___ .

5. The two groups of white blood cells, or ___leukocytes___ , are those with a lobed nucleus and cytoplasm with fine granules called ___granulocytes___ and those with a single nucleus and clear, nongranular cytoplasm called ___agranulocytes___ .

6. In the first group in the previous statement, there is a further classification, according to staining characteristics, as follows: ___neutrophils___ (red and blue staining granules), ___eosinophils___ (orange or yellow acid dye staining granules), and ___basophils___ (purple basic dye staining granules).

7. The white blood cells constitute an important element in protection of the body against invasion by microorganisms through their power to attack bacteria, called ___phagocytosis___ .

8. The force the heart exerts in pushing blood through the vessels of the body is ___blood pressure___ .

9. The contraction of the heart in measurement of the force mentioned in item 8 is called ___systolic pressure___

10. The ___diastolic___ pressure is the lowest because it is present during relaxation of the heart.

Exercise 9.2   *Matching*

__O__	1. cardiosclerosis	**A.**	decrease in lymphocytes
__F__	2. angiosclerosis	**B.**	decrease in granulocytes
__E__	3. erythropoiesis	**C.**	inner coat of blood vessel
__G__	4. granulocytopoiesis	**D.**	decrease of erythrocytes
__B__	5. granulocytopenia	**E.**	production of erythrocytes
__D__	6. erythropenia	**F.**	hardening of walls of a vessel
__J__	7. leukocytopenia	**G.**	production of granulocytes
__A__	8. lymphocytopenia	**H.**	relaxation of heart
__N__	9. tunica adventitia	**I.**	an upper chamber of the heart
__C__	10. tunica intima	**J.**	decrease of leukocytes
__I__	11. atrium	**K.**	contraction of heart
__K__	12. systole	**L.**	a lower heart chamber
__M__	13. sinoatrial node	**M.**	pacemaker
__H__	14. diastole	**N.**	external coat of blood vessel
__L__	15. ventricle	**O.**	hardening of heart tissues and vessels

Exercise 9.3   *Complete the following:*

1. The blood vessel that carries blood from the heart to the lungs is called the ___pulmonary___ artery.

2. The large artery that carries blood from the heart to all parts of the body is the ___aorta___ .

3. The three large arteries branching from the aortic arch are the ___innominate___ , ___left common cartoid___ , and ___left subclavian arteries___ .

4. The circulation from the abdominal digestive organs through the liver into the inferior vena cava is called ___hepatic portal___ circulation.

5. The arteries supplying right and left sides of myocardial muscle are the ___right and left coronaries___

6. The heart is divided into four chambers: two ___atria___ and two ___ventricles___ .

7. The Rh factor may be ___positive___ or ___negative___ .

8. Blood circulating from the left ventricle and returning to the right atrium is known as ___systemic___ circulation.

9. Blood passing from the right atrium into the right ventricle, to the lungs and back to the left atrium is known as ___pulmonary___ circulation.

10. ___low-density lipoprotein___ is commonly called "the bad cholesterol."

Exercise 9.4

The arrows in Figure 9.8 trace the flow of blood through the heart. The heart valves are labeled with numbers; the heart chambers, membranes, and vessels are labeled with letters. In the blanks provided below, place the name of the structure opposite the appropriate number or letter.

1. pulmonary valve
2. mitral valve

3. aortic valve
4. tricuspid valve

A. pulmonary vein
B. atrium
C. aorta
D. pulmonary artery
E. pulmonary vein
F. atrium

G. left ventricle
H. endocardium
I. pericardium
J. myocardium
K. right ventricle

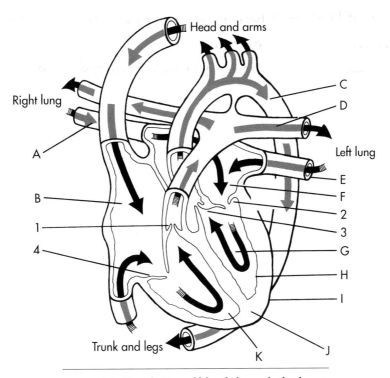

Figure 9.8 Circulation of blood through the heart.

Exercise 9.5   *Using the list of terms below, identify each structure in Figure 9.9 by writing its name in the corresponding blank.*

Aortic semilunar valve

Branches of right pulmonary vein

Left ventricle

Septum

Right atrium

Branches of left pulmonary artery

Coronary sinus

Mitral (bicuspid) valve

Superior vena cava

Arch of aorta

Branches of left pulmonary vein

Descending aorta

Myocardium

Tricuspid valve

Pulmonary artery

Branches of right pulmonary artery

Inferior vena cava

Right ventricle

Semilunar valve

Left atrium

1. _Superior vena cava_

2. _branches of right pulmonary artery_

3. _branches of right pulmonary vein_

4. _Semilunar valve_

5. _coronary sinus_

6. _right atrium_

7. _tricuspid valve_

8. _right ventricle_

9. _Inferior vena cava_

10. _arch of aorta_

11. _branches of left pulmonary artery_

12. _pulmonary artery_

13. _branches of left pulmonary vein_

14. _left atrium_

15. _aortic semilunar valve_

16. _mitral (bicuspid) valve_

17. _Septum_

18. _left ventricle_

19. _myocardium_

20. _descending aorta_

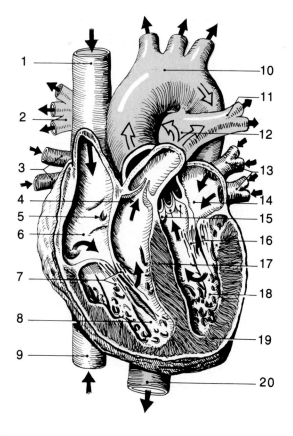

Figure 9.9 Frontal section showing the four chambers of the heart and the valves, openings, and major blood vessels. Arrows indicate direction of the blood flow. (The two branches of the right pulmonary vein continue from the right lung, behind the heart, to enter the left atrium.)

Exercise 9.6   *Using the list of terms below, identify each artery in Figure 9.10 by writing its name in the corresponding blank.*

Angular
Anterior tibial
Aorta
Aortic arch
Arcuate
Axillary
Brachial
Brachiocephalic
Celiac
Common iliac

Deep femoral
Deep medial circumflex
    femoral
Deep palmar arch
Digital
Dorsal metatarsal
Dorsal pedis
External carotid
External iliac
Femoral

Inferior mesenteric
Internal carotid
Internal iliac
Lateral thoracic
Left common carotid
Left coronary
Occipital
Peroneal
Popliteal
Posterior tibial

Pulmonary
Radial
Renal
Right common carotid
Right coronary
Splenic
Subclavian
Superficial palmar arch
Superior mesenteric
Ulnar

1. _angular_
2. _right common carotid_
3. _brachiocephalic_
4. _arch of aorta_
5. _right coronary_
6. _left coronary_
7. _aorta_
8. _celiac_
9. _Superior mesenteric_
10. _common iliac_
11. _internal iliac_
12. _external iliac_
13. _deep medial circumflex femoral_
14. _deep femoral_
15. _femoral_
16. _popliteal_
17. _anterior tibial_
18. _peroneal_
19. _posterior tibial_
20. _dorsal pedis_

21. _arcuate_
22. _dorsal metatarsal_
23. _occipital_
24. _internal carotid_
25. _external carotid_
26. _left common carotid_
27. _subclavian_
28. _pulmonary_
29. _lateral thoracic_
30. _axillary_
31. _brachial_
32. _splenic_
33. _renal_
34. _inferior mesenteric_
35. _radial_
36. _ulnar_
37. _deep palmar arch_
38. _superficial palmar arch_
39. _digital_

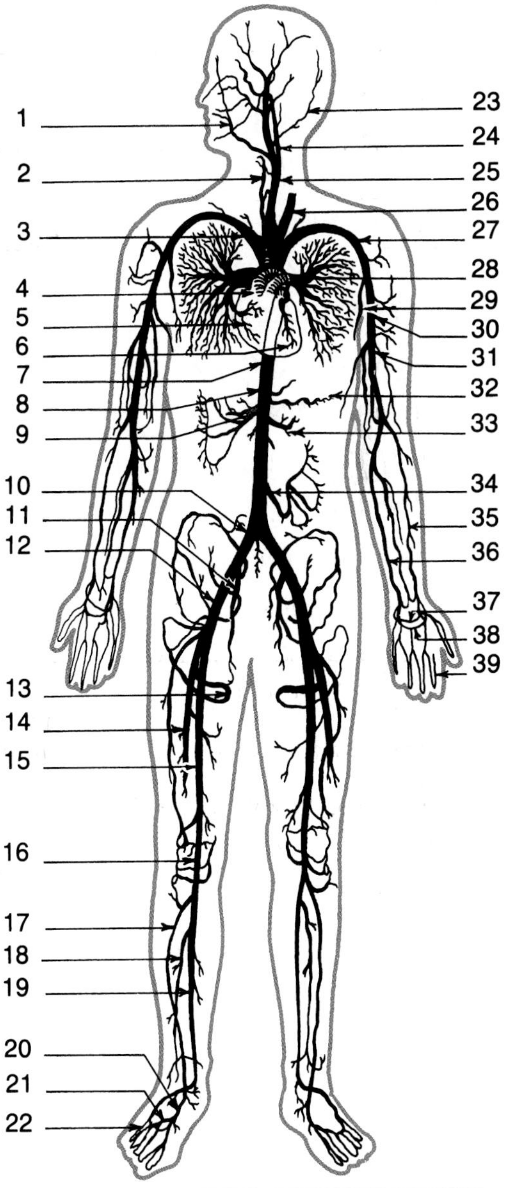

Figure 9.10 Principal arteries of the body.

Exercise 9.7   *Using the list of terms below, identify each vein in Figure 9.11 by writing its name in the corresponding blank.*

Angular	External jugular	Left coronary	Right pulmonary
Anterior facial	Femoral	Left pulmonary	Splenic
Anterior tibial	Great saphenous	Long thoracic	Straight sinus
Axillary	Hepatic	Median basilic	Subclavian
Basilic	Inferior mesenteric	Peroneal	Superior mesenteric
Cephalic	Inferior vena cava	Popliteal	Superior sagittal sinus
Cervical plexus	Inferior sagittal sinus	Portal	Superior vena cava
Common iliac	Internal iliac	Posterior tibial	Transverse sinus
Dorsal venous arch	Internal jugular	Right brachiocephalic	Volar digital
External iliac	Left brachiocephalic	Right coronary	

1. angular
2. anterior facial
3. internal jugular
4. right brachiocephalic
5. subclavian
6. superior vena cava
7. right pulmonary
8. right coronary
9. inferior vena cava
10. hepatic
11. portal
12. superior mesenteric
13. common iliac
14. superior sagittal sinus
15. inferior sagittal sinus
16. straight sinus
17. transverse sinus
18. cervical plexus
19. external jugular
20. left brachiocephalic
21. left pulmonary
22. cephalic
23. axillary
24. left coronary
25. basilic
26. splenic
27. media basilic
28. long thoracic
29. inferior mesenteric
30. internal iliac
31. external iliac
32. volar digital
33. femoral
34. great saphenous
35. popliteal
36. peroneal
37. posterior tibial
38. anterior tibial
39. dorsal venous arch

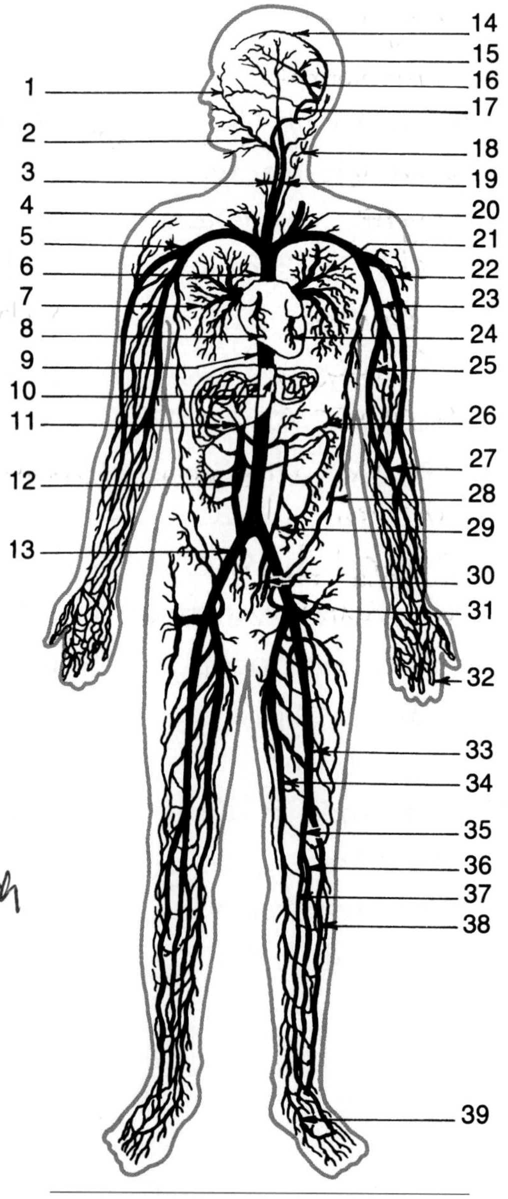

Figure 9.11 Principal veins of the body.

Exercise 9.8   *Multiple choice*

1. An excessive amount of blood in the body is called:
   a. erythremia
   b. polyemia
   c. hemophilia

2. Inflammation of serous membranes with serous effusion is called:
   a. polyarteritis
   b. thromboangiitis
   c. polyserositis

3. Effusion of blood into a cavity, such as the testis, is called:
   a. hematocele
   b. hematocolpos
   c. hematomyelia

4. Inflammation of an artery is called:
   a. aortitis
   b. arteritis
   c. phlebitis

5. Excision of a portion of an artery is called:
   a. angiotomy
   b. arteriectomy
   c. arteriotomy

6. Convulsive movements of the heart atrium or ventricle are called:
   a. congestive heart failure
   b. cardiac arrest
   c. fibrillations

7. Disease of lungs or their blood vessels produces heart disease called:
   a. aortic insufficiency
   b. cor pulmonale
   c. mitral insufficiency

8. Galloping rhythm of the heart might be described as:
   a. arrhythmia
   b. bradycardia
   c. blowing heart murmur

9. Stoppage of heartbeat might be described as:
   a. cardiac arrest
   b. fibrillation
   c. atrioventricular block

10. Paroxysmal thoracic pain characterized by feelings of suffocation and radiation of pain down the arm is specifically called:
    a. angina pectoris
    b. coronary heart disease
    c. congestive heart failure

Exercise 9.9 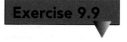   *Give the meaning of the components in the following words and then define the word as a whole. Suffixes meaning* pertaining to or state or condition, *shown following a slash mark (/), are not to be defined separately. Before reaching for your medical dictionary, check the Related Terms list in this chapter.*

1. Aortitis:

   aort _aorta_

   itis _inflammation_

   inflammation of aorta

2. Endocarditis:

   endo _end_

   card _cardium_

   itis _inflammation_

   inflammation of endcardium

3. Pericarditis:

   pericard _pericardium_

   itis _inflammation_

   inflammation of pericardium

4. Pyelophlebitis:

   pyelo _kidney pelvis_

   phleb _vein_

   itis _inflammation_

   inflammation of veins of kidney pelvis

5. Hematemesis:

   hemat _blood_

   emesis _vomiting_

   vomiting of blood

6. Hematoperitoneum:

   hemato _blood_

   peritoneum _peritoneum_

   accumulating of blood in the peritonedm

7. Hemophthalmia:

   hem _blood_

   ophthalm/ia _eye_

   accumulation of blood in the eye

8. Metrorrhagia:

   metro _uterus_

   rrhag/ia _hemorrhaghe_

   abnormal uterine bleeding

9. Arteriosclerosis:

   arterio _artery_

   scler/sis _hardening_

   hardening of an artery

10. Leukemia:

    leuk _white cells_

    emia _blood_

    malignant disease of the blood

CROSSWORD PUZZLE

CHAPTER 9

ACROSS

1. Innermost membrane covering heart

3. "Good" cholesterol

5. Upper border of heart

7. Minute blood vessles

9. Conduction node in heart

11. External covering of heart

12. Membrane lining pericardium

16. Undifferentiated stem cell

21. Wall between heart chambers

24. Red blood cells

25. Bicuspid valve

26. This term means iron

27. Major type of blood vessel

28. Valve separating right atrium and ventricle

DOWN

1. Very small veins

2. Positive or negative antigen

4. "Bad" cholesterol

6. Lower border of heart

8. Vines carrying oxygenated blood

9. Aortic _____

10. Relaxation part of cardiac cycle

12. Thrombocytes

13. Largest artery

14. Number of heart wall layers

15. Blood group

17. Heart muscle

18. Lower heart chambers

19. Upper heart chamber

20. The sinoatrial node

22. Liquid portion of blood

23. A leukocyte

26. The atrioventricular bundle

HIDDEN WORDS PUZZLE

Can you find the 20 words hidden in this puzzle? All hidden words puzzles have words running from top to bottom, left to right, and diagonally downward.

ERYTHROCYTES

CHOLESTEROL

SEMILUNAR

VISCERAL

SEPTUM

CIRCULATION

EPICARDIUM

ARTERIES

SYSTOLE

VALVES

ENDOCARDIUM

LEUKOCYTES

BICUSPID

BUNDLE

ATRIA

PERICARDIUM

AUTONOMIC

SYSTEMIC

MITRAL

NODE

```
F  J  H  R  K  S  J  L  Y  U  V  H  N  X  J  L  M  Y  Q  L  Z  D
O  Y  X  F  L  Y  T  A  Y  S  V  Y  P  V  J  F  Q  U  O  P  V  M
E  E  D  U  E  S  X  B  H  E  H  T  T  R  Q  G  Z  K  L  F  J  P
C  V  S  A  U  T  O  N  O  M  I  C  Y  H  W  H  Q  H  W  N  J  W
D  A  P  H  K  O  L  K  K  I  M  P  Y  V  R  M  H  O  C  Y  W  R
V  Y  W  S  O  L  Q  W  D  L  I  X  D  H  M  E  R  B  E  L  B  L
R  A  X  P  C  E  W  B  Q  U  D  T  R  O  L  W  D  X  Q  T  J  U
E  O  L  E  Y  D  K  Q  R  N  K  L  J  J  G  D  T  E  C  F  B  U
S  Y  Y  V  T  M  O  A  L  A  U  Y  D  M  U  S  R  O  N  Y  D  Y
L  F  R  L  E  P  I  C  A  R  D  I  U  M  M  S  N  I  E  Y  T  M
Z  R  P  I  S  S  E  I  C  S  A  S  I  Y  T  M  L  W  L  K  Y  N
G  B  I  E  C  B  N  R  A  E  T  Y  T  G  L  H  B  Y  U  W  P  K
H  D  A  W  R  H  D  C  Y  P  M  G  X  W  T  C  Q  W  L  D  N  W
B  A  B  R  V  I  O  U  S  T  G  T  Q  K  D  L  U  U  Q  B  T  V
C  M  K  G  T  F  C  L  I  U  H  Q  O  N  T  K  F  A  Y  X  Z  T
O  S  N  O  D  E  A  A  E  M  H  R  H  V  T  R  P  T  U  L  B  O
Z  T  Y  U  L  B  R  T  R  S  U  V  O  K  M  N  M  R  U  C  P  Z
J  V  J  S  X  C  D  I  Q  D  T  B  I  C  U  S  P  I  D  I  D  J
D  G  Q  M  T  B  I  O  E  F  I  E  X  S  Y  F  A  A  T  C  F  U
F  Q  B  U  C  E  U  N  X  S  B  U  R  Q  C  T  F  S  E  R  U  I
W  Q  W  R  H  G  M  N  Y  A  O  P  M  O  J  E  E  P  V  C  A  K
M  P  P  N  F  E  W  I  D  X  O  B  Y  V  L  O  R  S  U  T  U  L
A  X  E  K  W  I  E  B  C  L  G  Q  I  J  G  E  M  A  D  O  R  R
L  X  W  M  E  W  F  L  A  E  T  U  S  D  Z  V  T  L  V  I  N
```

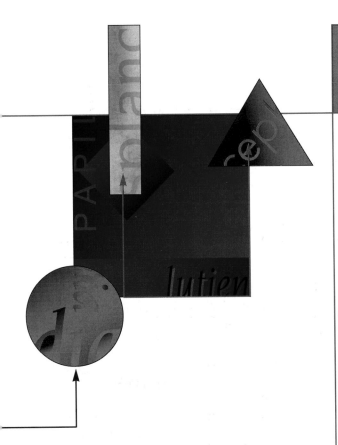

The Respiratory System

the breath of life

In this chapter the various parts of the respiratory system are presented, the system's interaction with the circulatory system is described, and the process of respiration is reviewed and illustrated.

STRUCTURES AND FUNCTIONS

The organs of the respiratory system include the *nose, pharynx, larynx, trachea, bronchi,* and *lungs,* and the *thorax* and *diaphragm,* which are accessory structures.

The process of respiration generally involves the *inspiration* (inhalation) of air that contains oxygen (O_2) for use by the cells of the body, and the **expiration** (exhalation) of carbon dioxide (CO_2), which has been removed as a waste product from the cells of the body.

The respiratory system depends on the circulatory system to complete the respiratory cycle, because oxygen inhaled by the lungs is transported via the blood to all parts of the body, and carbon dioxide is collected by the blood and brought back to the lungs to be exhaled.

It's a FACT

While asleep, some snorers reach a volume of 69 decibels, just slightly below the noise level of a pneumatic drill.

169

ORGANS OF THE UPPER RESPIRATORY TRACT

The Nose

The *nose* (Figure 10.1) is that part of the respiratory system serving as an entry for air and an exit for carbon dioxide. A ciliated, epithelial, mucous membrane *(mucosa)* lines the nose and much of the respiratory tract, serving as a filter for dust and other foreign matter. The nose warms and moistens entering air and has *olfactory* (sense of smell) receptors located in the nasal mucosa (the combining forms for nose are *naso* and *rhino*).

The Pharynx

The *pharynx* (throat) is a musculomembranous, saclike structure, about 5 inches (12 cm) in length, attached to the base of the skull above and continuous with the *esophagus* below, lined with a mucous membrane (see Figure 10.1). It communicates with the nasal chambers, mouth, larynx, and *eustachian tubes* and is divided into three parts: the *nasopharynx* (opening into the back of the nasal chambers and into the eustachian tubes), the *oropharynx* (opening into the back of the mouth), and the *laryngopharynx* (opening into the larynx and esophagus).

The pharynx is used by both the respiratory and digestive tracts as a passageway for air and food and has a role in the speech process.

The pharyngeal tonsils (adenoids) are located on the posterior wall of the nasopharynx, and the palatine and lingual tonsils are in the oropharynx. The tonsils and their functions are described in detail in Chapter 17.

The Larynx

The *larynx* (see Figure 10.1) is commonly called the voice box and is located just below the pharynx. The larynx also serves as a passageway for air and protects the airway against foods entering during swallowing. It plays an important role as the main organ of speech, since air, passing through the *glottis* during expiration, causes a vibration producing the sound of the voice. Other structures also play a part in this process.

The larynx is a musculocartilaginous structure lined with mucous membrane and moved by muscles of the hyoid group (named for the hyoid bone), which suspend the larynx from the hyoid, the base of the skull, and the mandible, anchoring it to the sternum. The movement of the larynx as a whole changes its size and shape to produce the complete range of sound between high and low notes. Other muscles of the larynx connect cartilages important to respiration, speech, and swallowing.

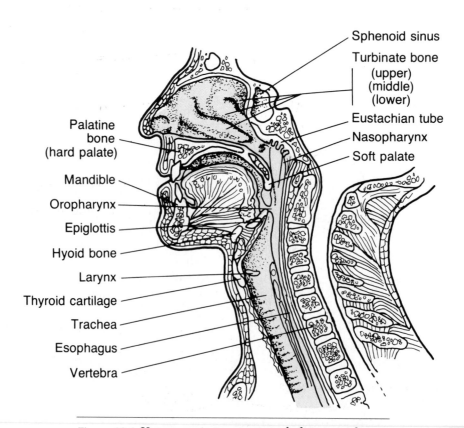

Figure 10.1 Upper respiratory tract, including some bones.

The larynx is made up of nine cartilages. The three largest are the *thyroid,* the *epiglottis,* and the *cricoid* (Figure 10.2), all of which are separate structures, and there are three pairs of accessory cartilages, the *arytenoid, corniculate,* and *cuneiform.*

The thyroid cartilage, largest of the three single cartilages, is shield shaped, forming the projection called "Adam's apple." The epiglottis cartilage, a leaf-shaped flap attached to the thyroid cartilage at one side, closes the trachea during swallowing to prevent food from entering it. The cricoid cartilage is ring shaped and is the lowest of the cartilages of the larynx.

The mucous membrane lining the larynx forms two pairs of folds, one pair above the other. The upper pair are called *false vocal cords,* which have no part in speech, whereas the lower pair, the *true vocal cords,* vibrate to create sounds as air passes out of the lungs. Three factors in determining the voice pitch are tension, elasticity, and rigidity of the vocal cords. Between the true vocal cords is a slit called the *glottis,* the most constricted area of the air passage of the larynx.

REVIEW 10.A

Complete the following:

1. The ___thorax___ and ___diaphragm___ are accessory structures of the respiratory system.
2. The main functions of the nose are to ___warm___ and ___moisten___ entering air.
3. The pharynx is divided into ___3___ parts.
4. The larynx is commonly called the ___voice box___.
5. The "Adam's apple" is formed by the ___thyroid___ cartilage.

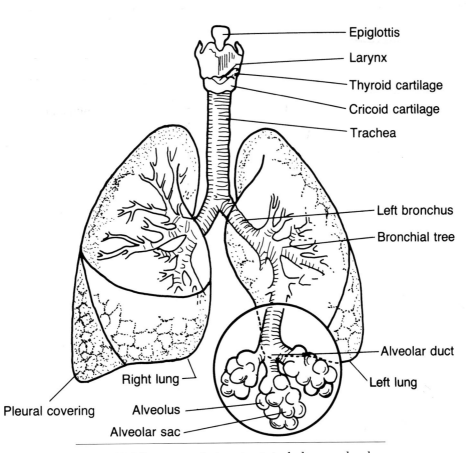

Figure 10.2 Lower respiratory tract, including an alveolus.

Epiglottis
Larynx
Thyroid cartilage
Cricoid cartilage
Trachea
Left bronchus
Bronchial tree
Alveolar duct
Left lung
Right lung
Pleural covering
Alveolus
Alveolar sac

ORGANS OF THE LOWER RESPIRATORY TRACT

The Trachea

The *trachea* (windpipe) is a tube formed of smooth muscle with 16 to 20 C-shaped rings of cartilage embedded in the muscle tissue (see Figure 10.2). It is approximately 4 inches (10 cm) long and 1 inch (2.5 cm) wide, stretching from the larynx to the bronchi and lined with mucous membrane. The main function of the trachea is to maintain its part of the airway.

The Bronchi

At its lower end the trachea separates into smaller airways called the right and left *primary bronchi* (singular—*bronchus*), with the right bronchus being slightly larger than the left. The bronchi, like the trachea, are lined with a ciliated mucous membrane and have C-shaped, cartilaginous rings in their walls, until entering the lungs when the rings become complete (O shaped). The two primary bronchi enter the lungs, one to the right lung and one to the left, dividing into smaller branches called *secondary bronchi,* which branch into *bronchioles.* The bronchioles continually branch into smaller and smaller bronchioles, finally becoming *alveolar ducts,* which have *alveolar sacs* at their termination. The walls of the alveolar sacs are composed of many *alveoli,* which are minute, squamous epithelial-lined spaces, allowing the lungs to achieve their main function, the exchange of oxygen and carbon dioxide.

As the bronchioles get smaller, the cartilage rings begin to disappear, until there are no rings in the alveolar ducts, sacs, or alveoli. The structure of the bronchi and their bronchioles resembles an upside-down tree, which is referred to as the *bronchial tree.*

The Lungs

The *lungs,* two large, cone-shaped, closed membranous sacs in the pleural cavity, are the organs of respiration (see Figure 10.2). Each sac contains millions of minute alveoli and blood capillaries lining its membranes. (It has been estimated that there are more than 300 million alveoli in a pair of lungs.) The lungs are encased in a serous membranous sac called the *visceral pleura,* and the *thoracic cavity,* in which the lungs are located, is lined with another serous membrane called the *parietal pleura.* These pleural membranes reduce friction during respiration. The space between the two membranes is called the *pleural cavity* or *potential space.*

Each lung occupies half the thoracic cavity, extending from a point slightly above the clavicles down to the diaphragm and separated from the other lung by the *mediastinum,* the space between the two pleural cavities. Because of the position of the heart, the right lung is larger than the left, with three lobes, *superior, middle,* and *inferior,* whereas the left has only two lobes, *superior* and *inferior.*

The functions of the lungs are distributing air to the alveoli and exchanging gases, produced by a cooperative effort of the alveoli and their blood capillaries. Early on the lungs are pink in color, but over time they become mottled and dark gray as a result of inhalation of dust and soot and sometimes tar and nicotine.

The Thorax

The *thoracic* (chest) *cavity* is lined with a layer of serous membrane, similar to that covering the lungs, allowing for lubrication of both surfaces during respiration. It is divided into three parts; the *right* and *left pleural cavities* and the *mediastinum,* which contains the heart, thymus, esophagus, trachea, bronchi, nerves, various arteries, veins, and lymphatic vessels and nodes.

The shape and slant of the ribs and their attachment to the spine allow them to be raised and lowered as the lungs expand and contract, creating a significant role for the thorax in the respiratory process. On inspiration particular muscles raise the thorax, making it larger and allowing the lungs to expand. On expiration the lungs empty, and the thorax is lowered and becomes smaller.

The Diaphragm

The *diaphragm,* a dome-shaped, musculomembranous partition separating the thoracic and abdominal cavities and attached to the lumbar vertebrae, lower ribs, and sternum is the chief muscle of respiration. (The action of the diaphragm is regulated by cervical spinal nerves 3, 4, and 5, a point remembered by some medical students with the rhyme "three, four, five, keep the diaphragm alive.")

During inspiration the diaphragm contracts, flattens, and lowers, increasing the capacity of the thoracic cavity, and allowing the lungs to fill with air and expand. On expiration the diaphragm relaxes and returns to its original position. This breathing process is also referred to as *pulmonary ventilation.*

REVIEW 10.B

Complete the following:

1. The trachea is also known as the __windpipe__

2. There are __2__ primary bronchi.

3. The sac encasing the lungs is called the __visceral__ .

4. The thoracic cavity is divided into three parts, the __right pleural cavity__ __left pleural__, and __mediastinum__.

5. The diaphragm separates the __thoracic__ and __abdominal__ cavities.

THE PROCESS OF RESPIRATION

The respiratory cycle is divided into three parts: *inspiration,* inhalation of air; *expiration,* exhalation of air; and *rest,* the interval between inspiration and expiration. Normally, the adult cycle is completed about 12 to 18 times per minute.

Respiration involves oxygen being passed throughout the body by the circulation and carbon dioxide wastes returning via the blood to the lungs to be exhaled. The bright red color of arterial blood results from the mix of oxygen and hemoglobin being carried to the tissues, whereas the dark red color of venous blood indicates that very little oxygen is present in the blood returning from the tissues.

The amount of oxygen retained by the tissues depends on need, since tissues do not store oxygen, and they will not take more oxygen than is needed. Increased activity of any tissue calls for more oxygen. During strenuous exercise, the use of oxygen may be more than doubled, with a significant increase in the amount of blood supplied to the muscles, consequently increasing the amounts of oxygen consumed and carbon dioxide discharged.

The flow of air into and out of the lungs depends entirely on changes in the capacity of the thoracic cavity. Inspiration and expiration are strictly in accordance with the pressure differences between the atmosphere and the air in the lungs caused by expansion or contraction of the thoracic boundaries. Approximate amounts indicated are for the average adult male (Table 10-1).

tidal volume (TV)—the volume of air inspired or expired during ordinary respiration (amounting to about 500 ml).

inspiratory reserve volume (IRV)—the maximum volume of air that can be forcibly inspired in ad-

TABLE 10.1 RESPIRATORY VOLUMES

Term	Meaning	Volume
tidal volume (TV)	air breathed during ordinary respiration	500 ml
inspiratory reserve volume (IRV)	air forcibly inspired in addition to tidal volume	3000 ml
expiratory reserve volume (ERV)	air forcibly expired in addition to tidal volume	1100 ml
residual volume (RV)	air trapped in the lungs at all times	1200 ml
vital capacity (VC)	TV + IRV + ERV	4600 ml
total lung capacity (TLC)	TV + IRV + ERV + RV	5800 ml

dition to tidal volume (about 3000 ml). The same principle applies to expiration.

expiratory reserve volume (ERV)—the volume of air that can be forcibly expelled in addition to the tidal volume (about 1100 ml). No matter how forcibly one exhales, some air will always remain trapped in the alveoli, because the intrathoracic pressure is below the atmospheric (normal air) pressure.

residual volume (RV)—the volume of trapped air in the alveoli (about 1200 ml).

vital capacity (VC)—the largest volume of air that can be moved in and out of the lungs. It is the sum of the inspiratory and expiratory reserve volumes plus the tidal volume (about 4600 ml).

total lung capacity (TLC)—the sum total of all the above volumes (about 5800 ml).

The respiratory center in the brain controls the movements of respiration. The nerves from the brain that pass down to the chest wall and diaphragm to control respiration are:

the *vagus* nerve—originating in the brain, sends branches to the larynx, heart, bronchi, esophagus, stomach, liver, and abdomen.

the *phrenic* nerve—originating in the cervical spine, passing to the diaphragm.

the *thoracic* nerves—originating in the thoracic spinal cord, are the nerves of the muscles of the thorax.

In summary, during inspiration, the thoracic cavity enlarges in all directions, the diaphragm con-tracts and descends, the ribs elevate, and air is drawn into the lungs. During expiration there is relaxation of the inspiratory muscles, and the thoracic framework resumes its original position. As the lungs contract, the diaphragm relaxes upward toward the thoracic cavity.

REVIEW 10.C

Complete the following:

1. The cycle of respiration is divided into three parts: __inspiration__ , __expiration__ , and __rest__ .

2. The volume of inhaled air during ordinary respiration is called __tidal__ volume.

3. The trapped air in the alveoli is called __residual volume__ .

4. The respiratory center is in the __brain__ .

5. The three nerves that control respiration are the __vagus__ , __phrenic__ , and __thoracic__ .

■ RELATED **TERMS** **THE RESPIRATORY SYSTEM** THE BREATH OF LIFE

ANATOMY

ala nasi winglike flare forming the outer side of each nostril.

alveolar ducts connecting passages between the bronchioles and the alveolar sacs.

alveoli (al-ve′o-lie) air cells of the lungs (singular—*alveolus*).

apex nasi tip of nose.

apex pulmonis pointed upper extremity of the lung.

arytenoid cartilage (ar″e-te′noid) small, jug-shaped cartilage of the larynx.

bridge upper portion of external nose, formed by nasal bones.

bronchial tree trachea, bronchi, and bronchioles.

bronchiole (brong′ke-ol) a small branch of the bronchi (plural—*bronchioli*).

bronchus (brong′kus) branch of the trachea going to each lobe of the lung (plural—*bronchi*).

carbon dioxide (CO_2) odorless, colorless gas formed in the tissues as a waste product, and expelled by the lungs.

choanae osseae (ko-a′ne) the openings between the nasopharynx and the nasal cavity (*choana* means funnel-shaped cavity).

cilia (sil′e-ah) tiny hairlike processes on epithelial tissue that filter out foreign matter (singular—*cilium*).

concha nasalis (kong′kah) shell-shaped structures of the nasal cavity and paranasal chambers (*concha* means shell).

cricoid cartilage cartilage of the larynx.

diaphragm (di′ah-fram) musculomembranous partition that separates the thoracic cavity from the abdominal cavity (commonly called *muscle of inspiration*).

ductus arteriosus (duk′tus ar-te″re-o′sus) fetal blood channel from the pulmonary artery to the aorta.

epiglottis (ep″i-glot′is) leaf-shaped, lidlike cartilage that covers the entrance to the larynx.

ethmoid sinus air spaces within the ethmoid bone that open into the nasal cavity (also called *ethmoidal air cells*).

expiration or **exhalation** breathing out; expelling air from the lungs.

expiratory reserve volume amount of air that can be forcibly expelled, beyond that exhaled during ordinary respiration.

frontal sinuses two air spaces in the frontal bone communicating with the nasal cavity by the nasofrontal duct.

glottis (glot′is) slit between the true vocal cords, helping to produce vocal sound.

hilus of lung depression on mediastinal lung surfaces for entry of bronchi, blood vessels, and nerves.

inspiration or **inhalation** breathing of air into the lungs.

inspiratory reserve volume amount of air that can be forcibly inhaled, beyond that inhaled during ordinary respiration.

laryngopharynx that part of the pharynx below the upper edge of the epiglottis, opening into the larynx and esophagus (also called *hypopharynx*).

larynx (lar′inks) musculocartilaginous structure, at the top of the trachea and below the root of the tongue and hyoid bone, housing the vocal cords (also called the *voice box*).

maxillary sinuses two air spaces in the maxilla, communicating with the middle opening of the nasal cavity on each side.

mediastinum space in the thorax between the two pleural sacs, containing the heart, blood vessels, etc.

mucous membrane epithelial lining of the respiratory tract.

nares (na′rez) the nostrils (singular—*naris*).

nasal septum membranous, skeletal partition between nasal cavities.

nasopharynx (na″zo-fahr′inks) that part of the pharynx, above the soft palate of the mouth, opening into the nose.

oropharynx (o″ro-fahr′inks) part of the pharynx between the soft palate and upper edge of the epiglottis.

oxygen (O_2) an element in air necessary for life, used by all cells of the body.

parietal pleura the lining of the thoracic cavity.

pharynx airway between the nasal chambers, the mouth, and the larynx; also a passageway for food.

phrenic nerve (fren′ik) nerve of the diaphragm.

pleura (ploor′ah) serous membrane, encasing the lungs, lining the thoracic cavity, and enclosing the pleural cavity (potential space).

pleural cavity *potential space* between the parietal and visceral layers of the pleura.

residual volume air remaining in the lungs after forced expiration.

respiration process involving inspiration and expiration, distribution of oxygen to the cells of the body, and the removal of carbon dioxide from these cells.

retropharynx back part of pharynx.

sphenoid sinuses two spaces in the anterior portion of the sphenoid bone, opening into the nasal cavity.

tidal volume air inhaled or exhaled in ordinary respiration.

total lung capacity the sum total of tidal, inspiratory reserve, expiratory reserve, and residual volumes.

trachea cartilaginous, muscular tube, extending from the larynx to the bronchi, also called the *windpipe.*

tracheal rings C-shaped rings of cartilage embedded in the muscle tissue of the trachea.

vagus nerve (va′gus) nerve extending from the brain to the pharynx, larynx, and thoracic and abdominal viscera (*vagus* means wandering).

vestibule front part of the nostrils and nasal cavity.

visceral pleura serous sac covering the lungs.

vital capacity largest amount of air that can be moved in and out of the lungs, the sum total of inspiratory and expiratory reserves plus tidal air.

vocal cords two pairs of membranous bands in the larynx; the superior pair (false vocal cords) not having any part in speech; and the inferior pair (true vocal cords), vibrating to produce sound.

windpipe trachea.

PATHOLOGIC CONDITIONS

Inflammations and Infections

The following infections primarily affect the lungs. Other infections that involve the lungs and other organs are described in Chapter 18.

arytenoiditis (ar-it″e-noi-di′tis) inflammation of a laryngeal arytenoid cartilage.

aspergilloma (as″per-jil-o′mah) granulomatous mass of the *Aspergillus* fungus in a pulmonary cavity or bronchus.

bronchiectasis (brong″ke-ek′tah-sis) chronic dilation of bronchi or bronchioles, as a consequence of an obstruction or an inflammation.

bronchiolitis (brong″ke-o-li′tis) inflammation of the bronchioles.

bronchitis (brong-ki′tis) inflammation of the bronchial membranes.

bronchopneumonia (brong″ko-nu-mo′ne-ah) inflammation of the lungs originating in the terminal bronchioles.

bronchosinusitis (brong″ko-si″nus-i′tis) simultaneous inflammation of the bronchi and sinuses.

chorditis (kor-di′tis) inflammation of a vocal cord.

coccidioidomycosis (kok-sid″e-oi″do-mi-ko′sis) several forms of respiratory fungal infection, of which the primary type is an acute, benign disease caused by the *Coccidioides immitis* fungus (also known as *valley fever, desert fever,* and *San Joaquin Valley fever*).

diphtheria (dif-the′re-ah) acute, infectious, contagious disease affecting the mucous membranes of the nose, throat, and/or bronchial tree, and marked by formation of a thin, gray-white, false membrane.

epiglottitis (ep″i-glot-ti′tis) inflammation of the epiglottis (also called *epiglottiditis*).

histoplasmosis (his′to-plaz-mo′sis) systemic fungal respiratory infection caused by the inhalation of spores of *Histoplasma capsulatum.*

influenza acute, contagious, respiratory disease transmitted by airborne viral droplet infection, occurring in epidemics (attacking many people in an area at the same time), with symptoms of headache, weakness, sore throat, and myalgia. Three general types of influenza are designated A, B, and C, with new strains emerging periodically and named for the geographic location first noted (Asian, Hong Kong, Chile, Panama, etc.) or the animal source (swine, equine, etc.), with only A and B types causing epidemics.

laryngitis (lar″in-ji′tis) inflammation of the larynx.

laryngopharyngitis (lah-ring″go-far″in-ji′tis) inflammation of the larynx and pharynx.

laryngophthisis (lar″ing-gof′thi-sis) tuberculosis of the larynx.

laryngotracheitis (lah-ring″go-trak″ke-i′tis) inflammation of larynx and trachea.

laryngotracheobronchitis (lah-ring″go-tra″ke-o-brong-ki′tis) inflammation of the larynx, trachea, and bronchi.

laryngovestibulitis (lah-ring″go-ves-tib″ul-i′tis) inflammation of the laryngeal vestibule.

legionnaires' disease acute form of bacterial pneumonia, with influenza-like symptoms, and a mortality rate of about 15%, caused by the *Legionella pneumophila* bacterium, which is believed to be waterborne; moist soil and air-conditioning cooling towers have been suspect (also called *legionellosis*).

mediastinitis (me"de-as"ti-ni'tis) inflammation of the tissues of the mediastinum.

nasopharyngitis (na"zo-far"in-ji'tis) inflammation of the nose and pharynx.

nasosinusitis inflammation of the nose and the paranasal sinuses.

pansinusitis (pan"si-nus-i'tis) inflammation of all the nasal sinuses.

pertussis whooping cough (also called *bronchocephalitis*).

pharyngitis inflammation of the mucous membranes of the pharynx.

pharyngolaryngitis (fah-ring"go-lar"in-ji'tis) inflammation of the membranes of the pharynx and larynx.

pharyngorhinitis inflammation of the mucous membranes of the pharynx and nose.

pleurisy inflammation of the pleura.

pleuropericarditis inflammation of the pleura and pericardium.

pleuropneumonia (ploor'o-nu-mo'ne-ah) pleurisy with pneumonia.

Pneumocystis carinii **pneumonia (PCP)** rare pneumonia condition usually seen in conjunction with AIDS (Chapters 17 and 18).

pneumonia (nu-mo'ne-ah) inflammation and congestion of the lungs (also called *pneumonitis*).

pneumopleuritis (nu"mo-ploo-ri'tis) pleurisy with presence of air in the pleural cavity.

psittacosis (sit-ah-ko'sis) respiratory viral infection (usually a pneumonia) transmitted to humans through contact with infected birds (also called *parrot fever*).

Q fever febrile rickettsial respiratory infection caused by *Coxiella burnetii*.

respiratory syncytial virus (RSV) respiratory *myxovirus* infection causing epidemics of acute bronchiolitis, bronchopneumonia, and the common cold in infants and young children, and serious, influenza-like symptoms in the elderly and adults with weakened immune systems.

rhinitis inflammation of the nasal mucous membranes (also called *coryza* or *common cold*).

rhinolaryngitis inflammation of the membranes of the nose and larynx.

rhinopharyngitis inflammation of the nasal and pharyngeal mucous membranes.

rhinosalpingitis inflammation of the mucous membranes of the nose and eustachian tubes.

sinusitis (sin"nus-i'tis) inflammation of the membrane lining a sinus.

tracheitis (tra"ke-i'tis) inflammation of the membrane lining the trachea.

tracheobronchitis inflammation of the membranes lining the trachea and bronchi.

tuberculosis infectious disease caused by the *Mycobacterium tuberculosis* organism, characterized by formation of tubercles in the lung tissues, with possible dissemination throughout the body.

Other Conditions and Diseases

allergic rhinitis any allergic response of the nasal mucosa.

aphonia loss of ability to speak.

apnea cessation of breathing. A special type called *sleep apnea* is a condition involving short periods of an inability to breath or maintain air flow during sleep.

asphyxia condition resulting from lack of oxygen.

asthma (az'mah) disease marked by recurring attacks of paroxysmal shortness of breath, wheezing, and coughing.

atelectasis (at'e-lek'tah-sis) collapse of the lung, or incomplete expansion of the lung at birth.

berylliosis (ber"il-le-o'sis) disease, marked by formation of granulomas, usually in the lungs, caused chiefly by inhalation of beryllium salts fumes.

broncholithiasis (brong"ko-li-thi'ah-sis) stone in a part of the tracheobronchial tree.

bronchoplegia (brong"ko-ple'je-ah) paralysis of the bronchial tube walls.

bronchorrhagia (brong"ko-ra'je-ah) bronchial hemorrhage.

bronchorrhea (brong"ko-re'ah) excessive discharge of mucus from the lung air passages.

bronchospasm (brong'ko-spazm) spasm of the muscles of the walls of the bronchi.

bronchostenosis narrowing of a bronchial tube.

chronic obstructive pulmonary disease (COPD) general term for pulmonary obstructive diseases, with breathing difficulties, such as *chronic bronchitis* and *emphysema.*

croup (kroop) condition occurring in young children marked by a laryngeal obstruction with a characteristic barking cough (also called *laryngostasis*).

deviated septum of nose nasal septum shifted to right or left, as a result of a congenital defect, disease, or trauma.

dysphonia (dis-fo′ne-ah) difficulty in speaking.

dyspnea (disp-ne′ah) difficulty in breathing.

emphysema (em″fi-se′mah) chronic pulmonary condition marked by abnormal increases in the size of the air spaces in the lungs, caused by alveolar dilation or destructive changes to alveoli walls.

epistaxis (ep″i-stak′sis) nosebleed.

hemopneumothorax blood and air in the pleural cavity.

hemoptysis (he-mop′ti-sis) spitting of blood.

hemothorax blood in the pleural cavity.

hiccup involuntary, spasmodic contraction of the diaphragm causing characteristic sounds in breathing (also called *hiccough*).

hyaline membrane disease respiratory distress condition affecting premature neonates, characterized by *atelectasis* (collapse of lung tissue).

hyperpnea (hi″perp-ne′ah) abnormal increased respiration.

hyperventilation abnormally prolonged, rapid, deep breathing.

hydropneumothorax collection of fluid and air in the pleural cavity.

hydrothorax fluid in the pleural cavity.

laryngalgia (lar″in-gal′je-ah) pain in the larynx.

laryngoplegia (lar″ing-go-ple′je-ah) paralysis of the larynx.

laryngoptosis (lah-ring″go-to′sis) dropping or displacement of the larynx from its normal position.

laryngorrhagia (lar″ing-go-ra′je-ah) hemorrhage from the larynx.

laryngospasm (lah-ring′go-spazm) spasmodic closing of the larynx.

laryngostenosis (lah-ring″go-ste-no′sis) narrowing of the larynx.

nasopharyngeal cyst saclike growth between the nose and pharynx.

orthopnea (or″thop-ne′ah) inability to breathe unless in an upright position.

pleuralgia (ploor-al′je-ah) pain in the chest (also called *pleurodynia* or *costalgia*).

pneumoconiosis (nu″mo-ko″ne-o′sis) chronic condition caused by inhalation of particulate substances into the lungs, such as *asbestosis*—asbestos fibers; *bagassosis*—sugar cane waste; *baritosis*—barium dust; *byssinosis*—cotton dust; *coal worker's pneumoconiosis (CWP)*, including *anthracosis*—coal dust; *silicosis*—stone, sand or flint containing silicon dioxide; *siderosis*—iron dust; *farmer's lung*—dust from moldy hay; and *stannosis*—tin dust; all of which are considered occupational and environmental diseases.

pneumohemothorax air and blood in the pleural cavity.

pneumohydrothorax air and fluid in the pleural cavity.

pneumolithiasis (nu″mo-li-thi′ah-sis) stone in the lungs.

pneumomalacia (nu″mo-mah-la′she-ah) softening of lung tissue.

pneumomediastinum air in the mediastinum.

pneumomelanosis (nu″mo-mel″ah-no′sis) blackening of the lungs by inhalation of coal dust or smoke.

pneumonocirrhosis (nu-mo″no-si-ro″sis) hardening of the lungs.

pneumopyothorax air and pus in the pleural cavity.

pneumorrhagia (nu″mo-ra′je-ah) hemorrhage from the lungs.

pneumothorax air in the pleural cavity.

pulmonary edema serous fluid accumulation in the air sacs and tissues of the lung.

pulmonary fibrosis progressive, usually fatal, fibrosis of the walls of the alveoli of the lungs (also called *diffuse interstitial pulmonary fibrosis*).

pyothorax collection of pus in the pleural cavity (also called *empyema*).

rales (rahlz) abnormal breathing sounds heard in the lungs.

rhinodynia (ri″no-din′e-ah) pain of the nose.

rhinolith stone in the nasal cavity.

rhonchus (rong′kus) whistling or rattling sound in the throat or bronchi.

tracheorrhagia (tra″ke-o-ra′je-ah) tracheal hemorrhage.

tracheostenosis (tra″ke-o-ste-no′sis) narrowing of the trachea.

vasomotor rhinitis a rhinitis caused by odors, substances, or temperatures, that produces dilation of blood vessels resulting in fluid leaking from the nose.

Oncology*

adenocystic carcinoma* malignancy of the mucous glands of the respiratory tract.

alveolar cell carcinoma* malignancy originating in the bronchioles and metastasizing to the alveolar surfaces (also called *bronchiolar carcinoma*).

bronchial adenoma* benign or malignant, slow-growing tumor of the mucous membranes of the bronchi.

bronchogenic carcinoma* malignancy that originates in the mucosa of the primary bronchi.

epidermoid carcinoma* malignancy in which the cells differentiate as they do in the epidermis, and become keratinized (also called *squamous cell carcinoma*).

glioma of nose (gli-o′mah) tumorlike mass of glial tissue at the base of the nose.

laryngeal papillomatosis (pap″i-lo-mah-to′sis) benign tumor of laryngeal epithelial mucous membranes, including warts, polyps, and condylomas, which may also occur on the trachea and other respiratory structures.

oat cell carcinoma* extremely malignant, bronchogenic, accounting for one third of lung cancers (also called *small cell carcinoma*).

polyp (pol′ip) tumor having a pedicle, commonly found in nose.

polyposis of nose multiple polyps in nose.

SURGICAL PROCEDURES

arytenoidectomy (ar″e-te″noid-ek′to-me) excision of an arytenoid cartilage of the larynx.

arytenoidopexy (ar″i-te-noi′do-pek″se) fixation of the arytenoid cartilage or muscle.

aspiration use of suction to remove fluid or gas from a cavity (also means breathing in).

bronchoplasty (brong′ko-plas″te) plastic repair of a bronchus.

bronchorrhaphy (brong-kor′ah-fe) repair of a bronchus by suturing.

bronchostomy (brong-kos′to-me) surgical creation of an opening into a bronchus.

bronchotomy incision of a bronchus.

cordectomy (kor-dek′to-me) excision of all or part of a vocal cord.

cordopexy (kor′do-pek″se) outward fixation of a vocal cord to relieve stenosis of the larynx.

cricoidectomy (kri″koi-dek′to-me) excision of the cricoid cartilage of the larynx.

cricotomy (kri-kot′o-me) incision to divide the cricoid cartilage of the larynx.

cricothyrotomy (kri″ko-thy′ro-to-me) emergency incision through the larynx and cricothyroid membrane to clear the airway.

epiglottidectomy (ep″i-glot′i-dek′to-me) excision of the epiglottis.

ethmoidectomy (eth″moi-dek′to-me) excision of all or part of the partition between the ethmoid sinuses.

intubation insertion of a tube into the airway to clear it of obstruction, named for the location of insertion (e.g., oral, nasal, endotracheal).

laryngectomy (lar″in-jek′to-me) excision of the larynx.

laryngopharyngectomy (lah-ring″go-far″in-jec′to-me) excision of the larynx and pharynx.

laryngoplasty (lah-ring′go-plas″te) plastic repair of the larynx.

laryngoscope (lah-ring′go-skop) instrument for the examination of the larynx.

laryngostomy (lar″ing-gos′to-me) creating a permanent opening in the larynx through the neck.

laryngotomy (lar″ing-got′o-me) incision of the larynx for repair of stenosis or removal of tumors (also called *laryngofissure*).

laryngotracheotomy (lah-ring″go-tra″ke-ot′o-me) incision of trachea and larynx to clear airway.

phrenicectomy (fren″i-sek′to-me) excision of part of the phrenic nerve.

phrenicotomy (fren″i-kot′o-me) division of the phrenic nerve.

pleuracotomy (ploor″ah-kot′o-me) creation of an opening into the chest wall for drainage (also called *thoracotomy* or *thoracostomy*).

pleurectomy (ploor-ek′to-me) excision of all or part of the pleura.

pleuracentesis (ploor′ah-sen-tee′sis) paracentesis (surgical puncture) of the thoracic cavity for drainage (also called *pleurocentesis*, *thoracentesis*, or *thoracocentesis*).

pleuroparietopexy (ploor″o-pah-ri′e-to-pek″se) fixation of the visceral pleura to the chest wall.

pneumocentesis (nu″mo-cen-tee′sis) puncture of lung for aspiration of fluid.

pneumonectomy excision of a lung.

pneumonorrhaphy (nu″mo-nor′ah-fe) suture of lung.

pneumonopexy (nu′mo-no-pek″se) fixation of lung to the chest wall.

*Indicates a malignant condition.

pneumonotomy (nu"mo-not'o-me) incision of lung.

rhinoplasty (ri'no-plas"te) plastic repair of the nose.

septectomy (sep-tek'to-me) excision of nasal septum.

sinusotomy incision into a sinus.

thoracentesis see *pleuracentesis.*

thoracoplasty (tho"rah-ko-plas'te) removal of ribs for collapse of the lungs.

thorascopic surgery procedure for lung volume reduction or resection for emphysema, in which a surgeon working through two chest incisions uses a television camera with a telescopic lens in a narrow tube inserted in a third incision, allowing for visualization of the operating field.

thoracotomy incision of the chest wall for lung biopsy, resection, or reduction.

tracheoplasty (tra'ke-o-plas"te) plastic repair of trachea.

tracheorrhaphy (tra"ke-or'ah-fe) suture of the trachea.

tracheostomy (tra'ke-os'to-me) creation of an artifical opening into the trachea through the neck (also called *tracheotomy*).

LABORATORY TESTS AND PROCEDURES

auscultation use of a stethoscope, an instrument that magnifies sounds within the chest cavity.

bronchogram x-ray of the bronchi and its branches, using a contrast medium.

bronchoscopy (brong'ko-sko-pee) examination of the bronchi by means of a bronchoscope (fiberoptic flexible tube or endoscope, inserted through mouth or trachea).

computerized tomography (CT) imaging device using x-rays at multiple angles through specific sections of the body, analyzed by computer to provide a total picture of the part being examined (also called *computerized axial tomography—CAT*).

chest x-ray examination to determine presence of lung disease.

endoscopy examination using an endoscope (flexible tube with a light and refracting mirrors) to examine the larynx and esophagus.

laryngoscopy examination of the larynx and upper trachea using a laryngoscope (an endoscope) to detect tumors and other abnormalities.

lung scan visualization procedures involving intravenous injection of radioactive material to diagnose pulmonary emboli and lung structure and function, and inhalation of radioactive gas to diagnose nonfunctioning lung areas and other abnormalities.

magnetic resonance imaging (MRI) noninvasive method of scanning the body by use of an electromagnetic field and radio waves, which provides visual images on a computer screen and magnetic tape recordings (also called *nuclear magnetic resonance—NMR*).

nuclear magnetic resonance (NMR) see *magnetic resonance imaging.*

percussion the use of light, sharp taps to the anterior and posterior chest surfaces to detect abnormalities by the sound produced.

pulmonary function tests group of tests, using a spirometer (instrument into which the patient breathes to provide measure of volume and rate of air inhaled and exhaled). Although not a comprehensive list, some of the tests are described in the following:

functional residual capacity (FRC) the volume remaining in lungs after ordinary exhalation.

inspiratory capacity (IC) maximum volume that can be inhaled after normal ordinary exhalation.

maximum expiratory pressure (MEP) pressure produced on exhalation.

maximum inspiratory pressure (MIP) pressure produced on inhalation.

residual volume (RV) volume remaining in lungs after maximal exhalation.

tidal volume (TV) volume of air in one inhalation or exhalation.

timed forced expiratory volume (FEV) volume of air that can be exhaled forcibly in 1 second, as a measure of total lung capacity.

total lung capacity (TLC) largest volume in lungs after maximal inhalation.

vital capacity (VC) maximum volume of air that can be expelled after maximal forced inhalation.

strobovideolaryngoscopy placement of a microphone near the larynx to trigger a stroboscopic (interrupted) light to illuminate and photograph the vocal folds for detection of small masses, scars, cancers, and other abnormalities not otherwise detectable under normal light.

throat culture incubation, in a growth medium, of material taken from throat surfaces, to determine presence and type of infection.

◤ E X E R C I S E S   THE RESPIRATORY SYSTEM THE BREATH OF LIFE

Exercise 10.1   *Complete the following:*

1. The process of respiration generally involves __inspiration__ and __expiration__.

2. The organs of the respiratory system are __nose__, __pharynx__, __larynx__, __trachea__, __bronchi__, and __lungs__.

3. The function(s) of the pharynx is(are) __to communicate between the nasal chambers, mouth, larynx, and eustachian tubes; to provide a passageway for food and air; to aid in the speech process__.

4. In respiration the functions of the larynx are __to provide an air passage and protect the airway against food enterily during swallowing__

5. The three large cartilages of the larynx are __thyroid__, __epiglottis__, and __cricoid__.

6. The two pairs of vocal cords are named __true__ and __false__.

7. The function of the trachea is to __maintain its part of airway__.

8. The __right__ lung is composed of three lobes.

9. The structure that separates the lungs from each other and divides the thoracic cavity into two parts is the __mediastinum__.

10. The diaphragm descends during the __inspiration__ phase of respiration.

Exercise 10.2   *Matching*

__H__	1. air sac of the lung	**A.** diaphragm
__G__	2. branch of the trachea going to each lobe of the lung	**B.** oxygen
__I__	3. warms and moistens entering air	**C.** carbon dioxide
__C__	4. odorless, colorless gas formed in tissues and excreted by the lungs	**D.** mucous membrane
		E. bronchiole
__J__	5. has a role in respiration, digestion, and speech	**F.** pleural cavity
__F__	6. potential space between the parietal and visceral pleural membranes	**G.** bronchus
		H. alveoli
__A__	7. muscular and membranous partition that separates the thoracic cavity from the abdominal cavity	**I.** nose
		J. pharynx
__D__	8. epithelial lining of the nose	
__E__	9. small branch of the bronchial tree extending from secondary bronchi	
__B__	10. gas present in air, necessary for survival	

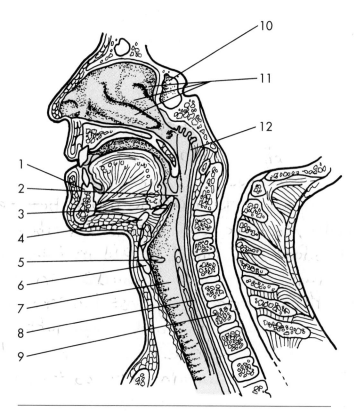

Figure 10.3 Upper respiratory tract, including some bones.

Exercise 10.3   *Using the list of terms below, identify each part in Figure 10.3 by writing its name in the corresponding blank.*

Oropharynx

Nasopharynx

Larynx

Vertebra

Thyroid cartilage

Sphenoid sinus

Epiglottis

Trachea

Mandible

Turbinate bones

Hyoid bone

Esophagus

1. mandible

2. oro pharynx

3. epiglottis

4. hyoid bone

5. larynx

6. thyroid cartilage

7. trachea

8. esophagus

9. vertebra

10. sphenoid sinus

11. turbinate bones

12. naso pharynx

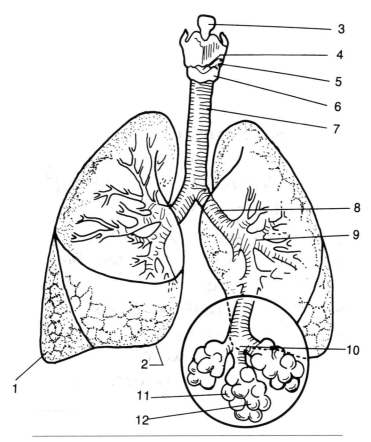

Figure 10.4 Lower respiratory tract, including an alveolus.

Exercise 10.4 *Name the structures in Figure 10.4 identified by the following numbers.*

1. pleural covering
2. right lung
3. epiglottis
4. larynx
5. thyroid cartilage
6. cricoid cartilage
7. trachea
8. left bronchus
9. bronchial tree
10. alveolar duct
11. alveolus
12. alveolar sac

Exercise 10.5 *In the blank following each pair of words, indicate whether their meaning is the same or opposite.*

1. expiration
   inspiration Opposite

2. visceral pleura
   pulmonary pleura Same

3. trachea
   windpipe Same

4. pharynx
   throat Same

5. tidal volume
   residual volume Opposite

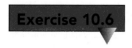

Exercise 10.6   *Give the meaning of the components in the following words and then define the word as a whole. Suffixes meaning pertaining to or state or condition are not to be defined separately and are shown following a slash mark (/). Before reaching for your medical dictionary, check the Related Terms list in this chapter.*

1. Nasopharyngitis:

   naso ___nose___

   pharyng ___Pharynx___

   itis ___inflammation___

   _____

2. Rhinitis:

   rhin ___nose___

   itis ___inflammation___

   _____

3. Anthracosilicosis:

   anthraco ___Coal___

   silic/osis ___silica___

   _____

4. Tracheobronchitis:

   tracheo ___trachea___

   bronch ___bronchi___

   itis ___inflammation___

   _____

5. Bronchostenosis:

   broncho ___bronchi___

   sten/osis ___narrowing___

   _____

6. Laryngoptosis:

   laryngo ___larynx___

   ptosis ___falling___

   _____

7. Tracheostenosis:

   tracheo ___trachea___

   sten/osis ___narrowing___

   _____

8. Bronchorrhagia:

   broncho ___bronchi___

   rrhag/ia ___hemorrhage___

   _____

9. Mediastinitis:

   mediastin ___mediastinum___

   itis ___inflammation___

   _____

10. Pharyngosalpingitis:

    pharyngo ___pharynx___

    salping ___eustachia tube___

    itis ___inflammation___

    _____

CROSSWORD PUZZLE   CHAPTER 10

ACROSS

2. Leaf-shaped lidlike cartilage
5. Musculomembranous partition
6. A nerve controlling respiration
8. Upside-down tree structure
10. Upper vocal cords
12. Pharyngeal tonsils
15. Small bronchi branches
16. Combining form for nose
18. Intake part of respiration cycle
22. Part of respiration cycle
24. Windpipe
25. Pleura lining thoracic cavity
26. A nerve controlling respiration
27. Volume of trapped air in alveoli

DOWN

1. Normal air breathed in and out
2. Exhalation
3. Pleural sac encasing lungs
4. Combining form for nose
7. Minute air spaces in lungs
9. The lung with two lobes
11. Membrane lining repiratory tract
13. A nerve controlling respiration
14. Space between pleural cavities
17. Number of cartilages in voice box
19. Space between lining of lungs and thoracic cavity
20. The largest bronchus
21. Throat
23. Shield-shaped cartilage

HIDDEN WORDS PUZZLE

Can you find the 20 words hidden in this puzzle? All hidden words puzzles have words running from top to bottom, left to right, and diagonally downward.

LARYNGOPHARYNX

EUSTACHIAN

BRONCHI

TRACHEA

THORAX

MEDIASTINUM

EXHALATION

GLOTTIS

LARYNX

VOLUME

NASOPHARYNX

INHALATION

PHRENIC

MUCOSA

CYCLE

RESPIRATION

OROPHARYNX

THYROID

PLEURA

VAGUS

```
C C R V G B A P J S H F R R Y W T I O Q X U O R W Y
D C R E U D U T Z J V M R G S O O J E E I P B X C L
V A G U S P K H H Y Q S O S F Y I X D W X J K L F X
S U M I E P R K D M X I T M H T O I N M G U Q R E L
M Y G U U B I X D C Q D E L L H R B S M A S P W K Y
P T K R S B S R I P Q H E I W O O L E U K G Z E U B
V F J T X M R F A N L M K Z T Q P P N C X I K U J K
F J C E V K S O F T H R P D K B H T Q O P E I M H S
Y V V S L O H E N U I A D R Q N A O R S R F T Q M V
V K C N Q X L L C C D O L H G N R V E A K N J L P G
S Y E G T V X U X Y H L N A T Z Y V E N C P T P D F
G U O Z U K G V M E D I A S T I N U M U C H O Y R F
E Q L Q X P D D D E G Q S R C I X T A E G R E T W I
R S V K E X H A L A T I O N Y Y O U K U M E H A U P
P G G R Q L W G U W B T P L G N C N Q S V N B P H W
I V P D M E N T F H K V H L N B G L O T T I S J O T
C B M D U Q M Z V Y L V A O E L X O E A H C S N C J
I F V W U I J Z R E M T R G R U D Z P C J Y G V R B
G Y N L S T G V B N D B Y C O A R X I H L A R Y N X
N X G L D G X J N W Z T N Y A L X A A I A N M O S M
N L C W D N L B E E K T X L E K F Y K A K R D R I E
O R J H D L R S A N Q M Y B G R P S J N T I Y E V D
F L Q Z H Z W B E G N H H U H X V X Y T P Y D N R C
E O L W S J B E W F Y N Q O W B N R L T L J P Z X Y
```

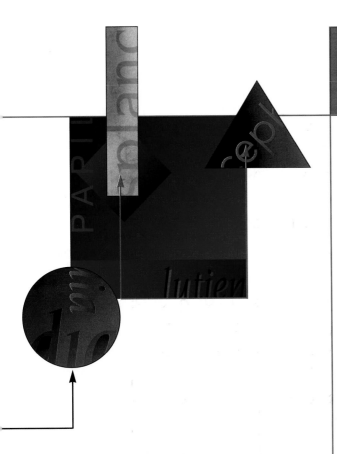

The Gastrointestinal System

the food processor

In this chapter the gastrointestinal system and its parts and functions are described and explained, with illustrations.

STRUCTURES AND FUNCTIONS

The organs of the gastrointestinal system, commonly called the *digestive* (or *alimentary*) tract, form a tube-like passage through the body cavities, extending from the *mouth* to the *anus* by way of the *pharynx, esophagus, stomach,* and *intestines.* The main functions of this system are to carry food for digestion, prepare it for absorption, and carry waste material for elimination. The accessory organs of digestion are the *teeth, salivary glands, liver, gallbladder,* and *pancreas.*

Food is chewed in the mouth and is swallowed by way of the pharynx and esophagus, passing through the neck and thorax into the abdomen, where it is received by the stomach. The stomach partially digests the food before it is passed on to the small intestine for further digestion and absorption, and the residue moves on to the large intestine, where it is retained

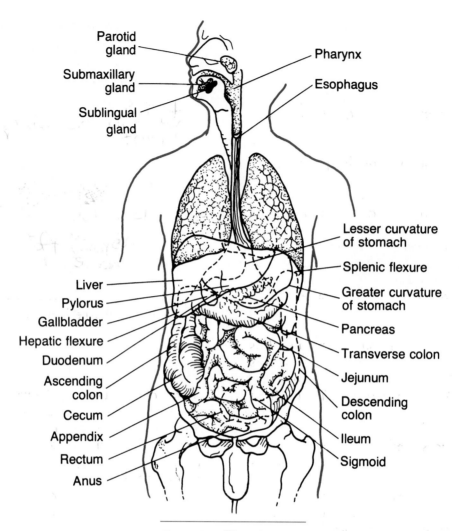

Figure 11.1 Digestive tract.

until it is excreted through the anus. All the organs of the digestive tract except the pharynx and esophagus are in the abdominal cavity (Figure 11.1).

The movement of contents through the digestive tract is aided by *peristalsis,* an involuntary wavelike movement produced by circular and longitudinal muscle fibers of the tubes of the body (e.g., intestines, blood vessels).

THE MOUTH

Lips

The *lips* (*labia* means lips) form the entrance to the mouth. They are covered on the outside by thin skin and on the inside by mucous membrane that extends to cover the surfaces of the oral cavity. In con-trast to the surrounding thick skin, the thin skin covering the lips reveals the underlying red blood in the capillary bed.

Oral Cavity

The *oral cavity* is formed by the arch of the upper and lower jaws. It contains the gums (*gingivae* means gums) and teeth (*dento-* and *donto-* refer to teeth) and divides the cavity into a vestibule between the teeth and lips and a mouth cavity behind the teeth. The structure forming the roof of the mouth is the *palate,* which is divided into the *hard* and *soft* palates.

Palates and arches. The *hard palate* is a rigid bony structure covered with mucous membrane. The *soft* *palate* is a partition between the mouth and na-sopharynx composed of muscle tissue shaped like an arch and covered with mucous membrane.

At the posterior border of the mouth the soft palate hangs in two curved folds, forming the *palatine arches*, between which the *uvula*, a soft, conical process, projects.

The *fauces* is the constricted opening between the arches and the second part of the pharynx, the *oropharynx*.

Cheeks. The *cheeks* are formed by buccinator muscles and a subcutaneous pad of fat, the buccal pad. The muscles keep the food between the teeth during the act of chewing, and the elastic tissue of the mucous membrane of the cheeks keeps the lining from forming folds that otherwise could be bitten during chewing.

Floor of the mouth. The *floor of the mouth* is formed by a series of structures under the mucous membrane, including the *sublingual gland*, the deep part of the *submaxillary gland*, and the *lingual nerve* and *vein*.

Tongue. The *tongue* is composed of skeletal muscle tissue covered by mucous membrane. It keeps food between the teeth during chewing and aids in swallowing by means of pressure against the hard palate. A thin mucous membrane, the *lingual frenulum*, anchors the underside of the tongue to the floor of the mouth.

The small elevations on the sides and upper surface of the tongue are called *papillae*, which are of three types: *filiform*, *fungiform*, and *vallate*, the latter two containing the taste buds (Figure 11.2).

Gingivae (gums). The *gingivae* consist of mucous membranes with supporting fibrous tissue, covering the surfaces of the maxilla and mandible (jawbones). Richly vascular but poorly innervated, the gums form a collar around each tooth.

Teeth. There are 32 permanent teeth at maturity (Figure 11.3), including the two upper and two lower third molars (commonly called *wisdom teeth*). In each jaw are two *central* and two *lateral incisors*, which are chisel shaped to aid in biting or cutting. On the outer side of each incisor is a pointed *canine* tooth, which aids in grasping and tearing food. Next to the canines are the *first* and *second premolars* and the *first, second,* and *third molars,* all of which are broad and are used to crush and grind the food.

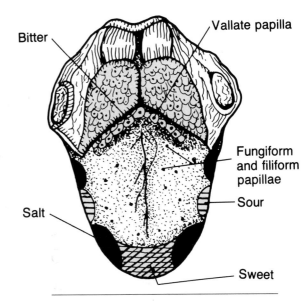

Figure 11.2 Tongue: location of taste buds.

Each tooth has a *crown*, the part projecting from the gumline; a *neck*, located in the gumline; and a *root*, which firmly fixes the tooth in the *alveolus (socket)* in conjunction with *cementum*, a bonelike connective tissue that covers the root and neck. *Periodontium*, a fibrous type of connective tissue, covers the root of the tooth, is embedded in the cementum, and attaches to alveolus walls. This periodontal tissue assists in holding the tooth in place and helps to cushion and support it against pressure produced in chewing and biting.

Teeth have three layers (Figure 11.4):

enamel—the hardest substance in the body, covering the crown of the tooth.

dentin—the bulk of the tooth, including the crown, neck, and root, and surrounding the pulp cavity.

pulp cavity—space within the tooth containing connective tissue, sensory nerves, and lymph and blood vessels.

Salivary glands. The mucous membranes of the mouth contain numerous small glands, the *submandibular, sublingual,* and *parotid glands* (see Figure 11.1) that secrete a thin, lubricating, serous fluid called *saliva.*

The chief functions of saliva are to dissolve or lubricate food to facilitate swallowing and to initiate digestion of some carbohydrates. The smell, sight, or thought of food causes the secretion of saliva.

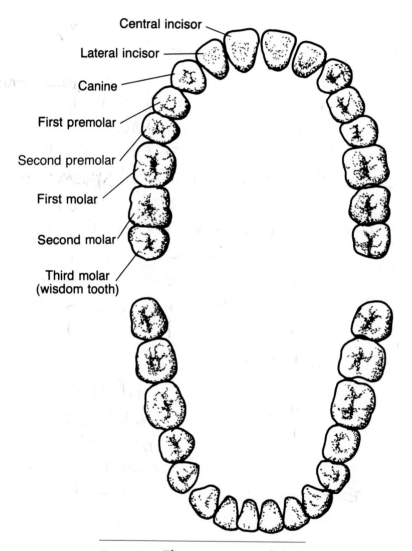

Figure 11.3 The permanent teeth (32).

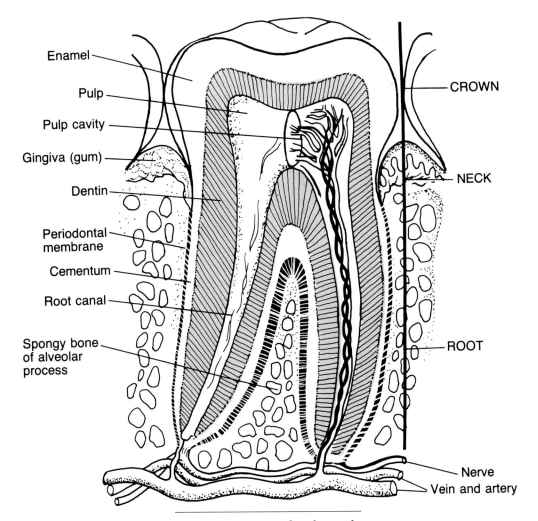

Enamel

Pulp

Pulp cavity

Gingiva (gum)

Dentin

Periodontal membrane

Cementum

Root canal

Spongy bone of alveolar process

CROWN

NECK

ROOT

Nerve

Vein and artery

Figure 11.4 Sectioned molar teeth.

THE PHARYNX

The *pharynx,* a musculomembranous, saclike structure, is described in Chapter 10 as part of the respiratory system, although it serves a dual purpose as an airway and as a passageway for food.

THE ESOPHAGUS

The *esophagus,* a narrow musculomembranous tube, about 10 inches (25 cm) long and about 0.5 inch (1 cm) in diameter, leads from the pharynx and descends in front of the vertebral column to enter the stomach. The walls of the esophageal tube are thick but are collapsible because they lack supporting cartilaginous rings such as those found in the trachea.

THE PROCESS OF SWALLOWING

There are three phases to the act of swallowing. Only the first is voluntary; the other two are instinctive reflexes. The voluntary phase is the passing of food from the mouth into the pharynx. This is followed by a second, involuntary (reflex) phase, which passes the food into the esophagus from the pharynx, and a third, involuntary (reflex) phase, which passes the food into the stomach from the esophagus (see Figure 11.1).

Because it functions as an organ of both the respiratory and digestive systems, the pharynx communicates with the oral and nasal cavities above and the larynx and esophagus below. When food enters the pharynx, all other openings are blocked to ensure its passage to the esophagus. This blocking is achieved by the tongue pressing against the hard palate to close off the oral cavity, the soft palate rising to block the nasal cavity, and contraction of the laryngeal opening. In addition, as previously noted (Chapter 10), the epiglottis cartilage closes the trachea during swallowing to prevent food from entering it. Swallowing also stimulates a momentary respiratory suspension that helps to guard against the passage of food into the respiratory tract. This process is an involuntary reflex action and is part of the second phase of swallowing.

The third phase of swallowing takes place in the esophagus, where the food is propelled by pharyngeal muscle contraction *(peristalsis)* through the sphincter muscle into the stomach.

THE STOMACH

The stomach (*gastro* refers to stomach), a musculomembranous, curved, pouchlike structure, is located toward the left side of the upper abdominal cavity, below the liver and diaphragm (see Figure 11.1), and is divided into three sections:

fundus—the rounded section above the esophageal opening.
body—the middle section.
pylorus—the lower, small end.

Curvatures

The right upper margin of the stomach is the *lesser curvature,* and the lower left margin is the *greater curvature.*

Sphincter Muscles

The ringlike muscles that contract to close an opening are called *sphincter* muscles. The *cardiac sphincter* muscle is located between the esophagus and the stomach, relaxing to allow food to enter the stomach and contracting while digestion takes place, preventing the stomach contents from *reflux* (backward flow). The *pyloric sphincter* muscle is located between the *pylorus of the stomach* and the *duodenum,* contracting to prevent the stomach contents escaping during digestion and then relaxing to allow the contents to enter the duodenum after the digestive process has been completed.

Gastric Coats and Glands

The stomach wall is made up of four coats, an outer *serous* coat, a *muscular* coat (consisting of *circular, longitudinal,* and *oblique fibers*), a *submucous* coat, and a *mucous lining* coat. The muscles of the stomach walls allow for expansion when food enters it and mix and churn these foods during the digestive process. Scattered throughout the mucosa of the stomach are innumerable microscopic, tubular, *gastric glands.* The gastric juice produced by these glands contains *enzymes, mucin, intrinsic factor* (necessary for absorption of vitamin B_{12}), and *hydrochloric acid*. The food in the stomach mixes with these secretions, forming a partially digested semiliquid called *chyme,* that is passed on to the *small intestine* for further digestion.

REVIEW 11.B

Complete the following:

1. The _pharynx_ serves a dual purpose in the respiratory and gastrointestinal systems.
2. The _esophageal_ tube is thick walled but collapsible.
3. There are _3_ phases to the act of swallowing.
4. The stomach is divided into the _fundus_, _body_, and _pylorus_.
5. The curvatures of the stomach are the _greater_ and the _lesser_ curvatures.

THE DIGESTIVE PROCESS

Food remains in the stomach from 1 to 4 hours after eating, and as the stomach contents liquefy, they pass into the *duodenum.* The chyme moves through the *jejunum* and *ileum* by means of the peristaltic waves and is further digested and absorbed. When the ileum empties into the *colon,* the contents contain water to be absorbed by the *large intestine* and waste to be eliminated from the body.

THE ABDOMINAL CAVITY

The stomach and the large and small intestines are enclosed in a space between the diaphragm and pelvis, the *abdominal cavity,* which is lined with a serous membrane, the *parietal peritoneum* (see Figures 11.1 and 11.5). A membranous fold of this peritoneum, the *mesentery,* connects a portion of the intestines to the posterior abdominal wall, and an extension of the peritoneum, the *visceral peritoneum,* covers all or part of many visceral (abdominal cavity) organs and helps to hold them in place.

A double fold of the peritoneum, the *omentum,* attaches to the stomach, connecting it with abdominal viscera. The *greater omentum* extends from the greater curvature of the stomach, covers the intestines, and is attached to the *transverse colon.* The *lesser omentum* extends from the lesser curvature of the stomach to the liver and the first part of the duodenum. Fat, distributed throughout the omentum, prevents abrasion and helps to keep the intestines warm.

The Small Intestine

The *small intestine* (*entero* refers to intestines) is the coiled 20-foot (about 6 m) muscular tube that occupies almost all the abdomen (see Figures 11.1 and 11.5) and is divided into three parts:

duodenum—attached to the pyloric end of the stomach, extending to the jejunum, approximately 10 inches (25 cm) long, crescent shaped, with both the pancreatic and common bile ducts emptying into it.

jejunum—the middle section of the small intestine, about 8 feet (2.5 m) in length, held in place by the mesentery and never very full because vigorous peristaltic waves rapidly move the fluid content into the ileum.

ileum—the longest part of the small intestine, about 12 feet (3.5 m) in length, located in the lower abdomen ending at the large intestine, in which most of the absorption of food takes place.

The intestinal digestive juice, containing mucus and many enzymes of digestion, is stimulated to flow by a hormone, *secretin,* which is produced by the intestinal glands when the chyme reaches the small intestine.

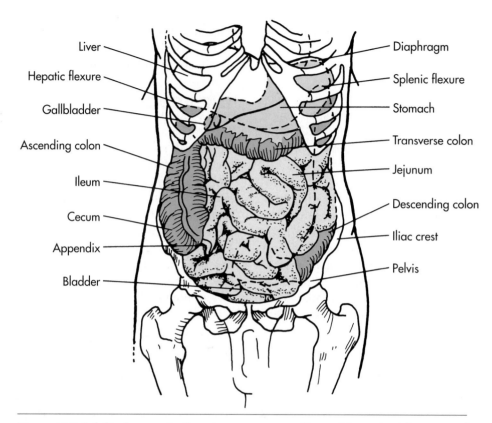

Figure 11.5 Subdiaphragmatic digestive tract organs. (Dotted lines show locations of hidden digestive organ structures.)

The digestive process is completed in the small intestine, and the digested food is then absorbed through the intestinal walls into the blood by the *villi,* countless threadlike projections in the mucous membrane lining the small intestine.

The Large Intestine

The *large intestine* is from 5 to 6 feet (1.5 to 1.8 m) in length and about 2½ inches (6 cm) in diameter at its widest point, decreasing in diameter as it progresses to the anus. It is divided into the *cecum* (with its *appendix*), *colon,* and *rectum* (see Figures 11.1 and 11.5).

Cecum. The first part of the large intestine, the *cecum,* located in the right lower quadrant of the abdomen, is 2 to 3 inches (5 to 8 cm) in length and forms a dilated, blind pouch that joins the *colon* just below the juncture of the *ileum* and the *colon.*

The *vermiform* (means wormlike) *appendix* is a narrow, tubelike projection about the size and shape of a worm, attached to the *cecum,* which can be surgically removed without any disturbance of body function.

Colon. The *colon* is divided into four sections:

ascending colon—lies vertically on the right side of the abdomen, reaches to the lower margin of the liver, and joins the *ileum* at the *cecal junction* (see Figure 11.5). The *ileocecal valve* allows matter to pass from the ileum into the colon but prevents a reversal of this process. The ascending colon turns and bends, becoming the

transverse colon—crosses the upper abdomen from right to left, below the stomach and liver, and above the small intestine.

descending colon—extends downward from below the stomach on the left side of the abdomen to the *iliac crest.*

sigmoid colon—an S-shaped curve from the *iliac crest* down to the *rectum.*

Rectum. The last segment of the large intestine, the *rectum,* is 7 to 8 inches (18 to 20 cm) in length and is lined with a mucous membrane with multiple upright folds called *rectal columns,* each of which is supplied with an artery and vein. The last section of the rectum, the *anal canal,* about 1 inch (2.5 cm) in length, terminates in the *anus,* which is protected by an *internal* (smooth muscle) *sphincter* muscle and an *external* (striated muscle) *sphincter* muscle.

THE PANCREAS

The *pancreas,* a large, elongated, lobulated gland, is divided into four parts: *head, neck, body,* and *tail.* It is located behind the stomach, its head and neck in the duodenal curve, its body extending transversely, and its tail touching the spleen (see Figure 11.1).

The pancreas is both an *exocrine gland* (secreting into ducts) and a ductless secreting *endocrine gland.* The exocrine cells secrete *pancreatic juice,* which contains enzymes necessary for digestion and is collected within the pancreas and transferred into the duodenum. Groups of endocrine cells, the *islands* or *islets of Langerhans,* secrete two major hormones, *insulin* and *glucagon,* which have opposing roles in carbohydrate metabolism (see Chapter 14).

THE LIVER

The largest gland in the body, the *liver* (*hepat* refers to liver), classified as an exocrine gland, weighs about 3 to 4 pounds (1.4 kg) and is located in the upper right abdomen under the diaphragm (see Figure 11.1). It is very soft and pliable and has a reddish-brown color because it contains numerous blood vessels. The liver has four major functions:

1. Secretes bile for use in the digestive process.
2. Essential to the metabolism of proteins, fats, and carbohydrates.
3. Filters and destroys foreign matter and neutralizes toxins.
4. Stores iron, glycogen, and vitamins A, B$_{12}$, and D.

The Biliary System

The *bile ducts* within the liver join together, forming the larger *right* and *left hepatic ducts,* emerging from the liver, and uniting to form a single *hepatic duct.*

This hepatic duct joins the *cystic duct* (emerging from the gallbladder), forming the *common bile duct,* which opens into the duodenum 3 to 4 inches (8 to 10 cm) below the pyloric opening of the stomach.

The Gallbladder

The *gallbladder* (*cholecyst* means gallbladder), a pear-shaped sac about 3 to 4 inches (8 to 10 cm) in length, the walls of which are composed of a serous, a muscular, and a mucous coat, is located on the inferior surface of the liver (see Figure 11.1).

The main function of the gallbladder is to store the concentrated bile deposited by the hepatic and cystic ducts and then to contract and expel the bile into the duodenum during digestion (*chol-* and *chole-* mean bile).

R E V I E W 1 1 . C

Complete the following:

1. The three divisions of the small intestine are the __duodenum__, __jejunum__, and __ileum__.

2. The large intestine is divided into the __cecum__, __colon__, and __rectum__.

3. The pancreas is divided into __head__, __neck__, __body__, and __tail__.

4. The hepatic and cystic ducts join to form the __common bile duct__.

5. The walls of the gallbladder have a __serous__, __muscular__, and __mucous__ coat.

■ RELATED TERMS THE GASTROINTESTINAL SYSTEM THE FOOD PROCESSOR

ANATOMY

alimentary or **digestive tract** passage from mouth to anus.

alveolus (al-ve'o-lus) tooth socket in the maxilla and mandible (also refers to air sac of lung).

ampulla (am-pul'lah) sac-shaped dilation of a canal or tube.

anal canal most distal portion of the alimentary tract.

antrum (an'trum) any partially closed cavity, and particularly the pyloric end of the stomach that is partly shut off, during digestion, by the sphincter.

anus (a'nus) distal opening of the alimentary canal.

appendix any appendage, especially the vermiform appendix attached to the cecum.

bicuspid (bi-kus'pid) premolar tooth.

bile secretion of the liver that aids in digestion.

biliary pertaining to bile.

body of pancreas part of pancreas extending from its neck to its tail.

buccal surface of tooth surface of the tooth next to the cheek.

cecum (se'kum) blind pouch that joins the colon just below the juncture of the ileum and colon and has vermiform appendix attached.

celiac (se'le-ak) pertaining to the abdomen.

cholecyst (ko'le-sist) gallbladder.

choledochus (ko-led'o-kus) common bile duct.

chyle (kile) milky fluid conveyed by lymphatic vessels from the intestine, after digestion, into the circulation.

chyme (kime) semifluid contents of stomach after digestion.

colon part of large intestine extending from cecum to rectum.

common bile duct duct formed by the junction of the cystic and hepatic ducts.

cuspid (kus'pid) canine tooth.

cystic duct duct extending from neck of gallbladder to join the hepatic duct to form the common bile duct.

dentin type of connective tissue surrounding the tooth pulp that is covered by enamel on the exposed tooth and by cementum on the part implanted in the jaw.

duodenal glands glands in the submucous layer of the duodenum (also called *Brunner's glands*).

duodenum (du"o-de'num) first portion of small intestine, extending from the pylorus of the stomach to the jejunum.

enamel hard, white substance (hardest in body) covering the dentin of the exposed part of the tooth.

epigastrium (ep"i-gas'tre-um) upper, middle portion of abdomen.

esophagus (e-sof'ah-gus) musculomembranous canal that extends from the pharynx to the stomach.

fauces (faw'sez) passage from the throat to the oropharynx.

flexure (flek'sher) bend, fold, or curved part of a structure.

gallbladder pear-shaped organ on the undersurface of the liver, for the storage of bile.

gastric glands glands of the stomach that secrete digestive chemicals.

gingivae (jin'ji-vie) gums of the mouth.

glossopalatine arch anterior fold of mucous membrane on either side of the oral pharynx, connected with the soft palate and enclosing the glossopalatine muscle (also called *palatine arch* or *pharyngopalatine arch*).

hypogastrium (hi"po-gas'tre-um) lowest, middle abdominal region.

ileocecal valve mucous membrane folds between ileum and cecum, to prevent reflux from colon into ileum (also called *ileocolic valve*).

ileum distal portion of the small intestine, extending from the jejunum to the cecum.

incisor (in-si'zer) any one of the four front teeth of either jaw.

intestinal glands tiny, tubular depressions in the intestinal mucous membrane (also called *Lieberkühn's glands).*

islands of Langerhans (lahng'er-hanz) irregular, microscopic formations of cells in the pancreas, secreting insulin and glucagon.

jejunum (je-joo'num) portion of the small intestine that extends from the duodenum to the ileum.

labia (la'be-ah) lips.

lingua (ling'gwah) tongue.

liver large, dome-shaped gland in the upper part of the abdomen under the diaphragm on the right side.

mesentery (mes′en-ter″e) peritoneal fold that attaches the intestine to the posterior abdominal wall.

omentum fold of peritoneum that connects the stomach with other visceral organs.

oropharynx section of pharynx that lies between the soft palate and the epiglottis.

palate roof of the mouth separating the oral cavity from the nasal cavity.

pancreas large, elongated, lobed gland, located behind the stomach, divided into four parts: head, neck, body, and tail.

parotid salivary gland large salivary gland located near the ear.

peptic glands glands of the mucous membrane of the stomach, secreting acid and pepsin.

peristalsis (per″i-stal′sis) wavelike movement by which the alimentary tract propels its contents.

peritoneum (per″i-to′ne-um) serous membrane lining the abdominal cavity, with a part of it covering viscera and holding them in place.

pharynx musculomembranous opening into the nasal cavities, mouth, larynx, and esophagus.

pylorus distal opening of stomach through which stomach contents enter the duodenum.

rectosigmoid lower portion of sigmoid and upper portion of rectum.

rugae (roo′guy) wrinkles, or folds, appearing on the surface of the mucous membrane of the stomach when the muscular coat contracts.

saliva (sah-li′vah) clear secretion of the salivary glands, containing the digestive enzyme *ptyalin amylase*.

salivary glands oral cavity glands that secrete saliva.

secretin hormone produced by glands of the duodenum that stimulates secretion of pancreatic juice.

sigmoid S-shaped flexure of colon, extending from the end of the descending colon to the upper part of the rectum.

sphincter (sfingk′ter) ringlike muscle that closes a natural opening.

stomach ovoid, musculomembranous digestive pouch below the esophagus.

sublingual salivary glands smallest of the salivary glands, located beneath the tongue on either side.

submandibular and **submaxillary salivary glands** salivary glands below the angle of the lower jaw on either side.

tongue freely moving, muscular organ of taste, located in floor of the mouth, that aids in mastication, swallowing, and articulation of sound.

uvula soft, conical, pendulum-like process hanging between the palatine arches.

villi threadlike projections covering the mucosa of the small intestine that aid in the absorption of digested matter.

PATHOLOGIC CONDITIONS

Inflammations, Infections, and Toxic Conditions

ancylostomiasis (an-si-lo-sto-mi′ah-sis) infection with hookworm, a member of the genus *Ancylostoma*.

anusitis inflammation of the anus.

aphthous stomatitis (af′thus) ulcer of the mucous membranes of the mouth, commonly called *canker sore.*

appendicitis inflammation of the appendix.

ascariasis (as″kah-ri′ah-sis) infection with parasitic intestinal roundworms, of the genus *Ascaris*.

cheilitis (ki-li′tis) inflammation of the lip.

cholangiolitis (ko-lan″je-o-li′tis) inflammation of the bile duct tubules.

cholangitis (ko″lan-ji′tis) bile duct inflammation.

cholecystitis (ko″le-sis-ti′tis) inflammation of the gallbladder.

colitis inflammation of the colon; may be episodic, as in *irritable bowel syndrome*, which includes *spastic colon* and *mucous colitis*, or chronic, as in *Crohn's disease* and *ulcerative colitis.*

Crohn's disease a chronic inflammatory disease affecting the ileum, cecum, and colon (also called *regional enteritis*).

cysticercosis (sis″ti-ser-ko′sis) infection with tapeworm larvae, of the genus *Cysticercus*.

distomiasis (dis″to-mi′ah-sis) infection with a trematode worm of the genus *Fasciola*.

diverticulitis (di″ver-tik-u-li′tis) inflammation of a pocket (*diverticulum*) in the intestine.

duodenitis inflammation of the duodenum.

dysentery (dis′en-ter″ee) any of a number of disorders that involve inflammation of the intestines, particularly the colon.

enteritis (en″ter-i′tis) inflammation of the intestines, particularly the small intestine.

enterobiasis (en"ter-o-bi'ah-sis) roundworm infection with nematodes of the genus *Enterobius vermicularis,* commonly called pinworm, seatworm, or threadworm (also called *oxyuriasis*).

enterocolitis (en"ter-o-ko-li'tis) inflammation of the colon and small intestine.

enterogastritis (en"ter-o-gas-tri'tis) inflammation of the intestines and stomach (also called *gastroenteritis*).

enterohepatitis (en"ter-o-hep-ah-ti'tis) inflammation of the intestines and liver.

esophagitis (e-sof"ah-ji'tis) inflammation of the esophagus.

food poisoning sudden illness caused by eating food contaminated with any one of a large group of bacterial or other toxic substances, including bacterial food poisoning and shellfish poisoning.

gastritis inflammation of the stomach (chronic gastritis is caused by *Helicobacter pylori* bacteria).

gastroduodenitis inflammation of the stomach and duodenum.

gastroenteritis inflammation of the stomach and intestine (an acute form, common in young children, with symptoms of fever, vomiting, and diarrhea is caused by a *rotavirus* that results in more than 3 million attacks per year in the United States alone).

gastroenterocolitis (gas"tro-en"ter-o-ko-li'tis) inflammation of the stomach, small intestine, and colon.

gastrohepatitis (gas"tro-hep-ah-ti'tis) inflammation of the stomach and liver.

gastroileitis (gas"tro-il-e-i'tis) inflammation of the stomach and ileum.

giardiasis (je"ar-di'ah-sis) a parasitic infection of the intestinal tract, caused by the protozoa *Giardia lamblia.*

gingivitis (jin"ji-vi'tis) inflammation of the gums.

glossitis (glos-si'tis) inflammation of the tongue.

hemorrhagic colitis gastrointestinal infection caused by ingestion of undercooked meat contaminated by a rare form of *Escherichia coli* bacteria.

hepatitis (hep"ah-ti'tis) inflammation of the liver resulting from toxic or viral causes, with symptoms of anorexia, nausea, jaundice, and enlargement and tenderness of the liver. Of the three major viral types, hepatitis A is spread through fecal-contaminated food or water; hepatitis B is spread by blood transfusion, sexual contact, and contaminated needles or instruments; and hepatitis C is transmitted by blood transfusion and contaminated needles. There are vaccines for types A and B; there is currently no vaccine for type C.

herpes simplex (her'peze) cold sore or fever blister of the mouth or nares caused by herpes virus.

ileitis (il"e-i'tis) inflammation of the ileum.

ileocolitis (il"e-o-ko-li'tis) inflammation of ileum and colon.

jejunitis (je"joo-ni'tis) inflammation of the jejunum.

jejunoileitis (je-joo"no-il"e-i'tis) inflammation of the jejunum and ileum.

linguopapillitis (ling"gwo-pap"i-li'tis) inflammation of the papillae of the tongue.

pancreatitis (pan"kre-ah-ti'tis) inflammation of the pancreas.

parotitis (par"o-ti'tis) inflammation of the parotid salivary gland (*mumps* is epidemic or infectious parotitis).

peptic ulcer disease inflammation of the stomach and/or duodenum, caused by the bacteria *Helicobacter pylori,* which destroys cells of the mucous membrane lining, resulting in ulceration by acid and/or enzymes.

perihepatitis inflammation of the serous covering of the liver.

periodontal disease inflammation affecting the tissue around a tooth, caused by bacteria, the most common being *Porphyromonas gingivalis,* resulting in tooth loss.

peritonitis (per"i-to-ni'tis) inflammation of the peritoneum.

proctitis inflammation of the rectum.

pulpitis inflammation of the dental pulp.

salmonellosis acute gastroenteritis due to ingestion of food and/or water contaminated with *Salmonella* bacteria, with symptoms of sudden onset of abdominal pain, nausea, vomiting, and fever (also called *Salmonella enteriditis*).

shigellosis infection caused by *Shigella* bacteria, with cramping, abdominal pain, watery diarrhea, high fever, and general muscle pain, transmitted by person-to-person contact and ingestion of contaminated food and water.

sialadenitis (si"al-ad"e-ni'tis) salivary gland inflammation.

strongyloidiasis (stron"ji-loi-di'ah-sis) infection with an intestinal roundworm *Strongyloides.*

trichuriasis (trik"u-ri'ah-sis) infection with an intestinal parasite of the genus *Trichuris.*

ulcerative colitis chronic inflammatory disease, with watery diarrhea containing blood, mucus, and pus, resulting in ulceration of the colon and rectum.

Vincent's stomatitis ulcerative, necrotizing inflammation of the gums or oral mucosa (also called *trench mouth*).

Hereditary, Congenital, and Developmental Disorders

aglossia absence of tongue.

annular pancreas developmental defect in which the pancreas lies in the bend of the duodenum, forming a ring encircling the duodenum, sometimes causing an intestinal obstruction.

ankyloglossia (ang″ki-lo-glos′e-ah) tongue-tie.

atresia (ah-tre′ze-ah) occlusion or absence of a normal body opening or tubular formation; may occur in the anus, the bile ducts, or the esophagus.

cleft palate incomplete closure in the midline of the palate.

congenital hypertrophic pyloric stenosis abnormal enlargement of the pyloric sphincter muscle of the stomach, creating an obstruction to the passage of gastric contents to the duodenum.

congenital megacolon developmental abnormality with loss of muscle function and hypertrophic dilation of the colon (also called *Hirschsprung's disease*).

glycogenosis group of hereditary disorders of glycogen metabolism.

harelip cleft in the upper lip.

Hutchinson's teeth tooth deformity with narrow-edged, grooved permanent incisors, caused by congenital syphilis.

hyperbilirubinemia (hi″per-bil″i-roo″bi-ne′me-ah) benign, familial disorders marked by excessive bilirubin in the blood (also called *Gilbert's disease*).

macrocheilia excessively large lips.

macroglossia excessively large tongue (also called *megaloglossia*).

macrostomia abnormally wide mouth.

Meckel's diverticulum residual pouch of the embryonic omphalomesenteric duct.

megalogastria (meg″ah-lo-gas′tre-ah) abnormally large stomach.

microgastria unusually small stomach.

microstomia unusually small mouth.

neonatal necrotizing enterocolitis (NEC) condition of a newborn in which the intestinal mucosa or submucosa becomes necrotic.

oligodontia developmental anomaly in which there are fewer than the usual number of teeth.

transposition of abdominal viscera reversal of normal position of the abdominal organs.

tyrosinemia rare, hereditary disorder of the liver in which the metabolism of amino acids is disrupted, resulting in liver failure.

Other Abnormalities

achalasia (ak′ah-la′ze-ah) failure to relax, especially in relation to sphincter muscles.

achlorhydria (ak″klor-hi′dre-ah) absence of hydrochloric acid in gastric secretions.

acholia (ah-ko′le-ah) absence of bile secretion.

achylia (ah″ki-le′ah) absence of digestive juices in the stomach.

aerophagia (aer″-o-fa′je-ah) swallowing of air, with belching (*eructation*).

anorexia lack of appetite.

ascites (ah-si′tez) accumulation of fluid in the abdominal cavity.

bulimia gorging food, followed by self-induced vomiting (also called *hyperorexia*).

cachexia (kah-kek′se-ah) generalized poor nutrition.

calculus formation of a stone (plural—*calculi*).

cholelithiasis (ko″le-li-thi′ah-sis) gallstones.

cholesteroleresis (ko-les″ter-ol-er′e-sis) increase in elimination of cholesterol in bile.

cholesterosis (ko-les″ter-o′sis) excessive deposits of cholesterol in tissues (also called *cholesterolosis*).

chylous ascites (ki′lus ah-si′tez) accumulation of chyle in the peritoneal cavity, due to thoracic duct obstruction.

cirrhosis (sir-ro′sis) liver disease with progressive destruction of liver cells.

colic acute, paroxysmal, abdominal pain.

constipation sluggish bowel with difficult or incomplete evacuation.

crepitus (krep′i-tus) flatulent discharge from bowels.

dental caries destruction of the enamel, dentin, or cementum of a tooth, resulting in tooth decay and cavities.

diabetes insipidus, diabetes mellitus see entry in Chapter 14.

diarrhea frequent discharge of abnormally liquid feces.

diverticulosis (di″ver-tik″u-lo′sis) presence of pouches within the intestines, protruding through the intestinal wall.

dyspepsia indigestion, caused by other disorder.

emesis vomiting.

enterocystocele (en″ter-o-sis′to-sel) hernia involving both the bladder and intestinal walls.

enterolith (en′ter-o-lith) stone in the intestines.

enteroptosis (en″ter-op-to′sis) dislocation of the intestines.

eructation belching.

fecalith (fe′kah-lith) stonelike fecal mass.

fistula abnormal opening between two organs, or between a hollow organ and the body surface, commonly found in the gastrointestinal system.

gastralgia pain in the stomach.

gastroesophageal reflux disorder (GERD) regurgitation of stomach contents into the esophagus.

gastrolith stone in the stomach.

gastroptosis (gas″trop-to′sis) downward dislocation of the stomach.

halitosis bad breath (caused by liver and kidney diseases, or bacterial infections of the mouth).

hemochromatosis (he″mo-kro″mah-to′sis) metabolic disorder with abnormal accumulation of iron in the body tissues, cirrhosis of the liver, and diabetes mellitus.

hemoperitoneum (he″mo-per″i-to-ne′um) escape of blood into the peritoneal cavity.

hepatomalacia (hep″ah-to-mah-la′she-ah) softening of the liver.

hepatomegaly enlarged liver.

hepatosplenomegaly enlarged liver and spleen.

hernia protrusion of an organ or part through its normal containing structures (also called *rupture*).

hiatal hernia (hi-a′tal) protrusion of part of the stomach through the esophageal opening of the diaphragm.

hydrops (hi′drops) abnormal accumulation of fluid in tissues or a body cavity (formerly called *dropsy,* an obsolete term).

hypercementosis (hi″per-se″men-to′sis) excessive development of cementum on the roots of the teeth.

hyperchlorhydria (hi″per-klor-hi′dre-ah) excessive hydrochloric acid in the gastric secretion.

hypercholesterolemia (hi″per-ko-les′ter-ol-e′me-ah) abnormal increase of cholesterol in the blood.

hypercholia excessive bile secretion.

hyperglycemia (hi″per-gli-se′me-ah) excessive concentration of glucose in the blood.

hyperinsulinism (hi″per-in′su-lin′izm) excessive pancreatic secretion of insulin (also called *insulin shock*).

hypersplenism (hi″per-splen′izm) abnormally increased hemolytic function of the spleen.

hypervitaminosis condition caused by excessive ingestion of vitamins, especially A and B.

hypochlorhydria deficiency of hydrochloric acid in the stomach.

hypocholesteremia (hi″po-ko-les′ter-e′me-ah) abnormal decrease of cholesterol in the blood.

hypochylia deficiency of chyle.

hypoglycemia (hi″po-gli-se′me-ah) low blood glucose level.

hypovitaminosis disease caused by deficiency of one or more of the essential vitamins.

ileus (il′e-us) mechanical obstruction of the intestines, with colic, vomiting, fever, and dehydration.

incontinence of feces inability to restrain fecal evacuation.

intussusception (in″tus-sus-sep′shun) prolapse of a portion of the intestine into the lumen of an immediately adjacent portion.

jaundice (jawn′dis) yellowish tinge of skin, sclerae, and other tissues, with deposits of bile pigments in the excretions.

leukoplakia (lu″ko-pla′ke-ah) development of white plaques (patches) on the mucous membranes.

malocclusion failure of proper closure of jaws because of malposition of teeth.

marasmus (mah-raz′mus) a type of protein and calorie malnutrition chiefly occurring in infants and children.

mucocele (mu′ko-sel) cyst or polyp containing mucus.

nausea sick sensation, often resulting in vomiting.

obstipation extreme constipation caused by intestinal obstruction.

oligopepsia lack of digestive tone.

oligotrophy insufficient nutrition.

pellagra (pel-lag′rah) niacin deficiency condition characterized by inflamed mucous membranes, dermatitis, and diarrhea.

phytobezoar (fi"to-be'zor) gastric mass composed of vegetable matter.

polydipsia extreme thirst.

polyphagia ravenous eating.

proctalgia pain in or near rectum and anus.

proctocele hernia of the rectum (also called *rectocele*).

proctoptosis (prok"top-to'sis) rectal prolapse.

pruritus ani chronic, intense itching of the anal region.

pylorospasm spasm of the pylorus of the stomach.

rickets vitamin D deficiency disorder, usually in infants and children, chiefly affecting calcification of bones, with resulting bending and deformation of the bones.

scurvy disease caused by vitamin C *(ascorbic acid)* deficiency, resulting in anemia, mucocutaneous bleeding, and hardening of the muscles of the legs.

splanchnoptosis (splank"nop-to'sis) prolapse of the viscera (also called *visceroptosis*).

sprue (sproo) chronic condition of malabsorption characterized by intolerance to certain foods, resulting in anorexia, anemia, diarrhea, and weight loss.

stenosis narrowing of an opening or passage.

tenesmus (te-nez'mus) painful, ineffective straining at stool.

ulcer lesion on the surface of a mucous membrane or the skin, caused by disintegration of inflamed necrotic tissue.

volvulus intestinal obstruction caused by twisting of the bowel.

vomiting forcible expulsion of gastric contents through the mouth.

Oncology*

Various types of tumors occur in other parts of the body, as well as in the gastrointestinal tract. Particular to the large intestine is a method of describing the stages of colorectal tumors called Dukes' classification (developed by and named for a British cancer specialist): Dukes'-A tumors are superficial, confined to mucosa and submucosa, with a high survival rate; Dukes'-B tumors have invaded the fat or muscle tissue but do not involve the lymphatic system and have a lower survival rate; Dukes'-C tumors involve greater penetration of the muscles and involve the regional lymph nodes; Dukes'-D tumors have metastasized to other organ tissues. C and D are associated with only a slight chance of survival. Some tumors of the gastrointestinal tract follow.

ameloblastoma (ah-mel"o-blas-to'mah) normally benign tumor of the jaw.

cementoma (se"men-to'mah) mass composed of cementum lying at the apex of a tooth, probably the result of trauma.

cholangiohepatoma (ko-lan"je-o-hep"ah-to'mah) tumor composed of hepatic cells and bile ducts in mixed masses.

cholangioma (ko-lan"je-o'mah) bile duct tumor.

dentigerous cyst (den-tij'er-us) cyst containing a tooth or teeth.

epulis any tumor of the gingivae such as an abscess or gumboil.

hepatoma* (hep"ah-toe'mah) malignant tumor of the liver (also called *hepatocarcinoma*).

odontogenic fibrosarcoma* malignant tumor of the jaw that develops from the formative components of a tooth.

odontoma (o-don-toe'mah) tumor of dental tissue.

polyp small, tumorlike growth on a mucous membrane surface, especially the throat or the intestines.

polyposis* (pol"e-po'sis) potentially malignant condition of multiple polyps in mucous membrane lining the intestine, particularly the colon.

signet ring cell carcinoma* malignancy most frequently found in the stomach and large intestine.

SURGICAL PROCEDURES

Because of the large number of surgical procedures applicable to the gastrointestinal system, they have been organized into groups involving excision *(-ectomy)*, fixation *(-pexy)*, incision *(-otomy)*, opening and anastomasis *(-stomy)*, puncture *(-centesis)*, repair *(-plasty)*, and suture *(-rrhaphy)*.

Excision to Remove All or Part of an Organ

alveolectomy partial excision of an alveolar process of a tooth.

appendectomy excision of the vermiform appendix.

cecectomy (see-kek"toe-me) excision of the cecum.

° Indicates a malignant condition.

° Indicates a malignant condition.

cholangiocholecystocholedochectomy (ko-lan"ge-o-ko"le-sis"to-ko"le-do-kek'to-me) excision of the gallbladder, hepatic duct, and common bile duct.

cholecystectomy excision of the gallbladder.

choledochectomy (ko"led-o-kek'to-me) excision of a portion of the common bile duct.

colectomy partial or total excision of the colon.

duodenectomy (du"o-de-nek'to-me) partial or total excision of the duodenum.

esophagectomy partial or total excision of the esophagus.

gastrectomy partial or total excision of the stomach.

gastropylorectomy (gas"tro-pi"lo-rek'to-me) excision of the pyloric portion of the stomach.

glossectomy surgical removal of part or all of the tongue.

hemorrhoidectomy excision of hemorrhoids.

hepatectomy excision of a portion or all of the liver.

ileectomy excision of the ileum.

jejunectomy excision of the jejunum.

omentectomy excision of a portion or all of the omentum.

omphalectomy (om"fah-lek'to-me) excision of the umbilicus (navel), or an attached tumor.

pancreatectomy surgical removal of all or part of the pancreas.

parotidectomy (pah-rot"i-dek'to-me) excision of the parotid gland.

pharyngectomy (far"in-jek'to-me) partial or total excision of the pharynx.

proctectomy excision of the rectum.

proctosigmoidectomy (prok"to-sig"moi-dek'to-me) excision of rectum and sigmoid flexure.

sialoadenectomy (si"ah-lo-ad"e-nek'to-me) excision of a salivary gland.

sigmoidectomy (sig"moi-dek'to-me) excision of the sigmoid flexure.

Fixation to Suspend or Fasten

cecopexy fixation of the cecum.

cholecystopexy fixation of the gallbladder.

colopexy fixation of the colon.

enteropexy fixation of the intestine to the abdominal wall.

gastropexy fixation of the stomach.

hepatopexy fixation of the liver.

mesenteriopexy fixation or attachment of a torn mesentery (also called *mesopexy*).

omentopexy fixation of omentum to the abdominal wall or an organ.

proctococcypexy (prok"to-kok'si-pek"se) fastening of the rectum to tissues in front of the coccyx.

proctopexy fixation of a prolapsed rectum to adjacent tissues.

sigmoidopexy attachment of the sigmoid colon to another structure.

Incision to Explore, Drain, or Remove a Foreign Body

celioenterotomy (se"le-o-en"ter-ot'-o-me) incision into intestine through abdominal wall (*celio* refers to abdomen).

celiogastrotomy (se"le-o-gas-trot'o-me) incision into the stomach through the abdominal wall.

celiotomy incision into the abdominal cavity.

cheilotomy incision into the lip.

cholangiotomy incision into the bile duct.

cholecystotomy incision into the gallbladder (also called *cholecystomy*).

choledocholithotomy (ko-led"o-ko-li-thot'o-me) incision into the common bile duct for removal of a stone.

choledochotomy (ko"led-o-kot'o-me) incision into the common bile duct.

cholelithotomy incision into the gallbladder for removal of stones.

colotomy incision into the colon.

duodenotomy incision into the duodenum.

enterocholecystotomy (en"ter-o-ko"le-sis-tot'o-me) incision into the intestine and gallbladder.

enterotomy incision into the intestine.

esophagotomy incision into the esophagus.

gastrotomy incision into the stomach.

hepatotomy incision into the liver.

ileotomy incision into the ileum.

jejunotomy incision into the jejunum.

laparotomy incision into the abdominal wall for exploratory purposes.

pancreatomy incision into the pancreas (also called *pancreatotomy*).

pharyngotomy incision into the pharynx.

proctotomy incision into the rectum (usually for rectal stricture).

pylorotomy incision into the pylorus.

sialoadenotomy (si"ah-lo-ad"e-not'o-me) incision and drainage of a salivary gland.

sialolithotomy removal of a stone from a salivary gland.

sigmoidotomy incision into the sigmoid.

sphincterotomy (sfingk"ter-ot'o-me) incision into a sphincter muscle.

Ostomies and Anastomoses

Ostomies are surgically created openings, usually in the intestines after partial resection to remove diseased or damaged parts, through which body waste is expelled. Anastomoses are surgically created openings, to produce communication between normally separated organs or spaces.

apicostomy (a"pe-kos'to-me) surgical creation of an opening through bone and gum to root portion of the tooth.

cecocolostomy (se"ko-ko-los'to-me) anastomosis between the cecum and colon (also called *colocecostomy*).

cecoileostomy (se"ko-il"e-os'to-me) anastomosis between the cecum and ileum (also called *ileocecostomy*).

cecostomy creation of an artificial opening into the cecum.

cholangioenterostomy (ko-lan"je-o-en"ter-os'to-me) anastomosis between intestine and bile duct.

cholangiogastrostomy (ko-lan"je-o-gas-tros'to-me) anastomosis between bile duct and stomach.

cholangiojejunostomy (ko-lan"je-o-je-joo-nos'to-me) anastomosis between a bile duct and the jejunum.

cholangiostomy creation of an opening into a bile duct.

cholecystenterostomy (ko"le-sis-ten"ter-os'to-me) anastomosis between the gallbladder and intestine (also called *enterocholecystostomy*).

cholecystocolostomy (ko"le-sis"to-ko-los'to-me) anastomosis between the gallbladder and colon (also called *cystocolostomy*).

cholecystogastrostomy (ko"le-sis"to-gas-tros'to-me) anastomosis between the gallbladder and stomach.

cholecystoduodenostomy (ko"le-sis"to-du"o-de-nos'to-me) anastomosis between the gallbladder and duodenum.

cholecystoileostomy (ko"le-sis"to-il'e-os'to-me) anastomosis between the gallbladder and ileum.

cholecystojejunostomy (ko"le-sis"to-je-joo-nos'to-me) anastomosis between the gallbladder and jejunum.

choledochocholedochostomy (ko-led"o-ko-ko-led'o-kos'to-me) anastomosis between two portions of the common bile duct.

choledochoduodenostomy (ko-led"o-ko-du"o-de-nos'to-me) anastomosis between the common bile duct and duodenum.

choledochoenterostomy (ko-led"o-ko-en"ter-os'to-me) anastomosis between the common bile duct and intestine.

choledochogastrostomy (ko-led"o-ko-gas-tros'to-me) anastomosis between the common bile duct and stomach.

choledochoileostomy (ko-led"o-ko-il-e-os'to-me) anastomosis between the common bile duct and ileum.

choledochojejunostomy (ko-led"o-ko-je-joo-nos'to-me) anastomosis between the common bile duct and jejunum.

choledochostomy (ko-led"o-kos'to-me) formation of an opening into the common bile duct for drainage.

colocolostomy (ko"lo-ko-los'to-me) anastomosis between two portions of the colon.

coloproctostomy (ko"lo-prok-tos'to-me) anastomosis between the colon and rectum (also called *colorectostomy*).

colosigmoidostomy (ko"lo-sig"moi-dos'to-me) anastomosis between the sigmoid and any other part of the colon.

colostomy formation of an artificial opening into the colon from the surface of the body.

duodenoenterostomy (du"o-de"no-en"ter-os'to-me) anastomosis between the duodenum and another part of the intestine.

duodenoileostomy (du"o-de"no-il"e-os'to-me) anastomosis between the duodenum and ileum.

duodenojejunostomy (du"o-de"no-je-joo-nos'to-me) anastomosis between the duodenum and jejunum

duodenostomy (du"od-e-nos'to-me) creation of an opening into the duodenum.

enteroanastomosis (en"ter-o-ah-nas"to-mo'sis) anastomosis between two sections of the intestine (also called *enteroenterostomy*).

enterocolostomy anastomosis between the small intestine and colon.

enterostomy (en"ter-os'to-me) creation of an opening into the intestine through the abdominal wall.

esophagoduodenostomy   (e-sof"ah-go-du"o-de-nos'to-me) anastomosis between the esophagus and duodenum.

esophagoenterostomy (e-sof"ah-go-en"ter-os'to-me) anastomosis between the esophagus and intestine.

esophagogastrostomy (e-sof'ah-go-gas-tros'to-me) anastomosis between the esophagus and stomach.

esophagojejunostomy (e-sof'ah-go-je-joo-nos'to-me) anastomosis between the esophagus and jejunum.

esophagostomy creation of an artificial opening into the esophagus.

gastroanastomosis (gas"tro-ah-nas"to-mo'sis) anastomosis between pyloric and cardiac ends of the stomach (also called *gastrogastrostomy*).

gastrocolostomy (gas"tro-ko-los'to-me) anastomosis between the stomach and colon.

gastroduodenostomy (gas"tro-du"o-de-nos'to-me) anastomosis between the stomach and duodenum.

gastroenterocolostomy (gas"tro-en"ter-o-ko-los'to-me) anastomosis between the stomach and intestines.

gastroenterostomy (gas"tro-en-ter-os'to-me) anastomosis between the stomach and colon.

gastroileostomy (gas"tro-il-e-os'to-me) anastomosis between the stomach and ileum.

gastrojejunostomy (gas"tro-je-joo-nos'to-me) anastomosis between the stomach and jejunum.

gastrostomy (gas-tros'to-me) creation of an opening into the stomach.

hepaticoduodenostomy (he-pat"i-ko-du"o-de-nos'to-me) anastomosis between hepatic duct and the duodenum (also called *hepatoduodenostomy*).

hepaticoenterostomy (he-pat"i-ko-en"ter-os'to-me) anastomosis between the hepatic duct and intestine (also called *hepaticocholangioenterostomy*).

hepaticogastrostomy (he-pat"i-ko-gas-tros'to-me) anastomosis between the hepatic duct and the stomach.

hepaticojejunostomy (he-pat"i-ko-je"joo-nos'to-me) anastomosis between the hepatic duct and the jejunum.

hepaticostomy creation of an opening into the hepatic duct.

hepatocholangiostomy (hep"ah-to-ko-lan'je-os'to-me) creation of an opening into the hepatic duct for drainage.

ileocolostomy (il"e-o-ko-los'to-me) anastomosis between the ileum and colon.

ileoileostomy (il"e-o-il"e-os'to-me) anastomosis between two different parts of the ileum.

ileoproctostomy (il"e-o-prok-tos'to-me) anastomosis between the ileum and rectum.

ileosigmoidostomy (il"e-o-sig"moid-os'to-me) anastomosis between the ileum and sigmoid colon.

ileostomy creation of an opening into the ileum through the abdominal wall.

jejunocolostomy (je-joo"no-ko"los'to-me) anastomosis between the jejunum and colon (also called *jejunoileostomy*).

jejunojejunostomy (je-joo"no-je"joo-nos'to-me) anastomosis between two parts of the jejunum.

jejunostomy creation of an opening through the abdominal wall into the jejunum.

pancreaticoduodenostomy (pan"kre-at"i-ko-du"o-de-nos'to-me) anastomosis of the pancreatic duct and the duodenum.

pancreaticoenterostomy (pan"kre-at"i-ko-en"ter-os'to-me) anastomosis of the pancreatic duct and the intestine.

pancreaticogastrostomy (pan"kre-at"i-ko-gas-tros'to-me) anastomosis of the pancreatic duct and the stomach.

pancreaticojejunostomy   (pan"kre-at"i-ko-je"joo-nos'to-me) anastomosis of the pancreatic duct and the jejunum.

proctostomy (prok-tos'to-me) creation of an opening into the rectum from the surface of the body (also called *rectostomy*).

pylorostomy (pi"lo-ros'to-me) creation of an opening through the abdominal wall near the pyloric end of the stomach.

sigmoidoproctostomy (sig-moi"do-prok-tos'to-me) anastomosis between the sigmoid flexure and the rectum (also called *sigmoidorectostomy*).

sigmoidosigmoidostomy (sig-moi"do-sig-moi-dos'to-me) anastomosis between two portions of the sigmoid.

sigmoidostomy creation of an artificial opening into the sigmoid flexure from the body surface.

Plastic Surgery for Repair

anoplasty (a"no-plas"te) repair of the anus.

cheiloplasty (ki'lo-plas"te) repair of the lip.

choledochoplasty (ko-led"o-ko-plas"te) repair of the common bile duct.

esophagoplasty (e-sof'ah-go-plas"te) repair of the esophagus.

gastroplasty repair of the stomach.

glossoplasty repair of the tongue.

hernioplasty repair of a hernia.

palatoplasty repair of palate, including cleft palate.

pharyngoplasty (fah-ring'go-plas"te) repair of the pharynx.

proctoplasty repair of rectum or anus.

pyloroplasty (pi-lo'ro-plas"te) repair to remove a pyloric obstruction and expedite emptying of the stomach.

sialodochoplasty (si"ah-lo-do'ko-plas"te) plastic repair of the salivary ducts.

sphincteroplasty (sfingk'ter-o-plas"te) repair of a sphincter.

stomatoplasty (sto'mah-to-plas"te) repair of mouth.

Puncture for Drainage or Aspiration

abdominocentesis (ab-dom"i-no-sen-te'sis) paracentesis of the abdominal cavity (also called *celiocentesis*).

colocentesis (ko"lo-sen-te'sis) paracentesis of the colon.

paracentesis surgical puncture of a cavity for fluid aspiration.

peritoneocentesis (per"i-to"ne-o-sen-te'sis) paracentesis of the peritoneal cavity.

Suture and Repair of Wounds, Lesions, Injuries, Ruptures, and Displacements

cecorrhaphy (se-kor'ah-fe) suture or repair of the cecum.

celiorrhaphy (se"le-or'ah-fe) suture or repair of the abdominal wall (also called *laparorrhaphy*).

cheilorrhaphy (ki-lor'ah-fe) suture or repair of the lip.

cholecystorrhaphy (ko"le-sis-tor'ah-fe) suture or repair of the gallbladder.

choledochorrhaphy (ko"led-o-kor'ah-fe) suture or repair of the common bile duct.

colorrhaphy (ko-lor'ah-fe) suture or repair of the colon.

duodenorrhaphy (du"o-de-nor'ah-fe) suture or repair of the duodenum.

enterorrhaphy (en"ter-or'ah-fe) suture or repair of the intestine.

gastrorrhaphy (gas-tror'ah-fe) suture or repair of the stomach.

glossorrhaphy (glo-sor'ah-fe) suture or repair of the tongue.

hepatorrhaphy (hep"ah-tor'ah-fe) suture or repair of the liver.

herniorrhaphy (her"ne-or'ah-fe) suture or repair of a hernia.

ileorrhaphy (il"e-or'ah-fe) suture or repair of the ileum.

jejunorrhaphy (je"joo-nor'ah-fe) suture or repair of the jejunum.

omentorrhaphy (o"men-tor'ah-fe) suture or repair of the omentum.

proctorrhaphy (prok-tor'ah-fe) suture or repair of the rectum.

Other Surgical Procedures

cholecystolithotripsy (kol"le-sis"to-lith'o-trip"se) crushing of stones in the gallbladder (also called *cholelithotripsy* and *cholelithotrity*).

choledocholithotripsy (ko-led"o-ko-lith'o-trip"se) crushing of a stone within the common bile duct.

exteriorize transpose an internal organ to the outside of the body.

proctotoreusis (prok"to-to-roo'sis) creating an artificial anus.

ptyalectasis (ti"ah-lek'tah-sis) dilation of a salivary duct.

pylorodiosis (pi-lo"ro-di-o'sis) dilating a stricture of pylorus with the finger, which is either inserted through a gastrotomy incision (*Loreta's method*), or the anterior stomach wall (*Hahn's method*).

LABORATORY TESTS AND PROCEDURES

biopsy insertion of needle to obtain sample of tissue in organs such as the liver, to detect abnormalities and diseases.

Blood Tests

amylase pancreatic enzyme elevated in disease of the pancreas or salivary glands.

Australian antigen detects serum hepatitis B, and differentiates between it and serum hepatitis A.

bilirubin a pigment of bile measurably present in liver and gallbladder diseases.

carcinoembryonic antigen to detect the presence of cancer in the colon and pancreas.

C-peptide test to determine the ability of diabetic individuals to make their own insulin.

glycated hemoglobin test measures percentage of glucose attached to red blood cells.

insulin test to determine amount of insulin secreted by the pancreas after fasting and again after receiving glucose.

Breath Tests

Halimeter device that measures the presence in the breath of volatile sulfur compounds.

Meretek UBT breath test diagnosis of a peptic ulcer (caused by *Helicobacter pylori*) using an ingested urea solution fortified with heavy carbon isotopes. If the bacteria are present, the urea is broken down and the carbon isotopes are detected.

Endoscope Examinations

A tubelike device with light and refracting mirrors is used to examine internal body areas for abnormalities and to remove tissue samples and small growths.

colonoscopy examination of the colon.

esophagoscopy examination of the esophagus.

gastroscopy examination of stomach and upper gastrointestinal tract.

proctoscopy examination of anus and rectum.

proctosigmoidoscopy examination of rectum and sigmoid colon.

sigmoidoscopy examination of sigmoid colon.

Gastric Fluid Analysis

Series of tests on fluid aspirated from the stomach, to detect various diseases.

Liver Function Tests

Tests to determine damage or disease, normal enzymes or injected chemicals are measured for elevation or retention in the blood serum.

aminotransferases levels are measured for elevation to detect liver disease:

aspartate aminotransferase—AST (formerly called *serum glutamic-oxaloacetic transaminase—SGOT*)

alanine aminotransferase—ALT (formerly called *serum glutamic-pyruvic transaminase—SGPT*).

argininosuccinic lyase normally present enzyme.

bromsulphalein injected and found retained in blood over a specified time period.

cephalin-cholesterol flocculation reaction of blood serum mixed with cephalin and cholesterol.

ceruloplasmin elevation of this protein indicates liver disease, while decreased levels indicate nutritional deficiencies and other forms of liver disease.

complement C3 elevated levels in cancer, decreased levels in liver disease.

guanase enzyme level elevated in hepatitis and other types of liver disease.

lactic dehydrogenase isoenzymes pattern of distribution is diagnostic for liver disease.

ornithine carbamoyl transferase level of this enzyme elevated in liver disease.

plasma volume elevated in liver and spleen disease.

protein elevated in liver disease.

total alkaline phosphatase increased levels indicate liver disease.

total cholesterol elevated or decreased in particular liver diseases.

transferrin iron-binding protein that decreases in liver disease.

Radiologic Studies

barium enema studies using contrast media to visualize the colon and rectum.

celiac angiography studies of the blood vessels of the liver, spleen, stomach, and pancreas, using contrast medium.

cholangiography studies of the gallbladder and its ducts.

cholecystography (oral) studies of the gallbladder after ingestion of a fatty meal, using contrast media to outline structures.

computerized tomography (CT) imaging device using x-rays at multiple angles through specific sections of the body, analyzed by computer to provide a total picture of the part being examined (also called *computerized axial tomography—CAT*).

focused appendix computerized tomography (FACT) a CT technique in which dye is introduced into the colon to diagnose the condition of the appendix.

gastrointestinal series x-ray studies of esophagus, stomach, and small intestine, after swallowing a contrast medium such as barium (upper gastrointestinal tract). The large intestine is visualized by use of a barium enema (lower gastrointestinal tract).

magnetic resonance imaging (MRI) noninvasive method of scanning the body by use of an electromagnetic field and radio waves, which provides visual images on a computer screen and magnetic tape recordings (also called *nuclear magnetic resonance—NMR*). Used to examine soft tissues such as visceral contents.

nuclear magnetic resonance (NMR) see *magnetic resonance imaging.*

percutaneous transhepatic cholangiography x-ray study of bile duct by use of dye injected to detect obstruction.

sialography x-ray studies of salivary glands using contrast medium.

splenoportography x-ray studies of spleen, liver, and blood vessels using a contrast medium.

x-ray scans x-ray studies of liver, spleen, and pancreas, to detect tumors or other abnormalities by use of radioactive substances injected intravenously.

Stool Tests

combined fatty acids test determine ability to digest fat.

guaiac test for detection of blood in intestinal tract.

mucus test elevation in stool indicates bowel abnormality.

parasites test microscopic examination of fecal matter to detect parasitic infection.

pus presence indicates intestinal tract infection.

stool culture fecal matter incubated in growth media to detect presence of microorganisms.

total nitrogen content measured to detect pancreatic insufficiency or poor protein digestion.

trypsin activity elevation indicates fibrocystic disease of pancreas.

urobilinogen metabolic product that decreases in liver and gallbladder diseases.

Urine Tests

amylase elevated in pancreatitis.

copper element found in elevated amounts in liver disease.

coproporphyrin elevated in liver and metabolic disease.

diacetic acid produced in metabolic diseases such as diabetes.

oral glucose tolerance test measurable level of sugar present indicates metabolic disorder.

qualitative glucose present in metabolic diseases such as diabetes.

5-hydroxyindoleacetic acid elevation indicates tumor in appendix or lower intestinal tract.

inulin clearance rate of excretion of inulin indicates presence of liver disease.

EXERCISES THE GASTROINTESTINAL SYSTEM THE FOOD PROCESSOR

Exercise 11.1   *Complete the following:*

1. The chief organs of the alimentary tract are __mouth__, __pharynx__, __esophagus__, __stomach__, and __intestines__

2. The accessory organs of the digestive tract are __teeth__, __salivary glds__ __liver__, __gall bladder__, and __pancreas__.

3. The organs in the digestive tract through which food passes as it travels from the mouth to the anus are, in order, __mouth__, __pharynx__, __esophagus__, __stomach__, __small intestine__ and __large intestine__

4. Five of the eight structures in the oral cavity are __gums__, __teeth__, __palatine arches__ __salivary glands__, and __tongue__, __uvula__, __fauces__

5. The two main functions of the tongue in the digestive system are __aid in swallowing__ and __keep food__.

6. The four types of teeth are __incisors__, __canines__, __premolars__ __between teeth__, and __molars__.

7. The thin, lubricating, serous fluid secreted by the salivary glands is called __saliva__.

8. The two chief functions of the secretions of the salivary glands are __dissolve food__ and __initiate digestion of carbs__.

9. The dual functions of the pharynx are __airway__ and __passageway for food__

10. The names of the curvatures of the stomach are __lesser__ and __greater__.

11. The names, in order, of the divisions of the small intestine are __duodenum__, __jejunum__, and __ileum__.

12. The process of digestion is completed in the __small intestine__

13. The __peritoneum__ is the serous membrane that lines the abdominal cavity.

14. Two hormones secreted by the islands of Langerhans are __insulin__ and __glucagon__.

15. Four important functions of the liver are __secrete bile for digestion;__ __metabolize fat protein and carbs; filter + destroy__ __foreign matter; store iron, glycogen and__ __vitamins A, B₁₂, and D__

16. The main function of the gallbladder is __store concentrated bile__.

17. Most of the water absorption of the body takes place in the __large intestine__.

18. The voluntary stage of swallowing is the __first__ stage.

19. The peritoneal fold that attaches the intestine to the posterior abdominal wall is called the __mesentery__.

20. The double fold of peritoneum attached to the stomach, connecting it with the abdominal viscera, is called the __omentum__.

Exercise 11.2 *Using the list of terms below, identify the parts in Figure 11.6 by writing the names in the corresponding blanks.*

Parotid gland	Appendix	Cecum
Esophagus	Submaxillary (or submandibular)	Lesser curvature of stomach
Gallbladder	gland	Splenic flexure
Liver	Pancreas	Ascending colon
Hepatic flexure	Pharynx	Pylorus
Rectum	Duodenum	Jejunum
Descending colon	Ileum	Sigmoid
Transverse colon	Anus	
Sublingual gland	Greater curvature of stomach	

1. *parotid gland*
2. *sub maxillary gland*
3. *sublingual gland*
4. *liver*
5. *pylorus*
6. *gall bladder*
7. *hepatic flexure*
8. *duodenum*
9. *ascending colon*
10. *cecum*
11. *appendix*
12. *rectum*
13. *anus*
14. *pharynx*
15. *esophagus*
16. *lesser curvature of stomach*
17. *splenic flexure*
18. *greater curvature of stomach*
19. *pancreas*
20. *transverse colon*
21. *jejunum*
22. *descending colon*
23. *ileum*
24. *sigmoid*

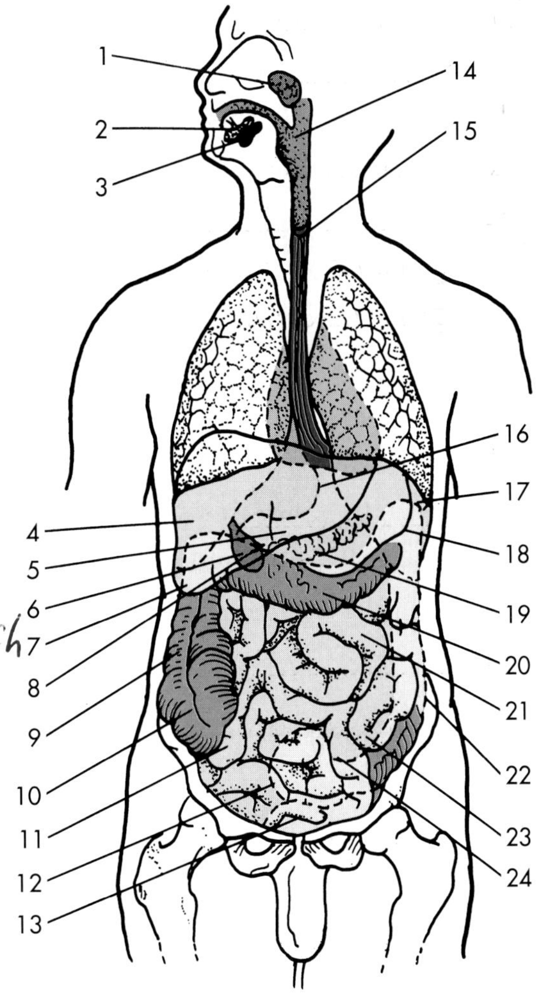

Figure 11.6 Digestive tract.

Exercise 11.3   *Matching*

___B___   1. rigid bony structure in the roof of the mouth

___A___   2. partition between the mouth and nasopharynx

___E___   3. constricted opening between arches and oropharynx

___F___   4. musculomembranous tube from pharynx to stomach

___M___   5. lower left margin of the surface of the stomach

___K___   6. upper right margin of the surface of the stomach

___L___   7. very hard substance that covers the exposed part of the tooth

___C___   8. chief substance of the tooth surrounding pulp

___J___   9. semifluid material produced by gastric digestion of food

___O___   10. threadlike projections covering the mucosa of the small intestine

___D___   11. any one of the four front teeth of either jaw

___H___   12. broad teeth used in grinding food

___I___   13. archlike structure formed by the soft palate at the posterior border of the mouth

___N___   14. pendulum of the soft palate

___G___   15. ringlike muscles that contract to close an opening

A. soft palate
B. hard palate
C. dentin
D. incisor
E. fauces
F. esophagus
G. sphincter
H. molars
I. palatine arch
J. chyme
K. lesser curvature
L. enamel
M. greater curvature
N. uvula
O. villi

Exercise 11.4   *Multiple Choice*

1. The peritoneal fold that attaches the intestine to the posterior abdominal wall is the:
   a. lesser curvature
   b. mesentery
   c. omentum

2. The part of the pancreas touching the spleen is the:
   a. neck
   b. tail
   c. head

3. The second part of the pharynx is called:
   a. nasopharynx
   b. fauces
   c. oropharynx

4. The dilated intestinal pouch that joins the colon below the juncture of the ileum and colon is the:
   a. appendix
   b. cecum
   c. anal canal

5. *Vermiform* is a name given to the:
   a. cecum
   b. appendix
   c. rectum

6. The number of coats in the stomach wall is:
   a. three
   b. four
   c. five

7. Another name for the gallbladder is:
   a. choledochus
   b. ductus choledochus
   c. cholecyst

8. The fluid secreted by the liver and poured into the intestines is called:
   a. chyle
   b. bile
   c. chyme

9. The involuntary, wavelike movement of the gastrointestinal tract is called:
   a. alimentary
   b. peristalsis
   c. gastritis

10. The bonelike connective tissue covering the root and neck of a tooth is called:
    a. periodontium
    b. enamel
    c. cementum

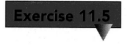

Give the meaning of the components in the following words and then define the word as a whole. Suffixes meaning *pertaining to* or *state or condition* shown following a slash mark (/) are not to be defined separately. Before reaching for your medical dictionary, check the Related Terms list in this chapter.

1. Cholangitis:
   chol _bile_
   ang _vessels_
   itis _inflammation_
   _____

2. Diverticulitis:
   diverticul _intestine, stomach_
   itis _inflammation_
   _____

3. Enterogastritis
   entero _diverticulum_
   gastro _stomach_
   itis _inflammation_

4. Gastroenterocolitis:
   gastro _stomach_
   entero _small intestine_
   col _colon_
   itis _inflammation_
   _____

5. Hepatitis:
   hepat _liver_
   itis _inflammation_

6. Ileitis:
   ile _ileum_
   itis _inflammation_
   _____

7. Ileocolitis:
   ileo _ileum_
   col _colon_
   itis _inflammation_
   _____

8. Linguopapillitis:
   linguo _tongue_
   papill _papillae_
   itis _inflammation_

9. Proctitis:
   proct _rectum_
   itis _inflammation_
   _____

10. Gastroduodenitis
    gastro _stomach_
    duoden _duodenum_
    itis _inflammation_
    _____

11. Glossitis:
    gloss _tongue_
    itis _inflammation_
    _____

12. Gingivitis:
    gingiv _gums_
    itis _inflammation_
    _____

CROSSWORD PUZZLE

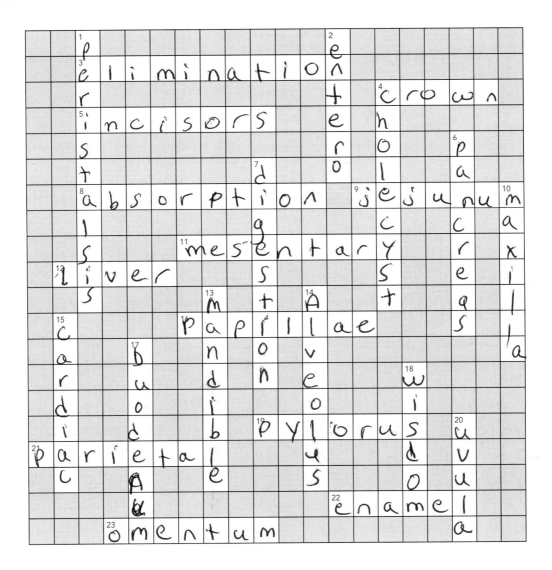

ACROSS

3. A function of the gastrointestinal system

4. Tooth part above the gum line

5. Chisel-shaped teeth

8. A function of the gastrointestinal system

9. A part of the small intestine

11. Connects intestines to abdominal wall

12. Largest gland in body

16. Small elevations on tongue

19. Lower small end of stomach

21. Peritoneum of abdominal cavity

22. Hardest body substance

23. Membrane attached to stomach

DOWN

1. Involuntary wavelike movement

2. Combining form meaning intestines

4. Root meaning gallbladder

6. Endocrine/exocrine gland

7. A function of the gastrointestinal system

10. Upper jawbone

13. Lower jawbone

14. Tooth socket

15. Entrance sphincter of stomach

17. Part of small intestine

18. Third molar teeth

20. Conical process between palatine arches

HIDDEN WORDS PUZZLE

```
H  C  N  T  O  F  X  Q  U  G  W  T  Q  P  I  D  T  B
C  X  O  I  I  A  S  O  O  I  T  O  Y  B  R  X  X  E
A  I  I  Y  L  O  L  F  F  N  D  H  Q  Q  H  B  U  L
Y  L  W  T  N  L  T  I  H  G  D  E  Y  D  V  O  L  O
H  J  V  X  S  F  N  B  A  I  P  P  U  W  P  X  T  M
M  K  C  E  C  U  M  N  C  V  K  A  P  D  C  N  H  A
N  P  V  N  O  X  Y  E  P  A  R  T  I  T  I  O  N  Y
G  A  L  L  B  L  A  D  D  E  R  I  T  G  F  K  X  T
C  P  L  F  V  Q  U  S  Y  W  R  C  P  J  X  M  N  T
M  I  U  I  U  I  S  S  U  B  L  I  N  G  U  A  L  W
I  L  E  H  M  N  S  P  H  I  N  C  T  E  R  G  J  Z
F  L  R  Q  M  E  D  C  A  R  P  A  R  O  T  I  D  K
F  A  C  O  L  O  N  U  E  L  C  T  F  D  N  N  Z  Z
R  E  C  T  U  M  G  T  S  R  A  S  I  U  P  E  S  P
M  T  Y  F  B  H  W  B  A  W  A  T  L  U  J  V  U  Z
H  X  J  C  G  R  O  J  L  R  V  L  E  N  A  I  Q  M
R  K  R  Z  H  Q  X  M  I  K  Y  W  U  S  V  G  W  U
T  M  R  B  I  E  E  O  V  U  J  O  M  B  L  L  K  K
G  Q  E  G  L  C  N  C  A  K  O  Z  T  E  Y  D  S  M
R  D  O  U  N  I  U  Z  R  V  M  T  V  R  C  N  D  L
L  D  P  M  F  J  K  Q  Y  Z  I  X  H  V  P  U  Q  D
X  N  M  P  U  G  Y  U  N  M  J  W  M  P  D  X  O  B
W  K  D  K  T  D  W  M  T  O  E  O  W  U  E  V  G  I
Z  L  H  V  T  L  Q  A  U  U  E  S  U  P  H  M  X  H
```

Can you find the 20 words hidden in this puzzle? All hidden words puzzles have words running from top to bottom, left to right, and diagonally downward.

GALLBLADDER	SALIVARY	COLON
PARTITION	PAROTID	SUBLINGUAL
PAPILLAE	CECUM	GINGIVAE
HEPATIC	PERITONEUM	ENZYMES
RECTUM	ALVEOLUS	PALATE
ALIMENTARY	VISCERAL	ILEUM
SPHINCTER	FUNDUS	

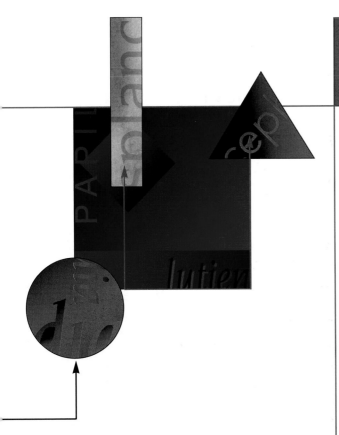

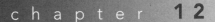

The Urinary System

liquid waste processing

The urinary systems in both sexes are very similar. In this chapter, the structures and functions of the various parts of the urinary system are presented and discussed. The organs that produce and excrete the waste substance urine from the body are the two *kidneys,* which filter the blood and remove waste products of metabolism in the form of urine; two *ureters,* which carry the urine from the kidneys; a *bladder,* which receives and stores the urine; and a *urethra,* which excretes the urine from the body. These organs are common to both sexes, with essentially the same structure.

THE KIDNEYS

The *kidneys* (Figure 12.1) are two bean-shaped organs (*nephro-* and *reno-* refer to kidney) located on both sides of the vertebral column, behind the parietal peritoneum, and just above the waist. An average kidney weighs 4 to 6 ounces (152 to 240 g), is about 4 inches (11 cm) long, 2 to 3 inches (5 to 7.5 cm) wide, and 1 inch (2.5 cm) thick. The left kidney is usually a

It's a **FACT**

There are more than 1 million little tubes in the average human kidney, and the total length of these tubes in both kidneys is about 40 miles.

little larger and is suspended a little higher than the right one. Renal fasciae (fibrous tissue) connecting to other structures, in conjunction with heavy encapsulating pads of fat surrounding the kidneys, hold them in place. Each kidney has a concave depression, the **hilus,** on its medial margin, for the entry of blood vessels, nerves, and its ureter.

Kidney Composition and Structure

The kidneys are dark reddish-brown and are solid organs except for the **renal sinus,** the space into which the hilus opens. Sectioning of the kidney shows it to be composed of an external **cortex** and an internal **medulla** (Figure 12.2).

The renal sinus contains the **renal pelvis,** blood vessels, nerves, and fat. The renal pelvis, a funnel-shaped reservoir that occupies most of the renal sinus, is made up of the major and minor **calyces** (singular—**calyx**), irregular saclike structures, that collect urine from all portions of the kidney. The broad portion of the renal pelvis lies within the renal sinus, and its apical portion passes out through the hilus to unite with the **ureter,** the outlet tube of the kidney extending to the bladder (see Figure 12.1).

Twelve to eighteen small, cone-shaped structures called **medullary pyramids,** which make up the medulla, stud the walls of the renal sinus, with their **bases** facing the cortex and their narrow ends, the **papillae,** extending into the renal pelvis calyces, where the urine collects through ducts in the papillae. The cortex extends between the pyramids, forming the **renal columns** (see Figure 12.2).

The Functional Unit of the Kidney

The **nephron** is the functional unit of the kidney, consisting of the **renal corpuscle** and the **renal tubule.** There are about 1 million nephrons in the human kidney. The renal corpuscle consists of a double-walled, cup-shaped structure called the **glomerular** or **Bowman's capsule,** which contains a twisted cluster of capillary channels called the **glomerulus,** forming a rounded body.

The renal tubule is divided into the **proximal convoluted tubule,** the **descending limb** of the **loop of Henle,** the **ascending limb** of the **loop of Henle,** the **distal convoluted tubule,** and the **collecting tubule** (see Figures 12.2 and 12.3).

The renal corpuscles and the attached proximal convoluted tubules into which they drain lie in the cortical portion of the kidney, with the tubules making up the largest part of the renal cortex. The loop of Henle follows the proximal convoluted tubule and is divided into a descending and an ascending limb, lying for the most part within the renal medulla. The

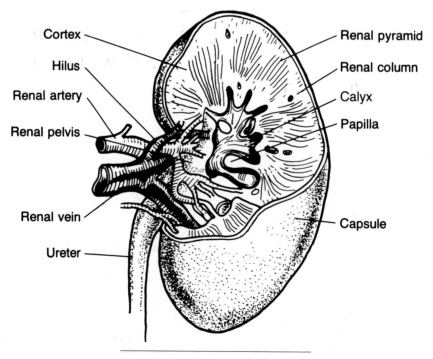

Figure 12.1 Structure of the kidney.

distal convoluted tubule resembles the proximal convoluted tubule in structure, except that it is much shorter when uncoiled, and drains into the collecting tubules, which convey the urine to the renal pelvis by way of the papillary ducts of the pyramids.

Functions of the Kidneys

The main function of the kidneys is to filter waste materials from the blood and excrete them in the urine. The waste products include nitrogenous wastes from the breakdown of proteins, toxic substances, mineral salts, excess glucose, and water (both ingested water and that produced during metabolism). In the blood-filtering process, water and solutes from blood in the glomeruli pass through the capillaries and the glomerular walls into the tubules. The tubules have the ability to select substances needed by the body and return them to the blood.

The speed at which the blood filters through the kidneys is affected by the blood pressure. If the systemic blood pressure drops, as in shock, it may cause filtration of blood to slow to a point where the kidneys stop functioning. Similarly, if the systemic pressure is too high, kidney damage may result, causing a loss of substances that normally would have been reabsorbed for use by the body.

The kidneys affect the rate of secretion of some hormones, synthesize other hormones, and maintain the pH of the blood so that it does not become too acid or too alkaline.

R E V I E W   1 2 . A

Complete the following:

1. The organs of the urinary system are the
   Kidneys , *ureters* ,
   bladder , and *urethra* .

2. The concave depression on the medial margin
   of the kidney is called the *hilus* .

3. The *nephron* is the
   functional unit of the kidney.

4. The main function of the kidneys is to
   filter waste from the blood.

5. The speed of blood filtering through the
   kidneys is affected by the *blood pressure*

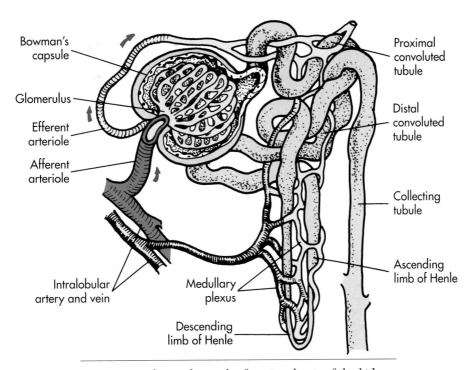

Figure 12.2 The nephron, the functional unit of the kidney.

Bowman's capsule

Glomerulus

Efferent arteriole

Afferent arteriole

Intralobular artery and vein

Medullary plexus

Descending limb of Henle

Proximal convoluted tubule

Distal convoluted tubule

Collecting tubule

Ascending limb of Henle

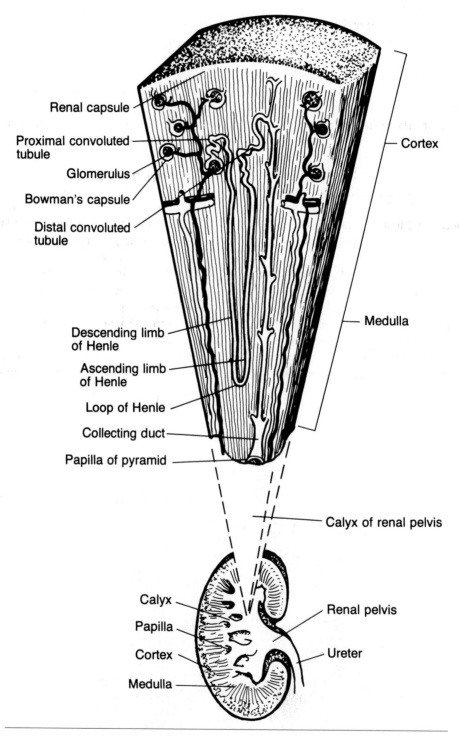

Renal capsule

Proximal convoluted tubule

Glomerulus

Bowman's capsule

Distal convoluted tubule

Cortex

Medulla

Descending limb of Henle

Ascending limb of Henle

Loop of Henle

Collecting duct

Papilla of pyramid

Calyx of renal pelvis

Calyx

Papilla

Cortex

Medulla

Renal pelvis

Ureter

Figure 12.3 Magnification showing renal corpuscles, proximal and distal convoluted tubules, and loops of Henle and collecting tubules.

THE URETERS

The *ureters*, one from each kidney, are about 15 to 18 inches (38 to 46 cm) long and are less than ½ inch (1.25 cm) in diameter, extending from the renal pelvis of the kidney down to the urinary bladder. The ureter on the left is slightly longer because of the higher position of the left kidney. The walls of the ureters are made up of an outer fibrous tissue layer, two center layers of smooth muscle, and a mucous membrane lining.

Urine enters the bladder through the ureters every 10 to 30 seconds, in spurts rather than in a continuous flow. The spurts are produced by the action of successive peristaltic waves, beginning in the renal pelvis and passing down throughout the extent of the ureters. Situated at the bladder entrance is a ureteral orifice, which opens for 2 to 3 seconds and then closes until a succeeding peristaltic wave opens it again, serving to prevent urine from flowing back to the ureters during bladder contraction.

THE URINARY BLADDER

The *urinary bladder* is an extremely elastic, musculomembranous sac, lying in the pelvis, formed of three layers of smooth muscle tissue lined with mucous membrane containing *rugae* (wrinkles or ridges). It contains two openings (to receive urine from the two ureters) and another opening into the urethra, through which urine is excreted. The bladder has two functions, to serve as a storage place for urine and to excrete urine through the urethra.

The average bladder will hold more than 250 ml of urine, but that amount will usually create a desire to empty the bladder. The contraction of the bladder and the relaxation of the internal sphincter muscle are involuntary actions, but the external sphincter muscle is controlled by voluntary action. The act of preventing or concluding voiding (urinating) is learned and voluntary in a mature, healthy human.

THE URETHRA

The *urethra* is a membranous, tubular canal that carries the urine from the bladder to the exterior of the body.

In the female, the urethra is approximately 1 to 1½ inches (2.5 to 4 cm) in length, extending from the neck of the bladder to the exterior surface of the body. The exterior opening of the urethra, called the *urinary meatus,* is located between the vagina and clitoris. In the female, the only function of the urethra is urination (Figure 12.4, *A*).

In the male, the urethra is approximately 8 inches (20 cm) long and is narrower than in the female. It extends from the neck of the bladder, through the

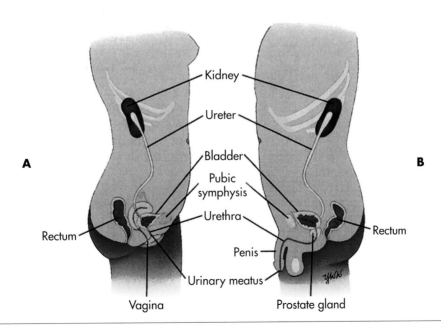

Kidney
Ureter
Bladder
Pubic symphysis
Urethra
Rectum
Penis
Urinary meatus
Prostate gland
Rectum
Vagina

A

B

Figure 12.4 **A,** Sagittal section of the female urinary system. **B,** Sagittal section of the male urinary system. (Modified from Thibodeau GA, Patton KT: *Anatomy and physiology,* ed 3, St Louis, 1996, Mosby, p 927.)

prostate gland, between the fascia connecting the pubic bones, and through the *penis* (external male reproductive organ). The male urethra is divided into three sections, *prostatic, membranous,* and *cavernous.* The exterior opening of the urethra in the male is also called the *urinary meatus.* In males, the urethra has a dual function, carrying both urine and the reproductive organ secretions (Figure 12.4, *B*).

Characteristics of Normal Urine

Normal urine is usually clear, pale amber in color, with a characteristic odor. It is approximately 95% water, containing many dissolved substances, such as nitrogenous wastes, electrolytes, toxins, pigments, hormones, and at times abnormal substances such as glucose, albumin, or blood.

The average urinary output in a 24-hour period ranges from 1000 to 2000 ml. The normal specific gravity of urine varies from 1.015 to 1.025, with an acid reaction.

REVIEW 12.B

Complete the following:

1. The ___left___ ureter is slightly longer than the other.
2. The wrinkles on the mucous membrane lining the bladder are called ___rugae___.
3. The ___urinary meatus___ is the exterior opening of the urethra.
4. The ___male___ urethra is longer than the ___female___ urethra.
5. Normal urine is ___pale ~~aber~~ amber___ in color.

RELATED TERMS   THE URINARY SYSTEM LIQUID WASTE PROCESSING

ANATOMY

bladder elastic musculomembranous sac for storing urine.

Bowman's capsule the glomerular capsule of the kidney containing the cluster of capillary channels *(glomerulus).*

calyx or **calix (ka'liks)** urine-collecting, irregular saclike structure of the renal pelvis.

collecting tubules terminal collection passages that carry urine to the renal pelvis.

distal convoluted tubules portion of the convoluted tubules between loop of Henle and the collecting tubules.

glomerulus coils of capillaries within Bowman's capsule (plural—*glomeruli*).

hilus concave depression on medial margin of the kidney through which the ureters, blood vessels, and nerves enter.

kidneys two glandular bodies that filter blood and secrete urine.

loop of Henle U-shaped turn in a convoluted tubule of the kidney, located between the proximal and distal ends, with both ascending and descending limbs.

nephron (nef'ron) functional and structural unit of the kidney, including a renal corpuscle and a renal tubule.

renal corpuscle glomerular or Bowman's capsule (also called *malpighian corpuscle*).

renal cortex (kor'teks) outer part of the kidney, extending between the renal pyramids to form the renal columns.

renal medulla inner part of the kidney composed of conical structures, called renal pyramids.

renal papillae the narrow, conical ends of renal pyramids.

renal pelvis the reservoir that collects urine, made up of the major and minor calyces (calices).

renal pyramid see *renal medulla.*

renal sinus kidney cavity containing renal pelvis, blood vessels, nerves and fat.

renal tubule minute tubule of the kidney that secretes, collects and transports urine, and forms part of the functional unit, the nephron (also called *uriniferous tubule*).

uresis normal passage of urine.

ureter tube that carries urine from the kidney to the bladder.

urethra tube that carries urine from the bladder to the surface of the body.

PATHOLOGIC CONDITIONS

Inflammations and Infections

balanitis (bal"ah-ni'tis) inflammation of the glans penis.

cystitis bladder inflammation.

glomerulonephritis (glo-mer"u-lo-ne-fri'tis) kidney disease with inflammation of the glomeruli, not caused by a kidney infection.

nephritis (ne-fri'tis) inflammation of the kidneys.

nephrotuberculosis tuberculosis of the kidney.

perinephritis (per"i-ne-fri'tis) inflammation of tissues surrounding the kidney.

pyelitis (pi"e-li'tis) inflammation of the kidney pelvis.

pyelocystitis (pi"e-lo-sis-ti'tis) inflammation of the kidney pelvis and bladder.

pyelonephritis (pi"e-lo-ne-fri'tis) inflammation of the kidney caused by infection (also called *nephropyelitis*).

pyonephritis (pi"o-ne-fri'tis) pus-producing inflammation of the kidney.

pyonephrosis (pi"o-ne-fro'sis) presence of pus in a kidney causing distention, usually because of obstruction.

ureteritis (u"re-ter-i'tis) inflammation of a ureter.

ureteropyelitis (u-re"ter-o-pi-e-li'tis) inflammation of a ureter and its kidney pelvis (also called *ureteropyelonephritis*).

ureteropyosis (u-re"ter-o-pi-o'sis) presence of pus in the ureter.

urethritis (u"re-thri'tis) inflammation of the urethra.

urethrocystitis (u-re"thro-sis-ti'tis) inflammation of the urethra and bladder.

Hereditary, Congenital, and Developmental Disorders

epispadias (ep"i-spa'de-as) urethral opening on dorsum of penis (*spadias* refers to cleft).

fused kidney one single kidney resulting from fusion during development.

horseshoe kidney fusion of the adjacent developing poles of the kidney so that the concavity formed faces upward, resembling a horseshoe.

hypospadias (hi"po-spa'de-as) urethra opens on the under surface of the penis or on the perineum.

renal ectopia displaced kidney.

supernumerary kidney developmental anomaly, with more than the normal two kidneys.

Other Abnormalities

albuminuria presence of albumin and other proteins in the urine.

anuria lack of urine being excreted (also called *anuresis*).

arteriolar nephrosclerosis (nef'ro-skle-ro'sis) scarring of a kidney caused by hypertension (also called *nephroangiosclerosis*).

azotemia (az"o-te'me-ah) presence of urea or other nitrogenous elements in the blood.

blennorrhea (blen"o-re'ah) excess mucus discharge from the urethra or vagina (also called *blennorrhagia*).

cylindruria (sil"in-droo're-ah) presence of cylindrical casts in the urine.

cystocele hernia of the urinary bladder through the vaginal wall.

dysuria painful or difficult urination.

glycosuria presence of sugar in the urine (also called *glucosuria* or *glycuresis*).

hematuria presence of blood in the urine.

hydronephrosis (hi"dro-ne-fro'sis) distention of a kidney caused by an obstruction of the ureter.

hypercalciuria (hi"per-kal'si-u're-ah) excessive calcium in the urine.

incontinence (in-kon'ti-nens) inability to control urination.

nephrolith (nef'ro-lith) kidney stone.

nephrolithiasis (nef"ro-li-thi'ah-sis) condition characterized by the presence of kidney stones (*renal calculi*).

nephromalacia (nef"ro-mah-la'she-ah) softening of the kidney.

nephromegaly (nef"ro-meg'ah-le) enlargement of the kidney.

nephroptosis (nef"rop-to'sis) downward displacement of the kidney.

nephrorrhagia (nef"ro-ra'je-ah) hemorrhage into or from the kidney.

nephrosis (ne-fro'sis) any disease of the kidney.

oliguria scanty urine output.

phosphaturia (fos"fat-u're-ah) excess of phosphates excreted in the urine.

polycystic kidney disease (PKD) multiple cysts of the kidney.

polyuria excessive urination.

pyelonephrosis (pi"e-lo-ne-fro'sis) any disease of the kidney pelvis.

pyuria pus in the urine.

renal colic pain caused by passage of a calculus in a kidney or ureter.

renal infarction ischemia of kidney resulting from thrombus or embolus.

retention keeping within the body a substance that is usually excreted, such as urine.

uraturia excess of urates in the urine.

uremia disturbed kidney function in which products of protein metabolism are found in the blood and produce a toxic condition.

ureteralgia pain in a ureter.

ureterectasis (u-re"ter-ek'tah-sis) dilation of a ureter.

ureterolith (u-re'ter-o-lith) stone in a ureter.

ureterolithiasis (u-re"ter-o-li-thi'ah-sis) formation of a stone in a ureter.

ureterolysis (u-re"ter-ol'i-sis) rupture or paralysis of a ureter.

ureterorrhagia (u-re"ter-o-ra'je-ah) hemorrhage of a ureter.

ureterostenosis (u-re"ter-o-ste-no'sis) ureteral stricture.

urethralgia pain in the urethra (also called *urethrodynia*).

urethremphraxis (u"re-threm-frak'sis) obstruction of the urethra.

urethrorrhagia (u-re"thro-ra'je-ah) urethral bleeding (also called *urethremorrhagia*).

urethrorrhea (u-re"thro-re'ah) abnormal urethral discharge.

urethrostaxis (u-re"thro-stak'sis) urethral oozing of blood.

urinary calculus (kal'ku-lus) stone or concretion in the kidney, ureter, or bladder.

Oncology*

The following list pertains specifically to tumors of the urinary system. Other tumors, both benign and malignant, occur in other parts of the body, as well as in the urinary system. Some of these are epidermoid carcinoma, sarcoma, fibrosarcoma, liposarcoma, leiomyoma, leiomyosarcoma, myxoma, myxosarcoma, and papillary carcinoma.

adenomyosarcoma* malignant tumor of the kidneys in young children (also called *Wilms' tumor, nephroblastoma,* and *embryoma of the kidney*).

renal cell carcinoma* malignancy of the kidneys invading all essential parts and frequently metastasizing (also called *hypernephroid carcinoma*).

transitional cell carcinoma* malignancy chiefly affecting the urinary bladder, ureters, and renal pelvis, arising from a transitional type of stratified epithelium.

SURGERY

cystectomy total or partial resection of the bladder.

cystendesis suturing of a wound of the urinary bladder.

cystidolaparotomy (sis"ti-do-lap"ah-rot'o-me) incision of the bladder through the abdominal wall.

cystidotrachelotomy (sis"ti-do-tra-kel-ot'o-me) incision of the neck of the urinary bladder (also called *cystotrachelotomy* or *cystauchenotomy*).

cystolithectomy (sis"to-li-thek'to-me) removal of a stone by incising the urinary bladder (also called *cystolithotomy*).

cystopexy (sis'to-pek"se) surgical fixation of the urinary bladder to a supporting structure such as the abdominal wall.

cystoplasty plastic repair of the bladder.

cystoproctostomy surgical communication of the posterior bladder wall to the rectum (also called *cystorectostomy*).

cystorrhaphy (sis-tor'-ah-fe) suturing of the urinary bladder.

cystostomy creation of an opening into the bladder.

cystotomy incision into the urinary bladder.

hemodialysis in cases of kidney failure, cleansing of waste from blood, using a dialysis machine, which filters the blood through a semipermeable membrane.

lithotripsy the use of shock waves to crush kidney stones, as a substitute for surgical removal.

nephrectomy (ne-frek'to-me) excision of a kidney.

nephrocapsectomy (nef"ro-kap-sek'to-me) excision of the renal capsule.

---

*Indicates a malignant condition.

*Indicates a malignant condition.

nephrocystanastomosis (nef"ro-sist"ah-nas"to-mo'sis) formation of a passage between a kidney and the urinary bladder, caused by ureteral obstruction.

nephrolithotomy (nef"ro-li-thot'o-me) removal of a kidney stone by incising the kidney.

nephropexy (nef'ro-pek"se) fixation of a floating kidney.

nephropyelolithotomy (nef"ro-pi"e-lo-li'thot'o-me) incising the substance of the kidney to remove a stone from its pelvis.

nephrorrhaphy (nef-ror'ah-fe) suturing the kidney.

nephrosplenopexy (nef"ro-sple'no-pek"se) fixation of the kidney and the spleen.

nephrostomy (ne-fros'to-me) creation of a permanent passage leading directly into the kidney pelvis.

nephrotomy (ne-frot'o-me) incision into the kidney.

nephrotresis (nef"ro-tre'sis) creating a passage into the kidney by stitching the parietal muscles to the edges of the kidney incision.

nephroureterectomy excision of the kidney and all or part of the ureter.

nephroureterocystectomy (nef"ro-u-re"ter-o-sis-tek'to-me) excision of the kidney, ureter, and a section of the wall of the bladder.

pyelocystostomosis (pi"e-lo-sis"to-sto-mo'sis) creation of a passage between the renal pelvis and the bladder (also called *pyelocystanastomosis*).

pyelolithotomy (pi"e-lo-li'thot'o-me) excision of a stone from the kidney pelvis.

pyeloplasty (pi'e-lo-plas"te) repair of the pelvis of the kidney.

pyelostomy creation of an opening into the pelvis of the kidney to temporarily divert urine away from the ureter.

pyelotomy incision of the renal pelvis.

pyeloureterolysis (pi"e-lo-u-re"ter-ol'i-sis) removal of adhesions near the attachment of the ureter and the renal pelvis.

pyeloureteroplasty plastic repair of the kidney pelvis and ureter.

ureterectomy removal of all or part of a ureter.

ureterocolostomy (u-re"ter-o-ko-los'to-me) transplantation of the ureter into the colon.

ureterocystanastomosis (u-re"ter-o-sis"tah-nas"to-mo'sis) creation of a new attachment between a ureter and the bladder (also called *ureterocystoneostomy*, *ureteroneocystostomy*, *ureterocystostomy*, and *ureterovesicostomy*).

ureteroenteroanastomosis (u-re"ter-o-en"ter-o-ah-nas"to-mo'sis) formation of an attachment between a ureter and the intestine (also called *ureteroenterostomy*).

ureterolithotomy (u-re"ter-o-li-thot'o-me) surgical incision for the removal of a calculus from a ureter.

ureterolysis freeing up of a ureter from adhesions or surrounding disease.

ureteroneopyelostomy (u-re"ter-o-ne"o-pi"e-los'to-me) excision of a urethral stricture and creation of an opening into the kidney pelvis for insertion of the newly formed end of the ureter (also called *ureteropelvioneostomy*).

ureteronephrectomy (u-re"ter-o-ne-frek'to-me) excision of an entire kidney and its ureter.

ureteroplasty (u-re"ter-o-plast"te) plastic repair of a ureter to widen a stricture.

ureteroproctostomy (u-re"ter-o-prok-tos'to-me) creation of an attachment between a ureter and the lower part of the rectum (also called *ureterorectoneostomy* and *ureterorectostomy*).

ureteropyeloneostomy (u-re"ter-o-pi"elo-ne-os'to-me) creation of a new passage to a ureter from the kidney pelvis (also called *ureteropyelostomy*).

ureteropyelonephrostomy (u-re"ter-o-pi"e-lo-ne-fros'to-me) surgical creation of an attachment between the kidney pelvis and the ureter.

ureteropyeloplasty repair of the ureter and renal pelvis.

ureterorrhaphy (u"re-ter-or'ah-fe) suturing a fistula of the ureter.

ureterosigmoidostomy insertion and attachment of a ureter into the sigmoid flexure.

ureterostomy (u"re-ter-os'to-me) creation of a passage by which a ureter may discharge its contents.

ureterotomy incision of a ureter.

ureterotrigonoenterostomy (u-re"ter-o-tri-go"no-en"ter-os'to-me) a ureter and a portion of its surrounding bladder wall, at its terminal point, is inserted and attached into the intestine.

ureterotrigonosigmoidostomy (u-re"ter-o-tri-go"no-sig"moid-os-'to-me) a ureter and a portion of its surrounding bladder wall, at its terminal point, is inserted and attached into the sigmoid flexure.

ureteroureterostomy (u-re"ter-o-u-re"ter-os'to-me) surgical end-to-end attachment of two parts of a transected ureter.

urethrectomy excision of all or part of the urethra.

urethrocystopexy (u-re"thro-sis'to-pek"se) fixation of the junction between the urethra and bladder and the bladder area above, to the back of the pubic bones, to relieve stress incontinence.

urethroplasty plastic repair of the urethra for a wound or defect.

urethrorrhaphy (u"re-thror'ah-fe) suturing of the urethra to close a urethral fistula.

urethrostomy creation of an opening passage into the urethra to relieve a stricture.

urethrotomy cutting of the urethra to relieve a stricture.

LABORATORY TESTS AND PROCEDURES

Addis count urine test to determine presence of kidney disease.

antideoxyribonuclease B blood test to determine the presence of a specific kidney disease, *poststreptococcal glomerulonephritis.*

catheterized urine specimen obtaining a urine specimen under sterile conditions, to check for microorganisms in the urinary system.

computerized tomography (CT) imaging device using x-rays at multiple angles through specific sections of the body, analyzed by computer to provide a total picture of the part being examined (also called *computerized axial tomography—CAT*).

concentration test to determine the kidney's ability to concentrate and dilute urine.

creatinine test urine test for creatinine, a metabolic product elevated in kidney function disturbance.

creatinine clearance, endogenous measure of the rate at which the kidneys remove creatinine from the blood, to evaluate kidney function.

cystogram x-ray study of the bladder.

cystoscope fiberoptic endoscope to examine the interior of the bladder.

Diodrast clearance used to evaluate kidney function: a blood test to determine the rate at which an injected substance is removed from the blood by the kidneys; and a urine test to determine the rate of excretion of the injected substance by the kidneys.

glucose urine test using paper strips impregnated with enzymes to determine the presence of glucose in the urine, (e.g., Clinistix, Diastix, and Tes-Tape)

hemoglobin urine test to determine the presence of hemoglobin in the urine, indicating an abnormal condition or disease of the urinary tract.

intravenous pyelogram (IVP) x-ray record of the kidneys and urinary tract after intravenous injection of a dye substance (also called *intravenous urography*).

magnetic resonance imaging (MRI) noninvasive method of scanning the body by use of an electromagnetic field and radio waves, which provides visual images on a computer screen and magnetic tape recordings (also called *nuclear magnetic resonance—NMR*).

nuclear magnetic resonance (NMR) see magnetic resonance imaging.

renal angiography and arteriography x-ray studies of the blood vessels surrounding the kidneys, the renal artery, and related blood vessels, after the injection of a contrast medium.

renal scan x-ray scan using intravenous injection of a radioactive substance to determine the size, shape, and exact location of the kidneys, and to diagnose abnormalities.

retrograde pyelogram x-ray record of the kidneys and urinary tract, using injection of a contrast medium directly into the bladder.

total volume measurement of urine excreted in a 24-hour period, to evaluate kidney function.

E X E R C I S E S   **THE URINARY SYSTEM** LIQUID WASTE PROCESSING

Exercise 12.1   *Complete the following:*

1. The urinary organs are __*kidneys*__, __*ureters*__, __*bladder*__, and __*urethra*__ .

2. Sectioning of the kidney shows it to have an external __*cortex*__ .

3. Sectioning of the kidney shows it to have an internal __*medulla*__ .

4. Within the renal sinus are irregular saclike structures called __*major and minor calyces*__ that collect the urine from all portions of the kidney.

5. The functional unit of the kidney is the __*nephron*__ .

6. The twisted cluster of capillary channels called the __*glomerulus*__ is contained in __*Bowman's*__ capsule.

7. The tubes extending down from the kidneys to the bladder for the passage of urine are called the __*ureters*__ .

8. The musculomembranous sac lying in the pelvis, which serves as a reservoir for urine, is called the __*bladder*__ .

9. In addition to the excretion of urine, the kidneys play a role in maintaining the __*ph*__ of the blood.

10. A __*ureteral orifice*__ prevents urine from flowing back to the ureters during bladder contraction.

11. The tube through which urine is voided in both sexes is called the __*ureter*__ .

12. The two functions of the bladder are __*storage*__ and __*excretion*__ .

Exercise 12.2   *Using the terms below, identify the parts in Figure 12.5 by placing the part name in the corresponding blank.*

Cortex	Renal artery	Ureter
Renal pyramid	Calyx (calix)	Capsule
Hilus	Renal pelvis	Papilla
Renal column	Renal vein	

1. _Cortex_
2. _hilus_
3. _renal artery_
4. _renal pelvis_
5. _renal vein_
6. _ureter_

7. _renal pyramid_
8. _renal column_
9. _calyx_
10. _papilla_
11. _capsule_

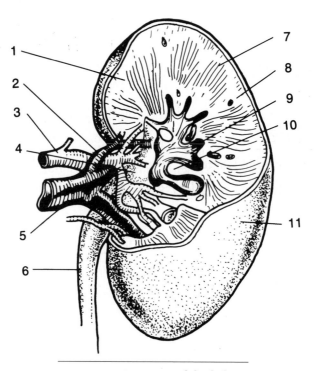

Figure 12.5 Structure of the kidney.

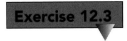

Give the meaning of the components in the following words and then define the word as a whole. Suffixes meaning *pertaining to or state or condition, shown following a slash mark (/),* are not to be defined separately. Before reaching for your medical dictionary, check the Related Terms list in this chapter.

1. Pyuria:

py ___pus___

ur/ia ___urine___

2. Balanitis:

balan ___glans penis___

itis ___inflammation___

3. Urethritis:

urethr ___urethra___

itis ___inflammation___

4. Pyelitis:

pyel ___kidney pelvis___

itis ___inflammation___

5. Cystitis:

cyst ___bladder___

itis ___inflammation___

6. Nephritis:

nephr ___kidney___

itis ___inflammation___

7. Ureteritis:

ureter ___ureter___

itis ___inflammation___

8. Nephropyelitis:

nephro ___kidney___

pyel ___kidney pelvis___

itis ___inflammation___

CROSSWORD PUZZLE

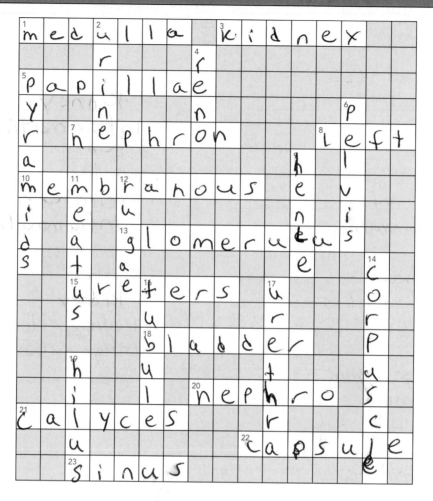

ACROSS

1. Internal part of the kidney
3. A bean-shaped organ
5. Narrow ends of cone-shaped structures
7. Functional unit of kidney
8. The longer ureter
10. One of three sections of the urethra in the male
13. Cluster of capillary channels
15. Tubes that excrete urine
18. Stores urine
20. Combining form meaning kidney

21. Irregular saclike structures that collect urine
22. Glomerular or Bowman's _____
23. Renal _____ , space into which the hilus opens

DOWN

2. Liquid waste
4. A combining form for kidney
5. Medullary _____ make up the medulla
6. Renal _____ , a funnel-shaped reservoir

9. Loop of _____
11. Urinary _____ , external opening of the urethra
12. Wrinkles or ridges in the bladder
14. Part of the functional unit of the kidney, the renal _____
16. Another part of the functional unit of the kidney, the renal _____
17. Tube from bladder to exterior of body
19. Concave depression on kidney

HIDDEN WORDS PUZZLE   CHAPTER 12

Can you find the 20 words hidden in this puzzle?
All hidden words puzzles have words running from
top to bottom, left to right, and diagonally
downward.

BLADDER

CALYCES

CAPSULE

CONVOLUTED

CORPUSCLE

CORTEX

GLOMERULUS

HILUS

KIDNEYS

MEATUS

MEDULLA

NEPHRON

PROSTATIC

PYRAMIDS

RENAL

RUGAE

TUBULE

URETERS

URETHRA

URINARY

```
D W S G L O M E R U L U S O
Q I L C A P S U L E R C Z U
Y I H O O E K M L E Z H B Q
B I L R P R O S T A T I C B
G Y F P R P T E X G U D U B
X N U U C M R E V U R L O H
Y O T S N S X T X R E N A L
K R P C O N V O L U T E D P
R H Y L N K K L H U H F J V
D P R E H X B I B R R J F L
M E A T U S L U D I A S P Y
C N M E D U L L A N M M X Q
S N I V S E Y M C A E W T T
Q B D B L A D D E R A Y E E
S L S L T V C A L Y C E S Q
```

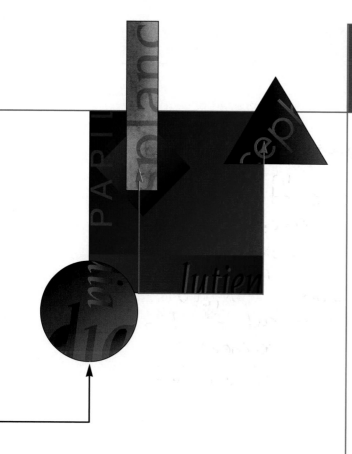

The Reproductive System

the cycle of life

In this chapter the reproductive systems and their structures and functions in both sexes are presented and discussed.

THE MALE REPRODUCTIVE ORGANS

The basic male reproductive organs *(gonads)* are the *testes.* The accessory organs are ducts, glands, and supporting structures. The ducts are the *epididymides, vas deferens, ejaculatory ducts,* and the urethra. The glands are the *seminal vesicles, prostate,* and *bulbourethral (Cowper's)* glands, with the *penis, scrotum,* and *spermatic cords* functioning as supporting structures (Figure 13.1).

The Testes

The *testes,* or *testicles,* are a pair of egg-shaped glands normally located in a saclike structure called the *scrotum.* Each testicle is enclosed in a fibrous white capsule that continues into the gland to divide it into nu-

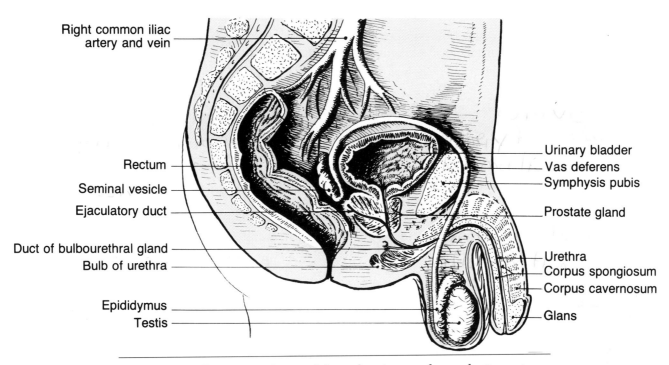

Figure 13.1 Midline sectional view of the male urinary and reproductive systems.

merous conical *lobules,* or compartments, each of which contains one or more coiled *seminiferous tubules* and *interstitial cells (Leydig cells).* The seminiferous tubules join into a cluster from which several ducts emerge and enter the head of the *epididymis.*

The testes have two functions, producing *spermatozoa* (sperm cells, the male reproductive cells; singular—*spermatozoon*) and secreting hormones. The sperm cells are produced by the seminiferous tubules. The chief hormone *testosterone* is an *androgen* (male sex hormone) that is secreted by the Leydig cells, which are specialized interstitial cells. Testosterone has several functions. It induces and maintains male secondary sex characteristics, such as hair growth and pitch of voice, as well as having an influence on growth of muscles and bones, accounting in part for the observed sex differences. Testosterone has an influence on general, as well as fluid and electrolyte metabolism, has an excitatory effect on kidney tubule reabsorption, and suppresses anterior pituitary secretion of gonadotropins.

The Epididymis

The *epididymides* (singular—*epididymis*), a pair of tightly coiled, tubelike structures, each about 20 feet

(6 m), lie along the posterior borders of each testis. The functions of each epididymis are to serve as a passageway for sperm from the testis to the body surface, store sperm before ejaculation, and secrete a part of the *semen* (seminal fluid).

The Vas Deferens (Ductus Deferens)

The *vas deferens* are a pair of tubes, each about ⅛ inch (0.3 cm) in diameter, a continuation of the epididymis. The vas extends from the epididymis up through the inguinal canal, where it is encased by the *spermatic cord,* into the abdominal cavity and down the posterior of the bladder where it connects with the seminal vesicle duct and forms the *ejaculatory duct.* The function of the vas deferens is to act as a duct for the testis and connect the epididymis with the ejaculatory duct.

The Ejaculatory Ducts

The *ejaculatory ducts* are two short tubes formed by the joining of the vas deferens with the ducts of the seminal vesicles. They pass through the prostate gland and extend to the urethra.

The Seminal Vesicles

The *seminal vesicles* are two twisted pouches lying along the lower posterior surface of the bladder, in front of the rectum. They secrete the mucid, liquid part of the semen, and prostaglandins.

The Prostate Gland

The *prostate gland* is composed of smooth muscle and glandular tissue, is doughnut shaped, about the size of a large walnut, and surrounds the urethra. The prostate secretes a viscous, alkaline substance that makes up most of the seminal fluid (semen). The alkalinity protects the sperm from acid present in the urethra of the male and the vagina of the female and increases its motility.

The Bulbourethral Glands

The *bulbourethral (Cowper's)* glands are two rounded, pea-sized bodies below the prostate gland, on either side of the membranous part of the urethra, and connected to it by a duct about 1 inch (2.5 cm) in length. These glands secrete an alkaline substance that has a protective action similar to that of the prostate secretion.

The Scrotum

The *scrotum* is a saclike, skin-covered structure that hangs from the perineal area. It is separated into two sacs internally, each containing one testis, one epididymis, and the inferior part of a spermatic cord.

The Penis

The *penis* is made up of three rounded masses of cavernous (erectile) tissue, encased in individual fibrous coats, and held together by an outer skin covering. The *glans penis (balanus)*, a slight bulge at the distal end of the penis, is covered with a retractable, loose, double fold of skin, the *prepuce (foreskin).*

The penis contains the urethra, which carries both reproductive tract secretions and urine, and is the organ by means of which sperm are introduced into the vagina.

The Spermatic Cords

The *spermatic cords* are formed of white fibrous tissue, encasing the vas deferens, blood and lymph vessels, and nerves. They are located in the *inguinal* (groin) *canals*, between the scrotum and abdominal cavity.

REVIEW 13.A

Complete the following:

1. The basic male reproductive organs are the
   testes .

2. The two functions of the male reproductive organs are *produce spermatozoa* and *secrete hormones* .

3. The coiled, tubelike passages for sperm, from the testes to the body surface, are the *epididymides* .

4. The doughnut-shaped, walnut-sized gland in the male reproductive system is the *prostate* .

5. The vas deferens are encased by the *spematic cords* .

THE FEMALE REPRODUCTIVE ORGANS

The basic female reproductive organs (gonads) are a pair of *ovaries.* The accessory organs consist of an internal group that include a pair of *fallopian (uterine) tubes* or *oviducts*, a *uterus*, and a *vagina*, and an external group consisting of the *vulva* (external *genitalia*) and a pair of *mammary glands* (breasts) (Figures 13.2 and 13.3).

The Ovaries

The adult *ovaries* are two almond-shaped and sized glands located on each side of the uterus, behind and below the *fallopian tubes.* Each ovary is connected to the uterus by a ligament. The end of each fallopian tube is suspended over the corresponding ovary so that the *fimbriated* (fingerlike) end of the tube does not come in contact with the ovary, making it a gland with an unattached duct (see Figure 13.2).

Structure. A single layer of epithelial cells forms the ovarian surface. The interior consists primarily of a network of connective tissue, in which are embedded countless numbers of microscopic formations, called *follicles*, containing *ova* (eggs) the female sex cells (singular—*ovum*) in different stages of development.

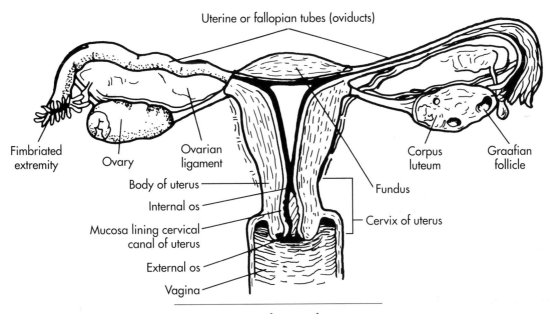

Figure 13.2 Female reproductive tract.

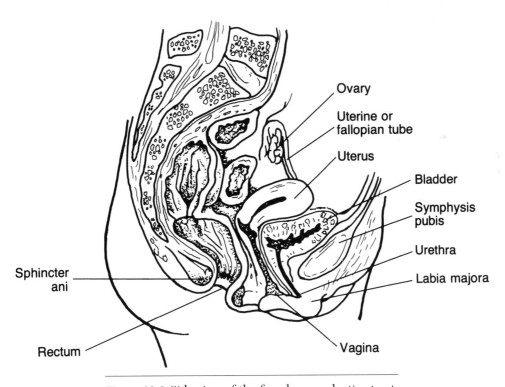

Figure 13.3 Side view of the female reproductive tract.

Functions. The functions of the ovaries are ovulation and hormonal secretion. The ova develop in the ovaries, and when an ovum matures, it is expelled by the ovary to be caught up by the fimbriated end of the fallopian tube over that ovary.

Estrogen and *progesterone* are the ovarian hormones. Estrogen is also produced in the adrenal cortex (male and female), the testes (male), and the fetal-placental unit (during pregnancy), and has a variety of functions in both sexes.

Ovarian estrogen has several functions. It induces the development of the female secondary sex characteristics and the cyclic (menstrual) changes in the uterus in preparation for the implantation and developmental support of a fertilized ovum. Progesterone, which is produced in the adrenal cortex and in the *corpus luteum* of the ovary and the placenta, also prepares the uterus to receive and nurture the fertilized ovum, in addition to having an effect on the female secondary sex characteristics.

The Fallopian (Uterine) Tubes

Structure. There are two fallopian tubes, each about 4 inches (10 cm) in length, consisting of an inner, ciliated mucous membrane layer; a middle, smooth layer; and an outer layer of serous tissue. The proximal ends of the fallopian tubes are attached to the uterus, and the distal ends, the *infundibula* (singular—*infundibulum*), are funnel shaped, with fringed, fingerlike processes called *fimbriae.* The fimbriated ends are suspended over, but not attached to, or touching, the ovaries (see Figure 13.2).

Function. The fallopian tubes act as ducts to the uterus for the ova produced by the ovaries. Normally, *fertilization* (ovum and sperm cell union) takes place in a fallopian tube.

The Uterus

The *uterus* is a thick-walled, hollow, pear-shaped organ (*metro-* and *hystero-* refer to the uterus), lying in the pelvic cavity between the bladder and rectum. The upper portion of the uterus, the *body,* has a rounded swelling, just above and between the entry points of the fallopian tubes, called the *fundus.* The lower, narrower portion of the uterus is the *cervix* (neck). The opening from the cervix of the uterus into the cervical canal is called the *internal os* (mouth or opening) and the opening from the cervical canal into the vagina is called the *external os* (see Figures 13.2 and 13.3).

Structure. The uterine walls are formed of three layers. The internal lining is a specialized epithelial mucous membrane called the *endometrium.* The middle layer, the *myometrium,* is formed of layers of smooth muscle, extending diagonally, crosswise, and lengthwise. The external layer, the *perimetrium,* is an extension of the parietal peritoneum serous membrane, which covers only the upper two thirds of the body of the uterus.

Functions. The uterus has several functions. During pregnancy the uterus maintains and supports the developing fetus. In labor the uterus completes childbirth by contracting and evacuating its contents. *Menstruation* provides a way to clear the uterus and build a fresh environment for a fertilized ovum.

The Vagina

The *vagina* is located in front of the rectum and behind the urethra and bladder, extending from the cervix of the uterus to the external genitalia (see Figure 13.3).

Structure. The vagina is an extremely elastic tube of smooth muscle, lined with a mucous membrane forming rugae. It is approximately 4 inches (10 cm) long at the back of the tube and 3 inches (8 cm) long at the front, because of the protrusion of the cervix into the upper portion of the anterior wall. In the virginal condition the external vaginal orifice may be partly occluded (blocked) by a fold of mucous membrane, the *hymen.*

Functions. The functions of the vagina in reproduction are to receive the fluid of the male sex organ and to provide passage out of the body for the menstrual flow, secretions of the uterus, and the neonate at birth.

The Vulva

The *vulva,* or external genitalia, includes the *mons pubis, labia majora, labia minora, clitoris, vaginal orifice,* and *Bartholin's* (or *greater vestibular*) *glands* (Figure 13.4).

The *mons pubis* is a pad of fat located in front of the *symphysis pubis,* which is covered by skin until after puberty, when hair grows in the area.

The *labia majora* (large lips) are two folds of fat-filled skin, covered with hair after puberty, and extending backward from the mons pubis. Within these two folds of skin are two smaller folds of thin-skinned mucous membrane called the *labia minora* (small lips), which unite anteriorly to enclose the clitoris, and contain numerous sebaceous glands in their lateral and medial surfaces. The area between the labia minora is known as the *vestibule.*

The *clitoris* is an organ formed of erectile tissue, located beneath the point of union of the labia minora, similar in structure to the glans penis of the male, and also covered with a prepuce (foreskin).

The *vaginal orifice* is located posterior to the urinary meatus. (Although the urinary meatus is located between the clitoris and the vaginal orifice, it is not a genital organ in the female.)

Bartholin's (greater vestibular) *glands* are two pea-sized mucus glands, on each side of the vaginal orifice, that secrete a lubricant.

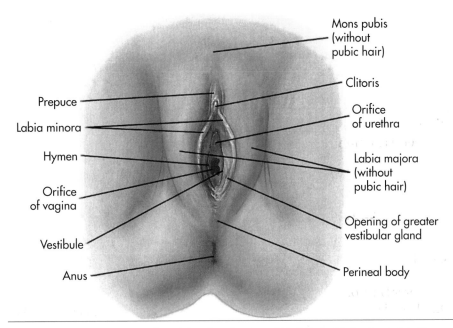

Mons pubis
(without
pubic hair)

Clitoris

Prepuce

Orifice
of urethra

Labia minora

Hymen

Labia majora
(without
pubic hair)

Orifice
of vagina

Opening of greater
vestibular gland

Vestibule

Anus

Perineal body

Figure 13.4 External genitalia of the female. (Modified from Thibodeau GA, Patton KT: *Anatomy and physiology,* ed 3, St Louis, 1996, Mosby, p 1017.)

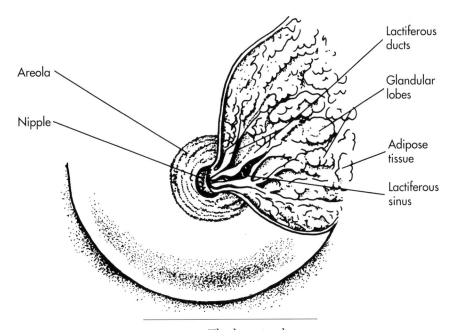

Lactiferous
ducts

Glandular
lobes

Areola

Nipple

Adipose
tissue

Lactiferous
sinus

Figure 13.5 The lactating breast.

The muscular, skin-covered area between the vaginal orifice and anus is called the *perineum.*

The Mammary Glands (Breasts)

The *mammary glands* (breasts) are the milk-producing glandular structures located over the pectoral muscles of the thorax, whose development is controlled by estrogen and progesterone, two hormones secreted by the ovaries.

Structure. Each breast is composed of connective and adipose tissue in lobes and lobules with milk-secreting cells around a duct. The individual ducts join with others to form larger ducts, which circle the nipple, ending in minute openings on the nipple surface. The halo of pigment surrounding the nipple is called the *areola* (Figure 13.5).

Function. The only function of the mammaries is to produce milk for the feeding of the neonate. Milk production is stimulated by the lactogenic hormone prolactin produced by the anterior lobe of the pituitary gland.

REVIEW 13.B

Complete the following:

1. The basic female reproductive organs are the
   ___ovaries___ .

2. Microscopic ___follicles___
   contain ova in different stages of development.

3. The rounded swelling at the top of the body of
   the uterus is called the ___fundus___ .

4. The smooth muscled, elastic tube extending
   from the uterine cervix to the external
   genitalia is the ___vagina___ .

5. The halo of pigment around the nipple is
   called the ___areola___ .

THE MENSTRUAL CYCLE

In the human female, secondary sex characteristics begin to develop and the ability to sexually reproduce is achieved at puberty, which may occur as early as age 9 and as late as age 16.

The onset of *menstruation* (also called *menarche*) occurs at puberty and normally continues for approximately 40 years, with variations caused by heredity, diet, and other factors. Cessation of menstruation is known as *menopause* (also called *climacteric*).

The female reproductive system undergoes cyclical changes about every 28 days to prepare the uterus to receive a fertilized ovum. At the beginning of each monthly menstrual cycle (*men-* means month), ova within the *graafian follicles* in the ovaries begin to develop. The follicles secrete estrogen and progesterone. One graafian follicle ruptures (*ovulation*), and its ovum is expelled from the ovary to the uterine tube. The ruptured follicle grows larger, filling with a yellow lipoid material, and becomes the *corpus luteum* (yellow body). The corpus luteum also secretes estrogen and progesterone. If fertilization occurs, the corpus luteum will continue to secrete these hormones. If fertilization does not take place, these secretions will slowly diminish and the reduced levels of the hormones will lead to a new menstrual cycle. This cycle of *menstruation* can be divided into four stages.

Stages of Menstruation

The stages of menstruation are the *menses* (menstrual period), the *postmenstrual* (preovulatory, proliferative, or follicular) stage, *ovulation,* and the *premenstrual* (postovulatory) stage, with individual variations as to time span (Figure 13.6).

Menses. The menstrual period occurs on days 1 through 5, during which the disintegrated endometrial lining of the uterus is sloughed off and evacuated with blood and other secretions through the vagina.

Postmenstrual stage. The endometrial lining of the uterus, which was sloughed off during the menses, builds up under the influence of the ovarian hormone estrogen, and the ova within the graafian follicles also grow at this time. This stage usually lasts from days 6 through 13.

Ovulation. Ovulation normally takes place midway between menstrual periods, on days 14 and 15, although the precise day is uncertain and is dependent on the postmenstrual phase. In the ovary the mature graafian follicle ruptures and the ovum is released and expelled into the fallopian tube.

Premenstrual stage. During the premenstrual stage, from days 15 through 28, the corpus luteum secretes progesterone and estrogen, which help to prepare the uterus to receive a fertilized ovum. If pregnancy does not occur, a new cycle will begin.

PREGNANCY

At conception the ovum is normally penetrated by one sperm cell while it is in the fallopian tube. After fertilization, the fertilized ovum begins to form a rounded mass of cells and slowly moves from the tube into the uterus, where it attaches itself to the endometrial lining and begins to develop. The *embryonic stage* lasts from the second through the eighth week of pregnancy, and the developing organism is called an *embryo.* The inner cells of the rounded cell mass form the embryo and its *amnion,* which is the thin, clear sac filled with *amniotic fluid* in which the embryo floats. The outer cells of the rounded cell mass (*chorion*) help to form the *placenta,* along with the endometrium of the uterus.

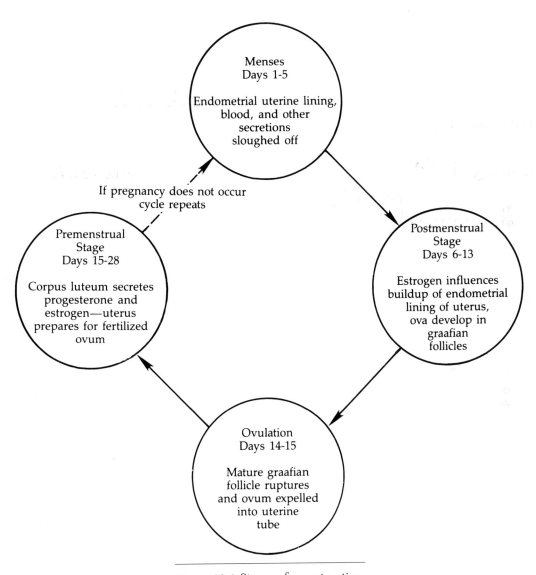

Figure 13.6 Stages of menstruation.

The placenta is the only connection between the mother and the developing *fetus.* The *fetal stage* lasts from the end of the eighth week until birth. Although the maternal and fetal circulations are independent of each other, the placenta carries nutrients, oxygen, and antibodies from the maternal blood to that of the fetus and carries fetal metabolic waste back to the maternal blood for disposal. The placenta secretes estrogen, progesterone, and *human chorionic gonadotropin (HCG),* which stimulates ovarian secretion of estrogen and progesterone.

REVIEW 13.C

Complete the following:

1. The onset of menstruation is called **menarche** .

2. The cessation of menstruation is called **climacteric** .

3. The menstrual stages are **menses, post menstrual, pre menstrual** .

4. The **embryonic** stage lasts from the second through the eighth week of pregnancy.

5. The only connection between the mother and the fetus is the **placenta** .

RELATED TERMS THE REPRODUCTIVE SYSTEM THE CYCLE OF LIFE

ANATOMY

Male Reproductive Organs and Associated Terms

bulbourethral glands glands located on either side of the urethra whose alkaline secretion has a protective function for sperm (also called *Cowper's glands*).

corpora cavernosa penis (kor'po-rah kav"er-no'sah) columns of erectile tissue of the penis, forming the sides and posterior portion that attaches to the pubic bone.

corpus spongiosum penis (kor'pus spun"je-o'sum) column of erectile tissue surrounding the urethra.

ejaculatory ducts two short tubes formed by the joining of the vas deferens and the ducts of the seminal vesicles, which pass through the prostate and extend to the urethra.

epididymis (ep"i-did'i-mis) pair of tightly coiled tube-like structures that secrete a part of the semen, serve as storage areas for sperm before ejaculation, and provide passageways for sperm from the testes to the body surface (plural—*epididymides*).

glans penis slight bulge at the distal end of the penis (also called *balanus*).

Leydig cells (li'dig) specialized interstitial cells that secrete the male sex hormone testosterone.

penis the male sex organ, containing the urethra, which carries both reproductive tract secretions and urine to the body surface.

prepuce (pre'puse) retractable, double fold of skin, covering the glans penis (also called *foreskin*).

prostate doughnut-shaped, walnut-sized gland surrounding the urethra, secreting a thick alkaline substance that makes up most of the seminal fluid.

scrotum (skro'tum) saclike, skin-covered structure, hanging from the perineal area, containing the testes, epididymides, and part of the spermatic cords.

semen thick, whitish secretion discharged by the male reproductive organs, containing the spermatozoa.

seminal vesicles two twisted pouches lying along the lower posterior surface of the bladder, in front of the rectum, which secrete the liquid part of semen, and prostaglandins.

seminiferous tubules (se"mi-nif'er-us) coiled tubules within the testes that produce sperm cells.

Sertoli's cells (ser"to'lez) cells in the testis that support and nourish the sperm germ cells.

spermatic cords white, fibrous tissue encasing the vas deferens, blood and lymph vessels, and nerves.

spermatid (sper'mah-tid) germ cell developing into a spermatozoon (also called *spermatoblast*).

spermatozoa (sper"mah-to-zo'ah) male reproductive (sperm) cells (singular—*spermatozoon*).

testis (tes'tis) egg-shaped male gland (also called *testicle*), that produces spermatozoa and secretes hormones (*orchis* refers to testis).

vas deferens excretory duct of the testis that joins the epididymis with the ejaculatory duct (also called *ductus deferens*).

Female Reproductive Organs and Associated Terms

areola (ah-re'o-lah) pigmented halo around the breast nipple.

Bartholin's glands (bar'to-linz) two pea-sized glands, one on each side of the vaginal orifice, which secrete a lubricant (also called *greater vestibular glands*).

cervix (ser'viks) neck of the uterus.

climacteric menopause.

clitoris (kli'to-ris) small mound of erectile tissue located beneath the point of union of the labia minora, similar to the penis, and also covered with a prepuce.

corpus (kor'pus) body (plural—*corpora*).

corpus cavernosum clitoridis (ka-ver-no'sum klitor'id-is) one of the two columns of erectile tissue that form the clitoris.

corpus luteum (lu'te-um) yellow body formed by the graafian follicle that has discharged its ovum (*luteum* means yellow).

ectopic pregnancy (ek-top'ik) fertilized ovum implanted outside uterus, most commonly in a uterine tube (*ectopic* means out of normal position).

endocervix mucous membrane lining the cervical canal, and/or the opening of the cervix into the uterus.

endometrium (en-do-me'tre-um) mucous membrane lining the uterus.

estrus cyclical period relating to sexual activity.

fallopian tubes pair of tubes extending from the uterus to the ovary on each side, which pick up and convey expelled ova to the uterus (also called *uterine tubes* and *oviducts*).

fimbria (fim'bre-ah) fringed fingerlike processes at the ends of the fallopian (uterine) tubes over the ovaries.

graafian follicles (graf'e-an) mature ovarian follicles.

hymen fold of mucous membrane partially blocking vaginal orifice.

labia majora (la'be-ah ma-jo'rah) two folds of skin that extend backward from the mons pubis.

labia minora two smaller folds of thin-skinned mucous membrane within the labia majora.

mammary glands breasts (also called *mammae*).

menopause (men'o-pawz) cessation of menstruation (also called *climacteric*).

menstruation (men"stroo-a'shun) flow of blood, tissue, and other secretions, evacuated through vagina, occurring monthly, after puberty, when an ovum has not been fertilized (*mensis* means month).

mons pubis (monz pu'bus) pad of fat located in front of the symphysis pubis.

myometrium (mi-o-me'tre-um) middle, muscular coat of the uterus.

oocyte immature ovum.

os mouth; the *internal os* is the opening from the cervix into the cervical canal, and the *external os* is the opening from the cervical canal into the vagina.

ovary female gland that produces ova (eggs).

ovum female reproductive cell (plural—*ova*).

pudendum (pu-den'dum) human external genitalia, especially referring to females.

Skene's gland (skenz) two ducts just within the meatus of the urethra that drain a particular group of glands into the vestibule (also called *paraurethral glands*).

uterus thick-walled, hollow, pear-shaped organ in the pelvic cavity of the female, that houses and nourishes the embryo and fetus.

Pregnancy and Associated Terms

amnion (am′ne-on) membrane containing the fetus floating in amniotic fluid.

chorion (ko′re-on) outermost layer of the fertilized ovum that helps form the placenta.

cyesis (si-e′sis) pregnancy (*cyema* means embryo).

decidua (de-sid′u-ah) mucosa of the uterus thrown off after birth.

ectoderm outer of three germ layers of the embryo.

embryo developing stage of an organism, from the second through the eighth week in humans.

endoderm innermost of three germ layers of the embryo (also called *entoderm*).

fetus developing offspring, from the end of the eighth week until birth in humans.

gravid (grav′id) pregnant.

gravida (grav′i-dah) pregnant female, referred to as gravida I in the first pregnancy, gravida II in the second pregnancy, and so forth.

lactiferous ducts (lak-tif′er-us) ducts that carry the milk secretions of the breast to and through the nipples (also called *galactophorous ducts*).

mesoderm middle of three germ layers of the embryo, lying between the ectoderm and the endoderm.

neonate newborn.

omphalus (om′fah-lus) see *umbilicus*.

para female who has produced living young (para I, para II, para III designate one, two, and three pregnancies, respectively, and so forth.).

parturition (par″tu-rish′un) process of giving birth.

placenta (plah-sen′tah) vascular fetal organ within the uterus that connects the fetus to the mother by way of the umbilical cord, for the exchange of nutrients, oxygen, antibodies, and waste products.

presentation the presenting part of the fetus, at birth.

primigravida female during her first pregnancy (also called *gravida I*).

primipara female who has had one pregnancy that resulted in viable young, or who is giving birth for the first time (also called *para I*).

umbilical cord communicating channel between the placenta and fetus.

umbilicus (um-bil′i-kus) scar that marks the site of the connection of the umbilical cord in the fetus (also called *navel* and *omphalus*).

zygote (zi-got) fertilized ovum.

PATHOLOGIC CONDITIONS

Inflammation and Infections

bartholinitis inflammation of Bartholin's gland.

cervicitis inflammation of the mucous membrane tissues of the uterine cervix, with frequent involvement of deeper tissues.

chronic cystic mastitis inflammation of the breast with fluid-filled cyst formation (also called *fibrocystic disease of the breast*).

decidual endometritis (de-sid′u-al en″do-me-tri′tis) inflammation of the decidual endometrial membranes of the uterus during pregnancy.

endometritis (en′do-me-tri′tis) inflammation of the endometrium.

epididymitis inflammation of the epididymis.

mammillitis (mam″i-li′tis) inflammation of the nipple.

mastadenitis (mas″tad-e-ni′tis) inflammation of the breast (also called *mastitis*).

metritis (me-tri′tis) inflammation of the uterus.

metroperitonitis (me″tro-per′i-to-ni′tis) inflammation of the peritoneum around the uterus.

metrophlebitis (me″tro-fle-bi′tis) inflammation of the uterine veins.

metrosalpingitis (me″tro-sal″pin-ji′tis) inflammation of the uterus and fallopian tubes.

myometritis (mi″o-me-tri′tis) inflammation of the uterine wall muscles.

oophoritis (o″of-o-ri′tis) ovarian inflammation.

oophorosalpingitis (o-of″o-ro-sal″pin-ji′tis) inflammation of an ovary and fallopian tube.

orchitis inflammation of one or both testicles.

perioophoritis inflammation of the covering of the ovary.

priapism persistent erection of penis, related to excessive amounts of androgens or to disease.

priapitis inflammation of penis.

prostatitis inflammation of the prostate gland.

pyocolpos (pi″o-kol′pos) accumulation of pus in the vagina.

pyometra (pi″o-me′trah) collection of pus in the uterine cavity.

pyosalpinx (pi″o-sal′pinks) accumulation of pus in a fallopian tube.

salpingitis (sal″pin-ji′tis) inflammation of a fallopian tube.

seminal vesiculitis inflammation of a seminal vesicle.

vaginitis inflammation of the vagina.

vulvitis inflammation of the vulva.

Sexually Transmitted Diseases (STDs)

This category covers diseases transmitted by sexual contact, formerly referred to as venereal diseases.

acquired immune deficiency syndrome (AIDS) see listing under the immune system (Chapter 17).

bacterial vaginitis vaginal infection caused by *Haemophilus vaginalis* or *Gardnerella vaginalis*, characterized by discharge, itching, and pain on urination.

chlamydia highly contagious, common infection, caused by *Chlamydia trachomatis* bacterium. A major cause of infection of the cervix and fallopian tubes, which, if untreated, may result in pelvic inflammatory disease (PID). Also may be transmitted to newborns in the birth canal, resulting in eye and ear, and possibly fatal lung, infections.

condyloma acuminatum (kon"di-lo'mah ah-ku"mi-nah'tum) infectious wart or papilloma, caused by the *human papilloma virus (HPV)*, a common STD source (see **carcinoma of cervix** entry under Oncology later in this chapter), usually found on the external genitalia, cervix, vagina, or anus (also called *venereal wart* and *genital wart*).

genital candidiasis fungal infection caused by *Candida albicans*, usually affecting moist cutaneous area, especially the vagina (also called *monilia* and *candidosis*).

gonorrhea (gon"o-re'ah) second most common STD, a contagious infection of genital mucous membranes by the gonoccocus *Neisseria gonorrhoeae*, usually contracted through sexual intercourse, but can be acquired by contact with exudates. It is a major cause of pelvic inflammatory disease *(PID)*.

herpes genitalis infection caused by the herpesvirus marked by clusters of herpes simplex vesicles on the genitalia, with no known cure (also called *genital herpes*). Treatment is palliative.

lymphogranuloma venereum (lim"fo-gran"u-lo'mah ve-ne're-um) infection usually caused by *Chlamydia trachomatis* bacteria (now considered the most common source of sexually transmitted diseases [STDs]), characterized by genital ulcerative lesions and hypertrophy of inguinal lymph nodes (also called *lymphopathia venereum* and *lymphogranuloma inguinale*).

pelvic inflammatory disease (PID) a bacterial infection usually caused by gonorrhea or *Chlamydia trachomatis*, with inflammation of fallopian tubes, ovaries, or other structures found in the pelvic cavity; a common cause of sterility.

syphilis acute, contagious infection caused by the spirochete *Treponema pallidum*, with a first symptom of chancre sore, progressing through primary, secondary, and tertiary stages. The latter involves many organ systems, such as the integumentary, skeletal, cardiovascular, and central nervous systems.

trichomoniasis (trik"o-mo-ni'ah-sis) protozoan infection, usually producing a leukorrhea of the vagina and vulva.

Hereditary, Congenital, and Developmental Disorders

anorchism (an-or'kizm) absence of one or both testes.

atresia of vagina (ah-tre'za-ah) absence of vaginal opening.

bifid clitoris clitoris divided into two parts.

cryptorchism (krip-tor'kizm) testes do not descend into the scrotum (also called *cryptorchidism*).

ectopia of testis one or both testes misplaced in other location.

hermaphroditism (her-maf'ro-di'tizm) individual having both ovarian and testicular tissue.

hypoplasia of cervix underdevelopment of the cervix.

ovotestis gonad that contains both ovarian and testicular tissue (see *hermaphroditism*).

polymastia more than two breasts.

polyorchism more than two testes.

polythelia more than the normal number of nipples, on the breast or elsewhere on the body.

pseudohermaphroditism presence of gonads of one sex, with physical characteristics of both sexes.

rudimentary uterus underdeveloped or imperfectly developed uterus.

supernumerary more than the normal number; referring, for example, to nipples, ovaries, or fallopian tubes.

synorchism (sin'or-kizm) the testes are fused together in the abdomen rather than the scrotum (also called *synorchidism*).

Other Abnormalities

abruptio placentae placenta that separates prematurely.

adenomyosis of the uterus (ad"e-no-mi-o'sis) benign invasion of the endometrium into the muscle wall of the uterus.

amenorrhea (ah-men"o-re'ah) absence of the menses.

aspermatogenesis (ah-sper"mah-to-jen'e-sis) failure to develop spermatozoa.

aspermia (ah-sper'me-ah) failure to form or emit semen.

benign prostatic hyperplasia enlargement of the prostate gland.

corpus hemorrhagicum blood clot in a corpus luteum, or blood in an ovarian follicle.

displacement of uterus retroflexion, retroversion, or anteflexion of the uterus.

dysmenorrhea (dis"men-o-re'ah) painful menstruation.

dyspareunia (dis"pah-roo'ne-ah) painful coitus (sexual intercourse or copulation) in women.

gynecomastia (jin"e-ko-mas'te-ah) unusual enlargement of male breast.

hematocele (hem'ah-to-sel) effusion of blood into a body cavity, canal, or part, such as the scrotum, testis, pelvis, or pudendum.

hematocolpos (hem"ah-to-kol'pos) menstrual blood collected in the vagina because of obstruction.

hematometra (hem"ah-to-me'trah) blood collected in the uterine cavity.

hematosalpinx (hem"ah-to-sal-pinks) blood collected in a fallopian tube.

hydatidiform mole (hi"dah-tid'i-form) abnormal pregnancy, with a mass of cystic tissue in the uterus resembling a bunch of grapes.

hydrocele collection of fluid in a testis.

hydrorrhea gravidarum (hi"dro-re'ah gra"vi-dah'rum) discharge of thin, watery fluid from the pregnant uterus.

hyperplasia of the endometrium overdevelopment of the lining of the uterus.

hysterolith (his'ter-o-lith) stone, or calculus, in the uterus.

hysterorrhexis (his"ter-o-rek'sis) rupture of the uterus (also called *metrorrhexis*).

impotence inability, in the male, to achieve or sustain penile erection.

kraurosis vulvae (kraw-ro'sis) shriveling of the skin of the vagina and vulva.

lactation secretion of milk.

leukorrhea (lu"ko-re'ah) whitish discharge from the vagina.

lithopedion (lith'o-pe'de-on) calcified dead fetus out of the uterus.

mammalgia (mam-mal'je-ah) pain in the breast (also called *mastalgia* and *mastodynia*).

mastoptosis (mas"to-to'sis) pendulous breast.

mastorrhagia (mas"to-ra'je-ah) hemorrhage from the breast.

menometrorrhagia (men"o-met"ro-ra'je-ah) excessive uterine bleeding during and between menstrual periods.

menorrhagia (men"o-ra'je-ah) profuse menstruation.

menoschesis (men"o-ske'sis, men-os'ke-sis) suppression of the menses.

menostasis (men-os'tah-sis) amenorrhea or absense of menses.

metratrophia (me"trah-tro'fe-ah) atrophy of the uterus.

metrorrhagia (me"tro-ra"je-ah) abnormal uterine bleeding, especially between menstrual periods.

metrostenosis (me"tro-ste-no'sis) narrowing of the uterine cavity.

nabothian cyst (nah-bo'the-an) cystlike formation in a nabothian gland (one of many small mucus-secreting glands) of the uterine cervix.

oligohydramnios (ol'i-go-hi-dram'ne-os) presence of less than normal amount of amniotic fluid.

oligomenorrhea (ol"i-go-men"o-re'ah) scanty menstruation.

oligospermia (ol"i-go-sper'me-ah) diminished amount of spermatozoa in the semen.

parovarian cyst cyst located beside the ovary.

phimosis (fi-mo'sis) constriction of the skin of the prepuce over the glans penis.

placenta accreta abnormal form of placenta adherence to the uterine wall.

placenta bipartita bilobate placenta.

placenta circumvallata cup-shaped placenta.

placenta previa placenta that develops in the lower segment of the uterus.

placenta tripartita trilobate placenta.

premenstrual syndrome (PMS) cyclical disorder involving physical and emotional symptoms preceding menstrual period, with fatigue, edema, tension, irritability, and depression.

prolapse of uterus protrusion of the uterus through the vaginal orifice.

prostatic hypertrophy enlargement of the prostate.

pruritus vulvae (proo-ri′tus) intense itching of the vulva.

puerperal eclampsia convulsions occurring in the female following delivery, associated with high blood pressure, edema, and protein in the urine.

salpingocele (sal-ping′go-sel) hernia of a fallopian tube.

salpingo-oophorocele (sal-ping″go-oof′or-o-sel) hernia of both an ovary and a fallopian tube.

spermatocele (sper′mah-to-sel) epididymal cyst with sperm cells.

spermaturia (sper″mah-tu′re-ah) discharge of semen in urine (also called *seminuria*).

spontaneous abortion premature discharge of an embryo or nonviable fetus from the uterus.

Stein-Leventhal syndrome female disorder characterized by facial hair, overweight, and infrequent or absent menstrual periods, caused by adrenal gland malfunction or excessive androgen secretion of the ovaries.

sterility inability to reproduce.

vaginismus (vaj″i-niz′mus) painful spasm of the vagina.

varicocele (var′i-ko-sel) varicose condition of the veins of the spermatic plexus that causes a swelling to form in the scrotum.

velamentous placenta placenta in which the umbilical cord is attached to the adjoining membranes.

Oncology*

The following list pertains only to tumors of the reproductive system, although other benign and malignant tumors, which occur in other parts of the body, also occur in the reproductive system. Some of these are fibrosarcomas, fibromas, adenocarcinomas, sarcomas, lipomas, medullary carcinomas, and lymphangiomas.

arrhenoblastoma (ah-re″no-blas-to′mah) ovarian neoplasm sometimes causing secondary male sex characteristics.

Brenner tumor ovarian tumor consisting of groups of epithelial cells lying in fibrous connective tissue.

carcinoma of cervix* malignant, epithelial tissue neoplasm, believed to be caused by the papilloma virus (STD-producing virus), also suspect in cancers of the vagina, vulva, and penis.

choriocarcinoma* highly malignant tumor that invades the myometrium and blood vessels (also called *chorioepithelioma*).

cystadenoma (sis″tad-e-no′mah) benign ovarian cystic tumor, with serous or pseudomucinous fluid.

dysgerminoma* (dis″jer-mi-no′mah) rare, malignant ovarian neoplasm derived from undifferentiated gonadal germ cells.

fibroadenoma benign tumor, of several different types, involving the mammary gland.

granulosa cell tumor* ovarian tumor, benign or malignant, that begins in the graafian follicle, and may produce estrogen, creating endometrial hyperplasia.

neomammary carcinoma* malignant tumor of breast (also called *medullary carcinoma*).

Paget's disease of the nipple* malignant tumor of the nipple, usually associated with deeper carcinomas.

prostatic carcinoma* malignant tumor of the prostate gland, with growth stimulated by male hormones, especially testosterone.

sclerosing adenosis benign nodular lesion of the breast, which may resemble carcinoma microscopically.

seminoma* malignant testicular tumor, similar to dysgerminoma.

teratoma* (ter″ah-to-mah) benign neoplasm of ovary, and malignant neoplasm of testis.

thecoma* (the-ko′mah) malignant ovarian tumor composed of theca cells.

SURGICAL PROCEDURES

abortion termination of pregnancy.

amniotomy (am″ne-ot′o-me) surgical rupture of fetal membranes to induce labor.

basiotripsy (ba′se-o-trip″se) surgical crushing of the head of a dead fetus to facilitate removal (also called *cranioclasis*).

cervicectomy excision of uterine cervix (also called *trachelectomy*).

cesarean section surgical incision through abdominal and uterine walls for delivery of neonate.

---

*Indicates a malignant condition.

*Indicates a malignant condition.

circumcision excision of all or part of the prepuce of the glans penis.

clitoridectomy (kli"to-rid-ek'to-me) excision of the clitoris.

colpectomy excision of the vagina.

colpocleisis (kol"po-kli'sis) closing of the vaginal canal (*cleisis* refers to closure).

colpohysterectomy (kol-po-his"ter-ek'to-me) removal of the uterus via the vagina.

colpohysteropexy (kol"po-his'ter-o-pek"se) fixation of the uterus via surgery through the vagina.

colpohysterotomy incision of the uterus via the vagina.

colpomyomectomy (kol"po-mi"o-mek'to-me) removal of a myoma through the vagina.

colpoperineoplasty (kol"po-per"i-ne-o-plast"te) surgical repair of the vagina and perineum.

colpoperineorrhaphy (kol"po-per"i-ne'or'ah-fe) suture to repair a torn vagina and perineum.

colpopexy (kol'po-pek"se) suturing of a relaxed vagina to the abdominal wall for support.

colpoplasty plastic repair of the vagina.

colpopoiesis (kol"po-poi-e'sis) creation of a vagina by plastic surgery.

colporrhaphy (kol-por'ah-fe) suturing repair of the vagina.

colpotomy surgical incision of the vaginal wall.

dilatation and curettage (D&C) (ku-reh-tahzh') cervical dilation and scraping of inside of uterus for diagnostic purposes, removal of endometrial tissue, or removal of uterine contents.

embryotomy (em"bre-ot'o-me) removal of a dead embryo or fetus from the uterus by means of dissection.

epididymectomy (ep"i-did"i-mek'to-me) excision of the epididymis.

epididymotomy (ep"i-did"i-mot'o-me) incision into the epididymis, usually for drainage purposes.

epididymovasotomy (ep-i-did'i-mo-vaz-o'to-me) anastomosis of the epididymis to the vas deferens.

episioplasty (e-piz'e-o-plas"te) repair of the vulva.

episiorrhaphy (e-piz'e-or'ah-fe) repair of torn vulva or an episiotomy.

episiotomy incision of the vulva to prevent tearing on delivery of neonate.

hymenectomy (hi"men-ek'to-me) excision of the hymen.

hymenotomy incision of the hymen.

hysterectomy removal of the uterus.

hysterolaparotomy (his"ter-o-lap"ah-rot'o-me) incision of the abdomen to remove or incise the uterus.

hysteromyotomy (his"ter-o-mi-ot'o-me) incision into the uterine muscle wall.

hysteropexy fixation of the uterus to correct misplacement or abnormal mobility.

hysterorrhaphy (his-ter-or'ah-fe) suturing of a torn uterus.

hysterosalpingostomy (his"ter-o-sal"ping-gos'to-me) surgical clearing of the lumen of a fallopian tube.

lumpectomy excision of a tumor leaving surrounding tissue and lymph nodes intact.

mamilliplasty (mah-mil'i-plas"te) plastic repair of the nipple (also called *theleplasty*).

mastectomy excision of the breast (also called *mammectomy*).

mastopexy (mas'to-pek-se) surgical reconstruction of a pendulous breast (also called *mastoplasty*).

mastotomy incision of the breast (also called *mammotomy*).

oophorectomy (o"of-o-rek'to-me) excision of one or both ovaries (also called *ovariectomy*).

oophorocystectomy excision of an ovarian cyst.

oophorohysterectomy (o-of'o-ro-his"ter-ek'to-me) removal of the uterus and ovaries.

oophoropexy (o-of'o-ro-pek"se) fixation of an ovary.

oophoroplasty (o-of'o-ro-plas"te) plastic repair of an ovary.

oophorosalpingectomy (o-of"o-ro-sal"pin-jek'to-me) removal of an ovary and a tube (also called *salpingo-oophorectomy* and *salpingoovariectomy*).

oophorotomy incision of an ovary.

orchidorrhaphy surgical fixation of an undescended testicle into the scrotum (also called *orchiopexy*).

orchiectomy (or"ke-ek'to-me) excision of one or both testes.

orchioplasty (or'ke-o-plas"te) plastic repair of a testicle.

ovariocentesis (o-va"re-o-sen-te'sis) puncture of an ovarian cyst or an ovary.

ovariostomy (o"va-re-os'to-me) creation of an opening in an ovarian cyst for purposes of drainage (also called *oophorostomy*).

ovariotomy incision of an ovary, usually for biopsy purposes.

panhysterectomy (pan"hist-er-ek'to-me) complete removal of the uterus and cervix.

perineal prostatectomy removal of the prostate gland through the perineum.

prostatectomy (pros"tah-tek'to-me) removal of all or part of the prostate gland.

prostatomy incision into the prostate gland (also called *prostatotomy*).

prostatovesiculectomy (pros"tah-to-ve-sik"u-lek"to-me) excision of the prostate gland and seminal vesicles.

radical mastectomy excision of the breast, pectoral muscle, axillary lymph nodes, skin, and other tissues.

retropubic prostatectomy excision of the prostate gland through the lower abdomen.

salpingectomy (sal"pin-jek'to-me) removal of a fallopian tube.

salpingopexy surgical fixation of a fallopian tube.

salpingorrhaphy (sal"ping-gor'ah-fe) suturing of a fallopian tube.

salpingostomatomy (sal-ping"go-sto-mat'o-me) procedure to create an opening in a fallopian tube when the fimbriated end is closed (also called *salpingostomy*).

salpingotomy incision into a fallopian tube.

scrotoplasty (skro'to-plas"te) repair of the scrotum.

tracheloplasty (tra'ke-lo-plas"te) plastic repair of the cervix.

trachelorrhaphy (tra"ke-lor'ah-fe) suturing of a torn cervix.

trachelotomy incision into the cervix.

transurethral resection of prostate (TURP) resection of the prostate gland through the urethra.

vasectomy excision of all or part of the vas deferens.

vasotomy incision into the vas deferens.

vesiculectomy (ve-sik"u-lek'to-me) excision of all or a portion of a seminal vesicle.

vesiculotomy (ve-sik"u-loto'-me) incision into the seminal vesicles to open them.

vulvectomy (vul-vek'to-me) excision of the vulva.

LABORATORY TESTS AND PROCEDURES

alpha-fetoprotein (AFP) blood test between the fourteenth and eighteenth weeks of pregnancy to screen for neural tube defects in the fetus.

amniocentesis (am"ne-o-sen"te'sis) aspiration of fluid from the amniotic sac for sampling of fetal cells after 5 months, to diagnose genetic defects and diseases and to determine sex of fetus.

chorionic villus sampling (CVS) biopsy technique, between the eighth and twelfth weeks of pregnancy, using a catheter to suction up a minute amount of the chorionic villi, which have the same cells as the fetus, to detect genetic defects and diseases (also called *chorionic villus biopsy—CVB*).

darkfield examination microscopic test of the fluid from the chancre lesion in the suspected primary stage of syphilis.

hysterostoscopy examination of the uterus using a fiberoptic endoscope.

karyotyping analysis of chromosomes of fetal cells or somatic cells of children and young adults to detect genetic diseases and abnormalities.

Papanicolaou smear microscopic examination of cell samples from the cervix and vagina to detect cancer and infections (also called *Pap smear*).

percutaneous umbilical blood sampling (PUBS) blood sample from fetal umbilical cord to detect genetic abnormalities, blood disorders, and infections.

prostatic acid phosphatase (PAP) blood test to detect a substance normally present, that increases when prostate cancer has spread.

prostate specific antigen (PSA) blood test to detect the presence of a specific antigen that increases in cases of prostate cancer and other prostate diseases.

seminal fluid tests series of tests of seminal fluid to determine the percentage and motility of spermatozoa, the makeup of the fluid, amount produced in ejaculation, etc.

Venereal Disease Research Laboratory test (VDRL) test for syphilis.

Pregnancy Tests

agglutination inhibition test (AIT) urine test as early as 10 days after conception, based on the the presence of the human chorionic gonadotropin (HCG), the hormone secreted by the female pituitary gland to stimulate ovaries, which indicates pregnancy.

radioimmunoassay (RIA) sensitive, reliable blood test, to detect the beta unit of human chorionic gonadotropin (HCG), which can diagnose pregnancy before the first menstrual period is missed.

radioreceptor assay (RRA) sensitive, reliable blood test to detect human chorionic gonadotropin (HCG) by means of a gamma counter to reveal radioactivity, taking about an hour to complete and being almost 100% reliable in detecting pregnancy as early as 1 week after conception.

Radiographic Studies

amniography (am″ne-og′rah-fe) an x-ray of the gravid uterus after injection of contrast media into the amniotic sac to visualize the contents.

computerized tomography (CT) imaging device using x-rays at multiple angles through specific sections of the body, analyzed by computer to provide a total picture of the part being examined (also called *computerized axial tomography—CAT*).

hysterogram x-ray of the uterus using contrast medium injected into the uterine cavity.

hysterosalpingography x-ray of uterus and fallopian tubes, using contrast medium.

magnetic resonance imaging (MRI) noninvasive method of scanning the body by use of an electromagnetic field and radio waves, which provides visual images on a computer screen and magnetic tape recordings (also called *nuclear magnetic resonance—NMR*).

mammography x-ray of breast tissue to detect tumors.

transrectal ultrasonography a procedure using ultrasound waves, made by an instrument inserted into the rectum, to visualize the prostate and nearby structures.

ultrasonography a procedure using ultrasound waves to visualize deep body structures, to monitor the fetus and placenta.

EXERCISES   THE REPRODUCTIVE SYSTEM THE CYCLE OF LIFE

Exercise 13.1   *Complete the following:*

1. The accessory organs of the male reproductive system are _ducts, glands, supporting structures_.

2. The supporting structures of the male reproductive system are _penis, scrotum, spermatic cords_.

3. The male reproductive cell is called _spermatozoa or sperm cells_

4. The chief male sex hormone is _testosterone_.

5. The accessory organs of the female reproductive system are _fallopian tubes, uterus, vagina, vulva, mammaries_

6. The fluid in the sac surrounding the embryo is called _amniotic_ fluid.

7. The functions of the ovaries are _ovulation_ and _hormonal secretion_.

8. The female cycle beginning with puberty is called _menstruation_

9. The cessation of this cycle is called _menopause_.

10. The female reproductive cells are called _ova_.

Exercise 13.2   *Using the following terms, identify each structure in Figure 13.7 by writing its name in the corresponding blank*

Bulb of urethra

Corpus cavernosum

Corpus spongiosum

Duct of bulbourethral gland

Ejaculatory duct

Epididymis

Glans

Prostate gland

Rectum

Right common iliac artery and
    vein

Seminal vesicle

Symphysis pubis

Testis

Urethra

Urinary bladder

Vas deferens

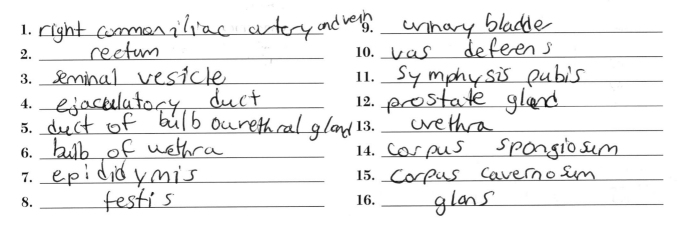

1. right common iliac artery and vein
2. rectum
3. seminal vesicle
4. ejaculatory duct
5. duct of bulb ourethral gland
6. bulb of urethra
7. epididymis
8. testis

9. urinary bladde
10. vas deferens
11. Symphysis pubis
12. prostate gland
13. urethra
14. corpus spongiosum
15. corpus cavernosum
16. glans

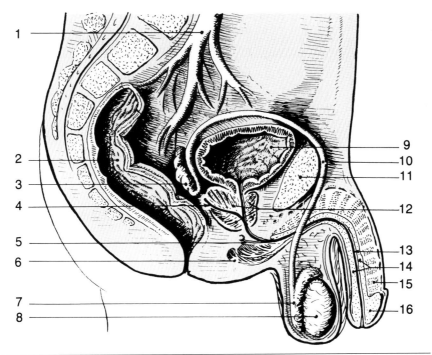

Figure 13.7 Midline sectional view of the male urinary and reproductive systems.

Exercise 13.3   *Using the terms below, identify each part in Figure 13.8 by writing the appropriate name in the corresponding blank.*

Corpus luteum

Fallopian, or uterine, tubes (oviducts)

Graafian follicle

Cervical canal of uterus

Ovary

Vagina

Ovarian ligament

External os

Body of uterus

Fimbriated extremity

1. ___fallopian tubes___

2. ___fimbriated extremity___

3. ___ovary___

4. ___ovarian ligament___

5. ___body of uterus___

6. ___cervical canal of uterus___

7. ___external os___

8. ___vagina___

9. ___corpus luteum___

10. ___graafian follicle___

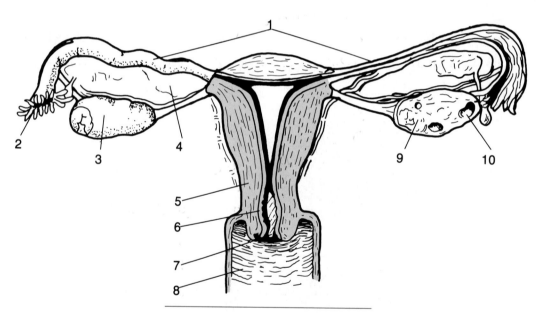

Figure 13.8 Female reproductive tract.

Exercise 13.4 *Using the terms below, identify each part in Figure 13.9 by placing its name in the corresponding blank.*

Vagina

Ovary

Fallopian, or uterine, tube (oviduct)

Uterus

Urethra

Labia majora

Rectum

Symphysis pubis

Bladder

Sphincter ani

1. Sphincter ani
2. rectum
3. ovary
4. fallopian tube
5. uterus
6. bladder
7. Symphysis pubis
8. urethra
9. labia majora
10. vagina

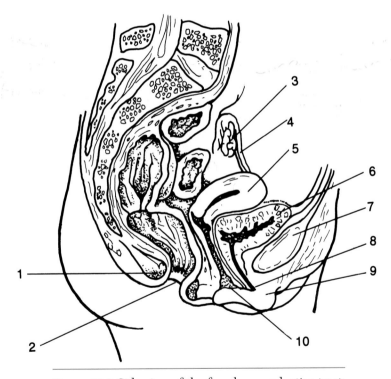

Figure 13.9 Side view of the female reproductive tract.

Exercise 13.5   *Matching*

___B___   **1.** pouches just above the prostate whose duct
                    unites with the vas deferens to form the ejacula-
                    tory duct
___R___   **2.** pair of tubes encased by spermatic cords
___M___   **3.** male gland producing spermatozoa
___E___   **4.** specialized interstitial cells secreting the male
                    sex hormone (testosterone), responsible for sec-
                    ondary sex characteristics
___D___   **5.** reproductive cells of the male
___L___   **6.** reproductive cells of the female
___S___   **7.** pigmented portion of nipple
___F___   **8.** mucous membrane lining of the uterus
___N___   **9.** early or developing stage of any organism
___C___   **10.** secretion discharged by male reproductive organ
___T___   **11.** developing human beginning with ninth week
___I___   **12.** fingerlike processes at ends of fallopian (uterine)
                    tubes
___J___   **13.** interior of cervix
___P___   **14.** foreskin of penis
___H___   **15.** pad of fat in front of symphysis pubis
___O___   **16.** external female genitalia
___Q___   **17.** elastic muscular tube below cervix, extending to
                    body exterior
___A___   **18.** saclike male structure
___G___   **19.** walnut-sized, doughnut-shaped male gland
___K___   **20.** neck of uterus

A. scrotum
B. seminal vesicles
C. semen
D. spermatozoa
E. Leydig cells
F. endometrium
G. prostate
H. mons pubis
I. fimbriae
J. endocervix
K. cervix
L. ova
M. testis
N. embryo
O. vulva
P. prepuce
Q. vagina
R. vas deferens
S. areola
T. fetus

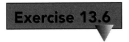 **Exercise 13.6**

Give the meaning of the components in the following words and then define the word as a whole. Suffixes meaning pertaining to or state or condition, shown following a slash mark (/), are not to be defined separately. Before reaching for your medical dictionary, check the Related Terms list in this chapter.

1. Ovotestis:

ovo ___ovary___

testis ___testis___

_____

2. Metrosalpingitis:

metro ___uterus___

salping ___fallopian tube___

itis ___inflammation___

_____

3. Hematometra:

hemato ___blood___

metra ___uterus___

_____

4. Oophorosalpingitis:

oophoro ___ovary___

salping ___fallopian tube___

itis ___inflammation___

_____

5. Metrocolpocele:

metro ___uterus___

colpo ___vagina___

cele ___hernia___

_____

6. Episiotomy:

episio ___vulva___

tomy ___incision___

_____

7. Hysterolaparotomy:

hystero ___uterus___

laparo ___abdomen.___

tomy ___incision___

_____

8. Oophorohysterectomy:

oophoro ___ovary___

hyster ___uterus___

ectomy ___removal___

_____

ACROSS

1. Mammary glands
2. Microscopic formations containing eggs
6. Passageways for sperm
9. An ovarian hormone
13. Basic reproductive organs
14. Male sex hormone
15. External saclike structure in the male
16. Female sex cells
18. Union of ovum and sperm
19. Cowper's glands
23. Neck of the uterus
24. Pear-shaped female pelvic organ
25. Glands producing sperm cells
27. Elastic tube extending from the cervix to the external genitalia
29. Male gland surrounding urethra

DOWN

1. Upper portion or uterus
3. Female reproductive organs
4. Female erectile tissue organ
5. Male reproductive cells
6. Internal uterine lining
7. Onset of menstruation
8. Developing organism from the second through the eighth week of pregnancy
10. Uterine tubes
11. Mouth or opening
12. Menopause
17. Fluid in which an embryo floats
18. Fringed, fingerlike processes of uterine tubes
20. Rupture of mature graafian follicle, releasing ovum
21. Root for uterus
22. Menstrual period
26. Foreskin
28. Pigmented halo around nipple

HIDDEN WORDS PUZZLE

CHAPTER 13

Can you find the 20 words hidden in this puzzle? All hidden words puzzles have words running from top to bottom, left to right, and diagonally downward.

ANDROGEN

BULBOURETHRAL

CAVERNOUS

CERVIX

ENDOMETRIUM

EPIDIDYMIS

ESTROGEN

FIMBRIAE

GONADS

LOBULES

MAMMARY

MENARCHE

OVARIES

OVULATION

PELVIS

PREPUCE

PROSTATE

SCROTUM

TESTES

UTERUS

```
E S T R O G E N N E C U P E R P
N M H X I S O V U L A T I O N R
D V S R S R V N Q T E S T E S O
O C X I V R E C A V E R N O U S
M L F J Y T K M R D N R U R I T
E P I D I D Y M I S S E U K O A
T W M I O G R N F Y V F G S Z T
R N B U L B O U R E T H R A L E
I F R O V A R I E S I N W Q Q H
U C I C Q N Z D N Q C K Y H W C
M L A Q P D Y B M I T R F N A R
Q C E S E R F V L C B R O V G A
S Q O Q L O B U L E S V L T W N
Y N T H V G T F W O G F T J U E
O E H S I E D Y S R A M M A M
G G R O S N B C Y O M Q T X O J
```

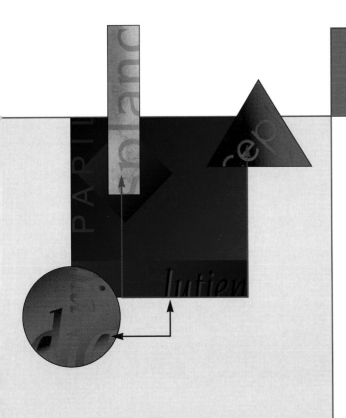

The Adaptive and Defense Mechanisms of the Body

This is the fourth of the five sections of *Learning Medical Terminology.* This section contains four chapters that describe those systems that aid the body in coordinating with and adapting to the external and internal environments and one chapter devoted to a listing of multiple-system diseases.

Chapter 14, the endocrine system, details the activity of the glands of internal secretion, and their regulation of body functions through chemical means.

Chapter 15, the nervous system, describes the separate divisions of this system and their functions in coordinating the complexities of human life.

Chapter 16 describes the special senses, through which the body receives stimulation from the world around it.

Chapter 17 presents the lymphatic and immune systems, which work together to protect and defend the integrity of the body.

Chapter 18 consists of a relatively comprehensive listing of pathologic conditions that affect more than one system of the body.

As in the previous section, there are drawings within the chapters illustrating the principal parts of the anatomy in that particular chapter. In addition, the color plates at the front of the text provide more vivid detail.

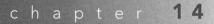

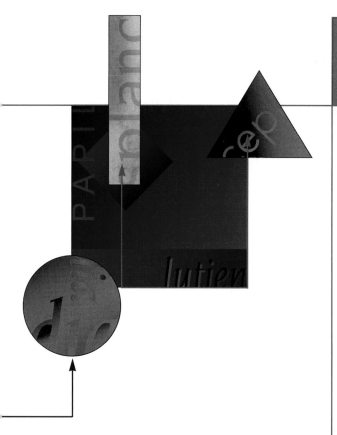

The Endocrine System

the chemical

stimulators

This chapter describes the ductless glands *(pituitary, hypothalamus, thyroid, parathyroids, adrenals, pineal, pancreas, ovaries, testes, and thymus)*, which constitute the endocrine system. The structure and function of the glands and their secretions are detailed narratively and in chart form.

The complex activities of the body are controlled by the endocrine and central nervous systems. The central nervous system acts directly and instantaneously, while the action of the endocrine system is more subtle, discharging its secretions slowly into the circulatory system and controlling organs from a distance.

The endocrine system (Figure 14.1) is made up of ductless glands of internal secretion, so-called because they have no ducts to carry away their secretions and depend on the capillaries and, to a certain extent, the lymph vessels, for this function. The secretions of these glands are called *hormones* (which means to rouse or set in motion). Although most hormones are excitatory in function, some are inhibitory.

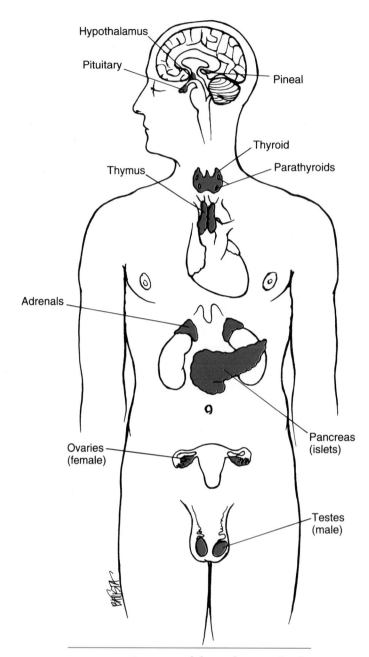

Figure 14.1 Location of the endocrine glands.

The secretion of hormones is controlled by a feedback mechanism. The presence and amount of a hormone, and any substances released by tissue excited by that hormone, regulate further secretion of that hormone by its gland. This ensures that the right amount of the hormone, no more and no less, will maintain the proper balance of bodily functioning.

THE PITUITARY GLAND

The *pituitary gland,* or *hypophysis,* despite all its important functions, is no larger than a pea. It is about ½ inch (1.3 cm) in diameter and weighs about 0.02 oz (0.5 g). It has been called the "orchestra leader" and "master gland" because it exerts control over all other glands.

Structure

The pituitary gland lies protected within the sphenoid bone in a saddle-shaped depression called the *sella turcica.* It is further protected by an extension of the *dura mater* (membrane covering the brain) called the *pituitary diaphragm.* A stemlike portion of the pitu-

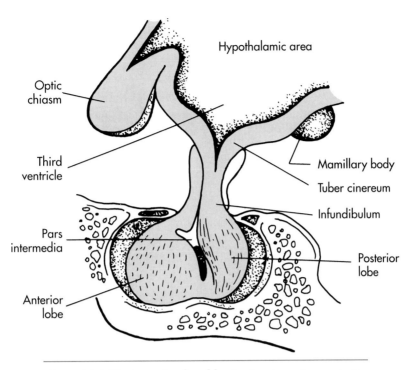

Figure 14.2 Pituitary gland and brain structures in proximity.

itary gland, the *pituitary stalk,* extends through the diaphragm and provides a connection (the *infundibulum*) to the *hypothalamus* portion of the brain, located on the underside.

The pituitary gland is actually made up of two separate glands with different embryonic origins and functions: the *anterior lobe,* or *anterior pituitary gland (adenohypophysis),* develops as an upgrowth from the embryonic pharynx, while the *posterior lobe,* or *posterior pituitary gland (neurohypophysis),* develops as a downward extension of the brain (Figure 14.2).

Functions of the Anterior Lobe

The master role is played by the anterior lobe, with its numerous anterior pituitary hormones influencing the actions of other endocrines. This internal regulation is further coordinated by the action of the hypothalamus on the anterior lobe, controlling the release of six major types of anterior pituitary hormones. The combining forms *-tropic* and *-tropin* mean influence or stimulation (see Table 14.1).

Growth hormone (GH), also called *somatotropin,* promotes bodily growth of both bony and soft tissues.

Thyroid-stimulating hormone (TSH), a *thyrotropic* hormone, influences the thyroid gland and causes secretion of the thyroid hormone.

Two *gonadotropic* hormones influence the ovaries and testes and are necessary for the proper development and function of the reproductive system:

Follicle-stimulating hormone (FSH) stimulates the growth of graafian follicles and the secretion of estrogen in the female and the development of the seminiferous tubules and sperm cells in the male.

Luteinizing hormone (LH) stimulates, in the female, ovarian follicle and ovum maturation, formation of the corpus luteum, secretion of estrogen, and ovulation. In the male this hormone stimulates the interstitial cells of the testes to produce and secrete testosterone.

Prolactin, or *lactogenic hormone,* is responsible for breast development during pregnancy and, as its name implies, for production of milk.

Adrenocorticotropic hormone (ACTH), or *adrenocorticotropin,* influences growth of the adrenal glands and also stimulates the adrenal cortex to synthesize and release corticosteroids. ACTH also appears to have a relationship to pigmentation of the skin.

Melanocyte-stimulating hormone (MSH), the last of the anterior pituitary hormones, stimulates formation of melanin pigment in the skin.

Functions of the Posterior Lobe

The posterior lobe of the pituitary gland secretes two hormones, which are actually made in the hypothalamus and passed through the infundibulum into the posterior lobe, where they are stored and secreted into the circulation.

Antidiuretic hormone (ADH), or *vasopressin,* limits the development of large volumes of urine by stimulating water reabsorption by the distal and collecting tubules of the kidneys.

Oxytocin stimulates both the ejection of breast milk into the mammary ducts and contraction of the uterus after pregnancy.

THE HYPOTHALAMUS

The *hypothalamus* is a part of the brain, made of neural tissue, but also has endocrine functions (see Chapter 15).

As previously noted, both *antidiuretic hormone* and *oxytocin* are produced by the hypothalamus and stored and released from the posterior pituitary. In addition, the hypothalamus produces hormones that cause stimulation or inhibition of the release of anterior pituitary hormones.

THE THYROID

The *thyroid gland* is composed of two pear-shaped lobes separated by a middle strip of tissue, the *isthmus,* which crosses in front of the second and third tracheal cartilages (Figure 14.3). The thyroid perches like a butterfly with wings extended on the front part of the neck below the larynx. The lobes are molded to the trachea and esophagus down as far as the sixth tracheal cartilage, and they extend upward to the sides of the cricoid and thyroid cartilages. The thyroid may be felt slightly and may even be visible as a swelling in some diseases of the gland.

Structure

The thyroid is a soft, highly vascular mass, brownish-red in color, consisting of tiny sacs, or follicles, that are filled with a gelatinous yellow fluid called *colloid.* The colloid contains the hormone secreted by the thyroid. It is stored in the colloid and passed into the capillaries to be sent to the tissues as required.

The thyroid weighs about 1 oz (28 to 30 g) in the average adult. It has a rich vascular supply from the inferior and superior thyroid arteries, with a wide capillary network for diffusion of blood to the veins, and a rich lymphatic system that drains the lymph spaces around

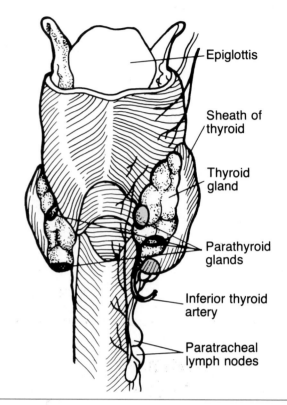

Figure 14.3 Posterior view of the thyroid and parathyroid glands.

the follicles. Although lymph vessels drain some of the hormones, the major portion is carried away by the capillaries. The hormone secreted by the thyroid is under the control of the anterior pituitary lobe.

Functions

The main function of the thyroid is the secretion of two iodine-laden hormones, *thyroxine* and *triiodothyronine,* which together are referred to as *thyroid hormone.* This hormone is high in iodine and vital for growth and metabolism; through variations in the activity of the gland, the thyroid hormone alters the metabolic rate in accordance with changing physiologic demands. Growth and differentiation of tissue during development is also regulated by the thyroid hormone.

Iodine is the essential element of the thyroid hormone. Most disorders of the thyroid are caused by either overproduction or underproduction of the thyroid hormone and its iodine-containing substance. The iodine in the thyroid hormone is combined with a protein in the blood, which is then referred to as *protein-bound iodine (PBI).* However, when the hormone enters the tissue, the separate components become unbound from the protein.

A secondary function of the thyroid gland is the secretion of *calcitonin*, which produces a decrease in the concentration of calcium in the blood, helping to maintain the balance of calcium necessary for a variety of bodily processes. This balance is achieved in conjunction with the functioning of the parathyroid glands.

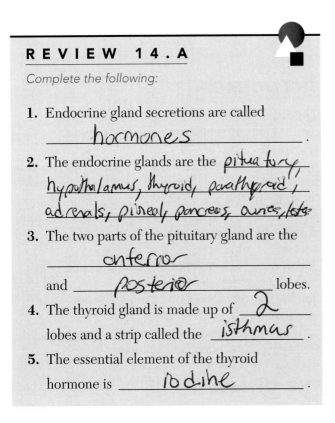

REVIEW 14.A

Complete the following:

1. Endocrine gland secretions are called
   _____hormones_____ .

2. The endocrine glands are the *pituitary,*
   hypothalamus, thyroid, parathyroid,
   adrenals, pineal, pancreas, ovaries, testes

3. The two parts of the pituitary gland are the
   _____anterior_____
   and _____posterior_____ lobes.

4. The thyroid gland is made up of _____2_____
   lobes and a strip called the _____isthmus_____ .

5. The essential element of the thyroid
   hormone is _____iodine_____ .

THE PARATHYROID GLANDS

The *parathyroid glands* (*para* means alongside of or next to) are small, reddish-brown, oval glands, about ¼ inch (6 mm) at their widest dimensions. There are usually two on each side, lying behind the thyroid gland and embedded in its posterior surface (see Figure 14.3). The blood supply of the parathyroid glands is from the inferior thyroid artery, and their functional activity is controlled by a hormone of the anterior lobe of the pituitary gland.

Parathyroid hormone (PTH), secreted by the glands, regulates the calcium and phosphorus content of the blood and bones. The regulation of calcium content is very important in certain tissue activities, such as blood formation and coagulation, milk production in pregnant females, and maintenance of normal neuromuscular excitability.

Parathyroid hormone promotes calcium absorption in the blood, increasing its calcium concentration.

This mechanism is antagonistic (opposite) to that of the hormone calcitonin from the thyroid gland. These two hormones together maintain calcium balance.

THE ADRENAL GLANDS

The *adrenal (suprarenal) glands* resemble small caps perched on the top of each kidney. They are flattened, yellowish bodies about 2 inches (52 mm) high, 1 inch (25 mm) wide, and ½ inch (13 mm) thick, slightly smaller in the female than in the male, and may vary in weight.

Structure

The adrenal glands are composed of two distinct parts, the *cortex* (outer part), and the *medulla* (inner part), with each having different glandular functions. The cortex is indispensable to life, but the medulla is not. The cortex, which is about ¼ inch thick (6 mm), makes up the bulk of the gland and is divided into three zones, *zona glomerulosa* (outer), *zona fasiculata* (middle), and *zona reticularis* (inner).

Functions

All the known adrenal hormones of the cortex are called *corticoids*, any of which can be manufactured synthetically. They are classified as:

Mineralocorticoids (MC), secreted by the outer zone, are concerned with the regulation of sodium and potassium and their excretion. The principal one is *aldosterone*, which is responsible for electrolyte and water balance by acting on the blood sodium and potassium concentration.

Glucocorticoids (GC), secreted mainly by the middle zone, including *cortisol (hydrocortisone)*, and *corticosterone.* The glucocorticoids affect literally all cells in the body, but their general effect is in the metabolism of carbohydrates, fats, and proteins, resistance to stress, antibody formation, lymphatic functioning, and recovery from injury and inflammation.

Sex hormones, secreted by the inner zone, which include, in both sexes, small amounts of the male hormone *androgen*, which stimulates the sex drive in the female, but, because of its relative insignificance in the male, compared to testosterone, has little influence.

The presence in the blood of adrenocorticotropin (ACTH), a pituitary hormone, is necessary for the anatomic integrity and functioning of the adrenal cortex in secreting androgens and cortisol.

The adrenal medulla secretes *epinephrine (adrenaline)* and *norepinephrine (noradrenaline).* Epinephrine, particularly, aids the body in meeting stressful situations, such as defense flight, attack, or pursuit. By stimulating or boosting the sympathetic nervous system, epinephrine aids in coping with stress. Norepinephrine is primarily a vasoconstrictor. The effects of these secretions include increases in heartbeat, blood pressure, blood glucose level, and rate of blood clotting.

THE PINEAL GLAND

The *pineal gland,* or *pineal body (epiphysis cerebri),* which derives its name from its resemblance to a pine cone, is a small, firm, oval body about ¼ inch (6 mm) long located near the base of the brain. Although exact functions have not been established, it secretes *melatonin,* a skin-lightening agent, which is believed to inhibit ovarian function and secretion of the pituitary luteinizing hormone, and may be related to the circadian (24-hour cycle) rhythms of the body.

THE PANCREAS

The *pancreas,* as part of the gastrointestinal system, is described in Chapter 11.

As an endocrine gland, microscopic, specialized cells of the pancreas, called the *islands* (or *islets*) *of Langerhans,* secrete *insulin, glucagon,* and *pancreatic polypeptide (PP)* into the circulation.

Insulin is necessary for the use and storage of carbohydrates and acts to decrease blood glucose levels, while glucagon acts to increase them. The level of glucose in the blood is also dependent on the action of many of the other endocrine secretions, such as the pituitary growth hormone, epinephrine, ACTH, and the glucocorticoids, all of which act to increase it, and the thyroid hormone, which acts to decrease it. Pancreatic polypeptide plays a role in the production of glucagon and gastric juices and has been identified as having additional functions in digestion and metabolism.

THE GONADS

The male and female *gonads,* as parts of the reproductive system, are described in Chapter 13.

As endocrine glands, the female ovaries produce the hormones *estrogen* and *progesterone,* and the male testes produce the hormone *testosterone.* All these hormones are important to the functioning of the reproductive system. These glands become active at puberty under the influence of the anterior pituitary lobe, producing both sexual behavior and secondary sex characteristics of pubic and axillary hair in both sexes, sperm development, deep voice and facial hair in the male, and breast development and the menstrual cycle in the female. Table 14.1 on pg. 263 and the Related Terms list in this chapter contain descriptions of the gonadal hormones.

THE THYMUS

The *thymus,* located in the mediastinum, produces the hormone *thymosin,* which plays an important part in the body's immune system (Chapter 17).

TABLE 14.1 THE ENDOCRINE GLANDS AND THEIR HORMONES

Gland	Hormone	Function
pituitary anterior lobe	growth hormone (GH) (somatotropin)	Promotes body and soft tissue growth
	thyroid-stimulating hormone (TSH) (thyrotropic hormone)	Stimulates thyroid gland production of thyroid hormone
	follicle-stimulating hormone (FSH)	Stimulates graafian follicle growth Stimulates secretion of estrogen in ovaries Stimulates development of seminiferous tubules in testes Stimulates development and production of sperm cells
	luteinizing hormone (LH)	Stimulates ovarian follicle and ovum maturation Stimulates formation of corpus luteum Stimulates secretion of estrogen Stimulates ovulation Stimulates interstitial cells of testes to produce and secrete testosterone
	prolactin (lactogenic hormone)	Stimulates breast development and milk production
	adrenocorticotropic hormone (ACTH) (adrenocorticotropin)	Influences growth of the adrenal glands Stimulates adrenal cortex to synthesize and release corticosteroids Affects skin pigmentation
	melanocyte-stimulating hormone (MSH)	Stimulates formation of melanin pigment in the skin
posterior lobe	antidiuretic hormone (ADH) (vasopressin)	Stimulates water reabsorption by kidney tubules
	oxytocin	Stimulates ejection of breast milk and uterine contractions after pregnancy
hypothalamus	antidiuretc hormone (ADH)	Passes hormone on to posterior pituitary
	oxytocin	Passes hormone on to posterior pituitary
	releasing and inhibiting hormones	Stimulate or inhibit production and release of anterior pituitary hormones

Continued

TABLE 14.1 THE ENDOCRINE GLANDS AND THEIR HORMONES—*cont'd*

Gland	Hormone	Function
thyroid	*thyroid hormone (thyroxine, triiodothyronine)*	Regulates growth, development, and metabolism
	calcitonin	Promotes calcium absorption in bones and reduces concentration in blood
parathyroid	*parathyroid hormone (PTH)*	Regulates phosphorus content of blood and bones Promotes calcium concentration in blood and reduces concentration in bones
adrenal cortex	*mineralocorticoids (e.g., aldosterone)*	Regulates sodium and potassium
	glucocorticoids (cortisol and corticosterone)	Metabolism of carbohydrates, fats, and proteins Resistance to stress, antibody formation, lymphatic functioning, recovery from injury and inflammation
	sex hormones (androgen)	Stimulate female sex drive
medulla	*epinephrine (adrenaline) and norepinephrine (noradrenaline)*	Stimulate sympathetic nervous system responses to stress
pineal	*melatonin*	Decreases skin pigmentation Inhibits ovarian function and secretion of the anterior pituitary luteinizing hormone
pancreas islands of Langerhans	*insulin*	Regulates use and storage of carbohydrates Reduces glucose in blood
	glucagon	Increases glucose in blood
	pancreatic polypetide (PP)	Stimulates production of glucagon and gastric juices Functions in digestion and metabolism

TABLE 14.1 THE ENDOCRINE GLANDS AND THEIR HORMONES—cont'd

Gland	Hormone	Function
gonads **ovaries**	estrogen and progesterone	Produces secondary sex characteristics and sexual behavior Produces menstrual cycle
testes	testosterone	Produces secondary sex characteristics and sexual behavior Promotes sperm development
thymus	thymosin	Functions in the immune system

REVIEW 14.B

Complete the following:

1. The parathyroid hormone regulates the _calcium_ and _phosphorus_ content of blood and bones.

2. The two little caplike glands on top of the kidneys are the _adrenal_ glands.

3. The pineal gland secretion is _melatonin_.

4. The islands of Langerhans in the pancreas secrete _insulin, glucagon, and pancreatic poly peptide_.

5. The gonads become active at puberty under the influence of the _anterior_ pituitary lobe.

RELATED TERMS THE ENDOCRINE SYSTEM THE CHEMICAL STIMULATORS

ANATOMY

acidophil (ah-sid'o-fil) acid-staining cell of the anterior lobe of the pituitary gland, which secretes growth and lactogenic hormones.

adenohypophysis (ad"e-no-hi-pof'i-sis) anterior lobe of the pituitary gland *(hypophysis)*, as distinguished from the posterior lobe *(neurohypophysis)*.

adrenal glands glands located at the top of each kidney (also called *suprarenal glands*).

adrenaline (ad-ren'ah-lin) adrenal medulla hormone, which stimulates smooth muscle, cardiac muscle, and glands, to assist the body in meeting stress (also called *epinephrine*).

adrenalopathy (ad-re"nal-op'ah-the) any adrenal gland pathology (also called *adrenopathy*).

adrenocorticotropin (ACTH) (ad-re"no-kor"tik-o-trop'in) hormone of the anterior pituitary gland that promotes growth and development of the adrenal cortex and stimulates the cortex to secrete glucocorticoids (also called *adrenocorticotrophin*).

aldosterone hormone of the adrenal cortex responsible for electrolyte and water balance.

androsterone (an-dros'ter-on) an androgen, or male sex hormone, secreted by the adrenal gland.

antidiuretic hormone (ADH) hormone secreted by the posterior pituitary, which stimulates water reabsorption by the distal and collecting kidney tubules (also called *vasopressin*).

basophils basic-staining cells of the anterior lobe of the pituitary, which secrete thyrotropin, a thyroid-stimulating hormone (TSH), adrenocorticotropin (ACTH), follicle-stimulating hormone (FSH), luteinizing hormone (LH), and melanocyte-stimulating hormone (MSH).

calcitonin hormone secreted by the thyroid that promotes calcium absorption in the bones and reduced concentration of calcium in the blood.

chorionic gonadotropin hormone secreted by the cells of the placental chorion.

chromophobe (kro'mo-fob) nonstaining cell of the anterior pituitary lobe.

colloid (kol'oid) gelatinous substance in the follicles of the thyroid glands that contains the hormone secreted by the thyroid.

cortex (kor'teks) outer portion of the adrenal gland that secretes mineralocorticoids, glucocorticoids, androgens, and some estrogen.

corticosterone (kor"ti-kos'ter-on) adrenocortical glucocorticoid hormone.

cortisol (kor'ti-sol) adrenocortical glucocorticoid hormone (also called *hydrocortisone*).

estrogenic hormones ovarian hormones that influence the development of secondary sex characteristics, sexual behavior, and the menstrual cycle.

euthyroid (u-thi'roid) normally functioning thyroid gland.

follicle-stimulating hormone (FSH) anterior pituitary hormone that stimulates the growth of graafian follicles, the secretion of estrogen in the female, and the development of the seminiferous tubules and sperm cells in the male.

glucocorticoid group of adrenocortical steroids that are concerned with protein, fat, and carbohydrate metabolism and aid the body in resisting stress.

gonadotropic hormones pituitary hormones that influence the gonads.

growth hormone (GH) hormone secreted by the anterior pituitary gland that promotes bodily growth (also called *somatotropin* and *somatotrophin*).

hormone chemical substance secreted by an endocrine gland.

hypophysis cerebri (hi-pof'i-sis) another name for pituitary gland.

infundibulum (in"fun-dib'u-lum) funnel-shaped passage with neural tracts from the hypothalamus of the brain to the pituitary gland.

iodine (i-o'din) essential element of the thyroid hormone.

islands of Langerhans (lahng'er-hanz) specialized pancreatic cells secreting insulin, glucagon, and pancreatic polypeptide (PP) into the circulation.

lactogenic hormone pituitary hormone responsible for breast development and milk production in pregnancy (also called *prolactin*).

luteinizing hormone (LH) anterior pituitary hormone that stimulates the formation of the corpus luteum, secretion of estrogen and progesterone in the female and the development and secretion of testosterone in the interstitial cells of the testes.

medulla inner portion of the adrenal glands producing epinephrine and norepinephrine.

mineralocorticoid adrenocortical steroid that affects sodium and potassium balance.

neurohypophysis posterior lobe of pituitary gland.

norepinephrine hormone secreted by the adrenal medulla (also called *noradrenaline*).

oxytocin (ok"se-to'sin) hormone of the posterior lobe of the pituitary gland that stimulates uterine contractions.

parathyroids glands, normally two on each side, behind or embedded in the thyroid gland.

parathyroid hormone (PTH) parathyroid gland secretion that regulates calcium and phosphorus content of blood and bones.

pineal body small gland located near the base of the brain.

pituicyte (pi-tu'i-sit) fusiform cell of the posterior lobe of the pituitary gland.

pituitary gland (pi-tu'i-tar"e) master gland, attached to the base of the brain, that exercises control over the other endocrine glands.

progesterone hormone produced by the corpus luteum, whose function is to prepare the uterus to receive the fertilized ovum by causing growth and development of the uterine endometrial lining (also called *corpus luteum hormone*).

prolactin see *lactogenic hormone*.

suprarenals adrenal glands.

testosterone hormone of the testis that induces and maintains secondary sex characteristics.

thyroid (thi'roid) large gland situated on the front part of the neck just below the larynx.

thyroid-stimulating hormone (TSH) hormone of the anterior pituitary gland that promotes growth and development of the thyroid gland and stimulates it to secrete thyroxine and triiodothyronine, which make up thyroid hormone (also called *thyrotropin* and *thyrotrophin*).

thyroxine (thi-rok′sin) one of two iodine-laden hormones making up the thyroid hormone whose main function is to regulate the metabolic rate and processes of growth and tissue differentiation (also called *thyroxin*).

triiodothyronine (tri″i-o″do-thi′ro-nen) second of two hormones that make up the thyroid hormone, containing less iodine than thyroxine, but having the same functions.

vasopressin see *antidiuretic hormone*.

PATHOLOGIC CONDITIONS

Inflammations and Infections

adrenalitis inflammation of the adrenal glands.

thyroiditis inflammation of the thyroid gland.

Hereditary, Congenital, and Developmental Conditions

acromegaly (ak″ro-meg′ah-le) disease caused by pituitary hypersecretion of the growth hormone after completion of bone development, characterized by enlargement of the bones of the hands, feet, and face.

adiposogenital dystrophy (ad″i-pi″so-jen′i-tal) developmental disorder of adolescent males caused by anterior pituitary tumor or malfunction of the hypothalamus, with symptoms of underdevelopment of genitals, female secondary sex characteristics, and adiposity of a feminine type (also called *Frohlich's syndrome*).

congenital adrenal hyperplasia congenital condition of hypersecretion of adrenocortical androgens in both sexes, causing virilization of females and underdevelopment of gonads in males.

congenital goiter goiter present at birth.

cretinism (kre′tin-izm) infantile hypothyroidism with symptoms including permanently stunted growth and mental development as a result of thyroid hormone deficiency, which may be related to maternal iodine deficiency (also called *infantile hypothyroidism*).

dwarfism developmental disorder caused by anterior pituitary growth hormone hypofunction (also called *Lorain-Levi syndrome*).

giantism developmental disorder caused by excessive secretion of growth hormone before completion of bone development, with overgrowth of the long bones producing excessively large stature.

Hashimoto's disease (hash″i-mo′toz) chronic lymphomatous thyroiditis of autoimmune origins, with marked hereditary pattern, predominantly affecting females, with hypothyroidism and degeneration of the secreting cells of the thyroid gland (also called *chronic lymphomatous thyroiditis* and *struma lymphomatosa*).

hypogonadism developmental disorder caused by inadequate secretion of pituitary gonadotropins, resulting in sexual immaturity and decreased functional activity of the gonads in males and females.

hypoparathyroidism insufficiency of the parathyroid glands, which may be familial or a result of excision, disease, or injury of the thyroid or parathyroid glands, resulting in hypocalcemia, with increased bone density caused by decreased bone resorption.

Other Abnormalities

Addison's disease life-threatening condition of adrenal insufficiency that may be caused by immune system processes, tumor, infection, or adrenal gland hemorrhage, characterized by darkening of the skin, severe weakness, progressive anemia, low blood pressure, anorexia, and digestive disturbance.

adrenocortical hyperfunction overfunctioning of the adrenal cortex.

adrenocortical hypofunction underfunctioning of the adrenal cortex.

adrenogenital syndrome developmental disorders caused by hyperplasia, or tumor, of the adrenal glands, with masculinizing symptoms such as hirsutism, deepening of voice, and absence of menses in females, and feminizing of males with gynecomastia and lack of sperm.

aldosteronism (al″do-ster′on-izm″) disorder caused by adrenocortical hyperfunction, with muscular weakness, tetany, and excessive thirst and urination (primary type also called *Conn's syndrome*).

anorexia (an″o-rek′se-ah) lack or loss of appetite, a symptom in some endocrine disorders.

cachexia (kah-kek′se-ah) general ill health and malnutrition, which may be symptomatic of some endocrine disorders.

Cushing's syndrome pituitary basophilism, with excessive secretion of adrenocortical hormone, characterized by obesity, moon-face, oligomenorrhea in women, and lowered testosterone levels in men (also called *hypercortisolism*).

diabetes insipidus (di"ah-be'tez in"sip'i-dus) metabolic disorder characterized by polyuria and excessive thirst as a result of insufficient production of antidiuretic hormone (ADH).

diabetes mellitus metabolic disease caused by a deficiency of production of the insulin hormone by the islands of Langerhans, with symptoms of sugar in the urine, loss of electrolytes and water, and degeneration of blood vessels. This disease appears in two forms: an insulin-dependent condition (formerly called juvenile-onset type) treated by insulin injections, and a non–insulin-dependent condition (formerly called adult-onset type) treated by diet control.

exophthalmos (ek"sof-thal'mos) protruding eyes, a symptom of one type of goiter.

fibrous thyroiditis enlarged thyroid with progressive fibrosis of the normal tissue, with the gland adhering to adjacent structures (also called *ligneous thyroiditis* and *Riedel's struma*).

goiter (goi'ter) enlargement of the thyroid, having a characteristic swelling at the front of the neck (also called *struma*).

Graves' disease hyperplasia of the thyroid gland (also called *Basedow's disease*).

hirsutism (her'sut-izm) abnormal hairiness, which may occur in some endocrine disorders.

hyperparathyroidism hyperfunction of the parathyroid gland: a primary type caused by neoplasms or unknown causes; and a secondary type caused by a metabolic disorder, producing calcium imbalance, with osteoporosis and deposition of calcium in tissues.

hyperthyroidism overproduction of the thyroid hormone.

hypophyseal cachexia (kah-kek'se-ah) hypofunction of the anterior pituitary gland caused by trauma, lesions, or tumors, resulting in generalized ill health with weakness, and overall insufficiency of adrenal, thyroid, and gonadal functions (also known as *Simmonds' disease* and *pituitary cachexia*).

hypothyroidism underfunction of the thyroid gland.

myxedema form of adult hypothyroidism, with metabolic slowdown resulting from deficient thyroid hormone secretion, producing symptoms ranging from milder forms with skin dryness, intolerance for cold, and some intellectual slippage, to severe forms with obesity, slowness of motor function, and severe intellectual dullness.

parathyroid tetany muscular cramps and spasms, resulting from hypocalcemia caused by excision of, or injury to, the parathyroids.

polydipsia excessive thirst, a symptom of diabetes.

polyuria excessive urination, a symptom of diabetes.

seasonal affective disorder (SAD) dysfunction linked to pineal gland production of melatonin, which is produced in darkness (night), and inhibited in daylight, becoming a problem for people residing in areas of extended darkness, such as in polar regions, producing symptoms of depression, known as "winter blues."

Sheehan's syndrome hypopituitarism as a result of a postpartum circulatory collapse, sometimes related to uterine hemmorhage, resulting in pituitary necrosis.

tetany muscle spasm and cramp, a symptom of hypoparathyroidism.

thyroid crisis exacerbation of preexisting hyperthyroidism as a result of trauma, surgery, or severe adrenocortical insufficiency (also called *thyrotoxic crisis* or *thyroid storm*).

thyrolytic pertaining to substances destructive to thyroid tissue.

thyropathy any disease or disorder of the thyroid gland.

thyroprivia (thi"ro-priv'e-ah) condition caused by lack of thyroid hormone.

virilism (vir'i-lizm) masculinization of a female, at birth or later in life, because of adrenocortical or gonadal dysfunction, or hormonal treatment.

Oncology*

adrenal cortical carcinomas* large, malignant, metastasizing tumors of the adrenal cortex, which produce virilism or Cushing's syndrome.

basophilic adenoma pituitary gland tumor whose cells stain with basic dyes.

chromophobic adenoma (kro'mo-fob-ik) benign tumor of pituitary gland whose cells resist staining with dyes.

*Indicates a malignant condition.

craniopharyngioma of pituitary gland (kra″neo-o-fah-rin″je-o′mah) tumor arising from the epithelium of the pituitary stalk.

eosinophilic adenoma of pituitary gland tumor of the eosinophilic cells of the anterior hypophysis, associated with acromegaly and giantism.

feminizing adenocarcinoma of adrenal gland* malignant tumor that produces female secondary sex characteristics in the male.

feminizing adenoma of adrenal gland benign tumor causing development of female secondary sex characteristics in the male.

glioma of pineal gland benign tumor of neuroglial tissue in the pineal gland.

Hürthle cell adenoma of thyroid gland (her′tel) adenoma containing Hürthle (large eosinophilic) cells.

Hürthle cell carcinoma of thyroid gland* malignant tumor of the thyroid.

pheochromocytoma (fe′o-kro-mo-si-to′mah) tumor of the adrenal medulla, usually benign.

pinealoma rare tumor of the pineal gland, sometimes associated with hydrocephalus or precocious puberty.

virilizing adenocarcinoma of adrenal gland* malignant tumor of the adrenal gland, with development of male secondary sex characteristics in the female.

virilizing adenoma of adrenal gland tumor of the adrenal glands, with development of male secondary sex characteristics in the female.

SURGICAL PROCEDURES

adrenalectomy (ad-re″nal-ek′to-me) excision of the adrenal glands.

hemithyroidectomy partial excision of the thyroid gland.

hypophysectomy (hi″po-fiz-ek′to-me) excision of the hypophysis, or anterior pituitary gland.

isthmectomy excision of the thyroid isthmus.

lobectomy excision of a lobe of the thyroid gland.

parathyroidectomy excision of a parathyroid gland.

pinealectomy (pin″e-al-ek′to-me) excision of the pineal body.

thyroidectomy excision of the thyroid gland.

thyroidotomy incision of the thyroid gland for exploration or drainage of an abscess or cyst.

°Indicates a malignant condition.

LABORATORY TESTS

aldosterone assay twenty-four hour urine or blood collection test to determine the presence of the hormone aldosterone, which is normally present and necessary for electrolyte balance.

catecholamine test urine test to measure amounts of adrenaline (epinephrine) and noradrenaline (norepinephrine), which are elevated in tumors of the adrenal gland (see also *vanillylmandelic acid*).

computerized tomography (CT) imaging device using x-rays at multiple angles through specific sections of the body, analyzed by computer to provide a total picture of the part being examined (also called *computerized axial tomography—CAT*).

cortisol tests tests of blood plasma and urine to measure levels of cortisol, to detect disorders of the adrenal glands.

estrogen receptor test test to determine whether hormonal therapy will be useful in cancer treatment, by measuring the response of the cancer to estrogen.

Goetsch's skin reaction test for hyperthyroidism involving localized reaction to epinephrine injection.

17-hydrocorticosteroid test (17-OCHS) twenty-four hour urine collection to determine the functioning of the adrenal glands to diagnose hyperadrenalism or hypoadrenalism.

17-ketosteroids tests (17-KS) twenty-four hour urine test to measure the levels of a group of adrenal cortex hormones involved in Addison's disease, Cushing's syndrome, stress, precocious puberty disorders, feminization in males, and virilization in females.

luteinizing hormone (LH) assay blood or urine test to determine the amount of pituitary hormones, follicle-stimulating hormone (FSH), and luteinizing hormone (LH) present, to detect gonadal failure or insufficiency, precocious puberty, testicular feminization, anorchia, and menopause.

magnetic resonance imaging (MRI) noninvasive method of scanning the body by means of an electromagnetic field and radio waves, which provides visual images on a computer screen and magnetic tape recordings (also called *nuclear magnetic resonance—NMR*).

protein-bound iodine (PBI) test test of thyroid function in which blood protein-bound iodine is measured to estimate the amount of available thyroid hormone in peripheral blood.

radioactive iodine uptake (RAIU) or thyroid ^{131}I uptake test thyroid function is evaluated by introducing radioactive iodine orally or intravenously during a selected time period, and measuring its absorption by the thyroid with a gamma ray detector.

thyroid hormone tests Group of blood tests to determine thyroid hormone levels and diagnose disorders of the thyroid.
triiodothyronine (T₃)
thyroxine (T₄)
thyroxine-binding globulin (TBG)

thyroid scan intravenous injection of radioactive substance for organ imaging to detect abnormalities in the size, shape, location, and function of the thyroid gland.

thyroid stimulation test anterior pituitary thyroid-stimulating hormone (TSH) is injected to determine if thyroid problems are due to pituitary or thyroid dysfunction.

thyroid ultrasonography noninvasive procedure to detect cysts and tumors of the thyroid by directing ultrasonic pulses at the gland that are reflected back for display on an oscilloscope.

vanillylmandelic acid (VMA) assay twenty-four hour urine test to detect VMA (a metabolite of catecholamines), to evaluate adrenal function.

EXERCISES THE ENDOCRINE SYSTEM THE CHEMICAL STIMULATORS

Exercise 14.1 *Complete the following:*

1. The thyroid gland is located in _front part of neck below the larynx_.
2. The normal location of the parathyroid glands is _behind the thyroid and embedded in its post. surf._
3. The part of the brain that has an endocrine function is the _hypothalamus_.
4. The function of the hormone secreted by the parathyroids is to _regulation of calcium_.
5. The pituitary gland is located _w/in depression of sphenoid bone_.
6. The connection between the hypothalamus and the pituitary gland is called the _infundibulum_.
7. The pituitary is called the "master gland" because it _exerts control over all the endocrine glands_.
8. The _posterior_ lobe of the pituitary gland secretes an antidiuretic hormone that stimulates water reabsorption by tubules of the kidneys.
9. The two distinct parts of the adrenals whose functions differ are the _cortex_ and the _medulla_.
10. The _cortex_ of the adrenal gland is indispensable to life.
11. The _cortex_ of the adrenal gland secretes glucocorticoids, mineralocorticoids, and sex hormones.
12. The _medulla_ of the adrenal gland secretes epinephrine and norepinephrine.
13. The endocrine system is made up of _ductless_ glands of internal secretion.
14. The secretions of the endocrine glands are called _hormones_.
15. The secretion of the thymus is called _thymosin_.

Exercise 14.2   *Matching*

A. growth hormone
B. mineralocorticoids
C. melatonin
D. oxytocin
E. prolactin
F. thyrotropic hormone
G. somatotropin
H. releasing and inhibiting hormones
I. luteinizing hormone

J. estrogen and progesterone
K. pancreatic polypeptide
L. glucagon
M. posterior lobe
N. anterior lobe
O. follicle-stimulating hormone (FSH)
P. calcitonin
Q. testosterone

R. glucocorticoids
S. antidiuretic hormone
T. adrenocorticotropic hormone
U. thymosin
V. parathyroid hormone
W. epinephrine
X. insulin
Y. melanocyte-stimulating hormone (MSH)

___Y___ **1.** Pigmentation hormone of the anterior lobe of the pituitary gland

___C___ **2.** A hormone of the pineal gland that decreases skin pigmentation

___B___ **3.** Hormones of the adrenal cortex that regulate sodium and potassium levels

___H___ **4.** Hormones of the hypothalamus that act on the anterior pituitary

___F___ **5.** Thyroid-stimulating hormone (TSH) of the anterior lobe of the pituitary gland that stimulates it to secrete thyroxine and triiodothyrine

___P___ **6.** Thyroid hormone that helps to regulate calcium levels in the blood

___G___ **7.** Growth hormone secreted by the anterior lobe of the pituitary gland

___D___ **8.** Hormone secreted by the posterior lobe of the pituitary gland that stimulates uterine contractions

___E___ **9.** Hormone responsible for development of the breast in pregnancy

___I___ **10.** Hormone from the anterior lobe of the pituitary gland that stimulates formation of the corpus luteum and secretion of testosterone by interstitial cells of the testis

___L___ **11.** Hormone, secreted by islands of Langerhans, which increases blood glucose

___K___ **12.** Functions in production of glucagon and gastric juices

___N___ **13.** Pituitary lobe that is an upgrowth of the embryonic pharynx

___M___ **14.** Pituitary lobe that is a downward extension of the brain

___J___ **15.** Ovarian hormones that promote menses after puberty

___O___ **16.** Anterior pituitary hormone that stimulates the growth of graafian follicles and secretion of estrogen in the female and the development of sperm cells in the male

___U___ **17.** Hormone that plays an important part in the immune system

___W___ **18.** Hormone secreted by the adrenal medulla that helps the body to meet stresses by stimulating the sympathetic nervous system

___R___ **19.** Adrenal cortex hormones concerned with fat, protein, and carbohydrate metabolism

___Q___ **20.** Male hormone producing secondary sex characteristics

___V___ **21.** Hormone regulating calcium and phosphorus in blood and bone

___T___ **22.** Meaning of the initials ACTH

___S___ **23.** Meaning of the initials ADH

___X___ **24.** Hormone that reduces glucose in the blood

___A___ **25.** Meaning of the initials GH

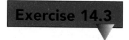

Exercise 14.3   *Using the list of terms below, identify each part in Figure 14.4 by writing the name in the corresponding blank.*

Adrenal gland

Ovary (female)

Pineal gland or body

Thyroid gland

Pituitary gland (hypophysis)

Parathyroid glands

Testis (male)

Pancreas

Thymus

Hypothalamus

1. _hypothalamus_
2. _pineal body_
3. _pituitary gland_
4. _thyroid gland_
5. _parathyroid glands_
6. _thymus_
7. _adrenal gland_
8. _pancreas_
9. _ovary_
10. _testis_

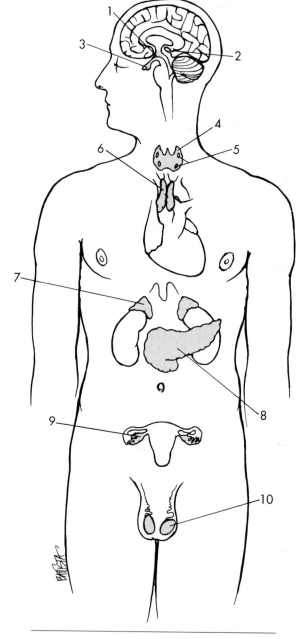

Figure 14.4 Location of the endocrine glands.

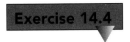 **Exercise 14.4** *Give the meaning of the components in the following words and then define the word as a whole. Suffixes meaning* pertaining to *or* state or condition, *shown following a slash mark (/), are not to be defined separately. Before reaching for your medical dictionary, check the Related Terms list in this chapter.*

1. Adrenalitis:

adrenal _____adrenals_____

itis _____inflammation_____

_____

2. Acromegaly:

acro _____extremities_____

megaly _____enlarged_____

_____

3. Adiposogenital dystrophy:

adiposo _____fat_____

genital _____genitalia_____

dys _____difficult_____

trophy _____nourishment_____

_____

4. Hypothyroidism:

hypo _____under_____

thyroid/ism _____thyroid_____

_____

5. Hypoadrenocorticism:

hypo _____under_____

adreno _____adrenal_____

cortic/ism _____cortex_____

_____

6. Hypogonadism:

hypo _____under_____

gonad/ism _____gonads_____

_____

7. Hyperthyroidism

hyper _____increased_____

thyroid/ism _____thyroid_____

_____

8. Adrenal hyperplasia:

adrenal _____adrenal_____

hyper _____over_____

plas/ia _____growth or development_____

_____

9. Thyrotoxicosis:

thyro _____thyroid_____

toxic/osis _____toxic_____

_____

10. Eosinophilic adenoma:

eosinophil/ic _____eosinophil cells_____

aden _____gland_____

oma _____tumor_____

_____

11. Hemithyroidectomy:

hemi _____partial_____

thyroid _____thyroid_____

ectomy _____surgical incision_____

_____

12. Isthmectomy:

isthm _____isthmus_____

ectomy _____excision_____

_____

CROSSWORD PUZZLE

CHAPTER 14

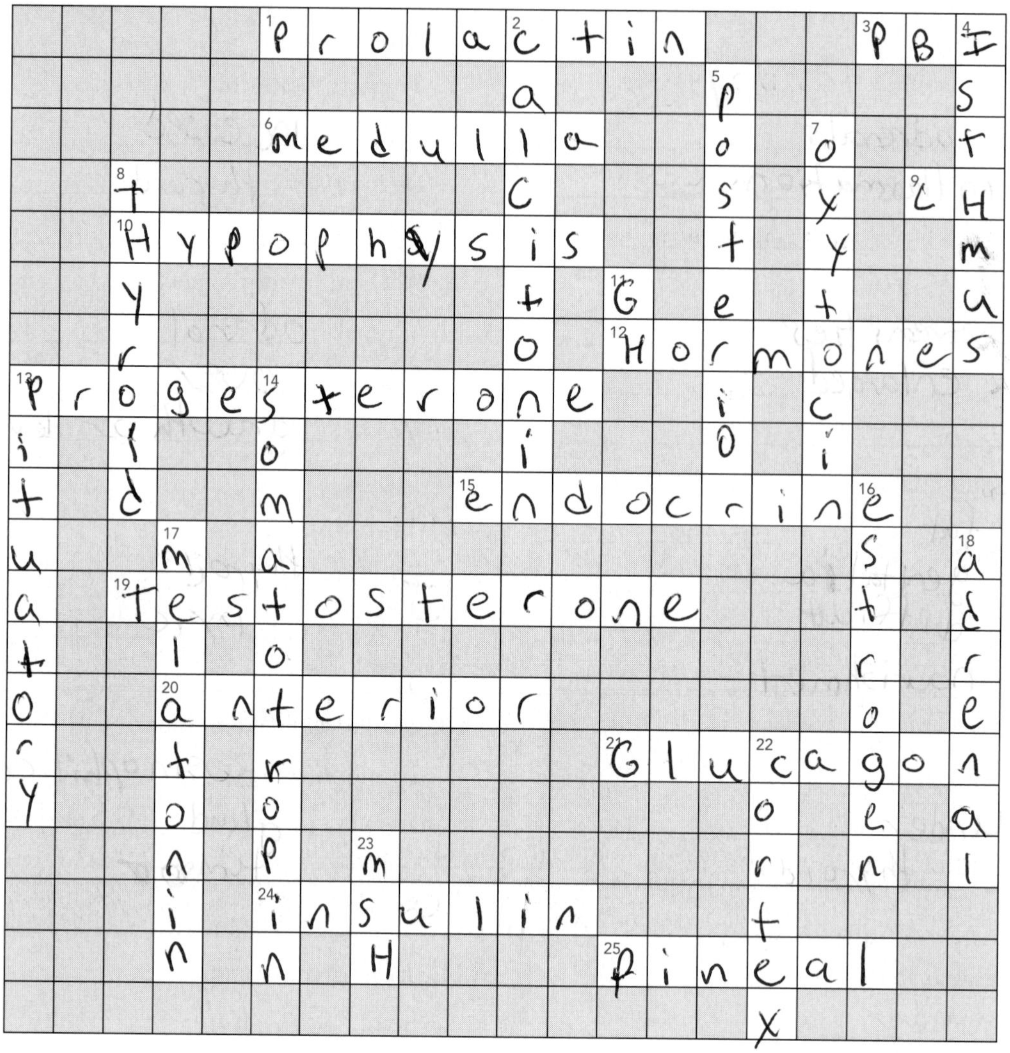

ACROSS

1. Hormone of milk production
3. Element in thyroid hormone combined with protein in blood
6. Inner part of adrenals
9. Hormone that stimulates ovaries and testes
10. Pituitary gland
12. Endocrine secretions
13. Female sex hormone
15. Ductless gland
19. Male sex hormone
20. A pituitary lobe
21. Increases blood glucose
24. Reduces blood glucose
25. Gland resembling pine cone

DOWN

2. Thyroid hormone promoting calcium absorption in bones
4. Separating strip of thyroid
5. A pituitary lobe
7. Hormone stimulating ejection of breast milk
8. Butterfly-shaped gland in neck
11. Abbreviation for hormone also known as somatrotropin
13. Master gland
14. Hormone promoting body and soft tissue growth
16. Female sex hormone
17. Skin-lightening agent
18. Gland resembling small cap on kidney
22. Outer part of adrenals
23. Hormone stimulating skin pigment

HIDDEN WORDS PUZZLE

```
T F J P V Z W K Q E Z K W D I C D S P H T N L F V U L
G O N A D S D N P Q B O J B X Y N Q V C O N U Y A C I
L R E N H B S G O W H N C J W Q C S Y H W J I R K R R
N O G C K Y G T H Y R O I D F S S H J M B P Q D Y O S
D I B R T Q P C C O W V E G K T P A U Q A D A V D Q Y
P E P E S T R O G E N A Y D L P N U M U Q X C A X N E
I M J A G T T L P H N R C O U G E P Y E L B K G L I O
T A N S M N G L O H N I K C W I C B I I D B K H D S L
Z K V N O O B O D O Y E R R I Q M F H N W K V T S H H
K V W S K H R I H M A S T E R P J W T T U W T S K F S
H N M H W E P D E R V Q I V L A F S O W I G M V S P C
B H U C W U K B S I B X D S D R Q H Q T K F O J S Y D
G N N Y V S R T O E U I K O J A I N V E R M U C Z S B
Q N S L N A Z Z T H R F J M S T A C Q R O K Y B U X B
B E Z K R Q S R H E P N U A E H U J M O B P H X W H V
Q P R F J P T O S H P M O T C Y Y L B N N T Y H W Y W
N N G O G J T H P D H E A O R R I P S S Q Q Y W T L B
N M P W E I H Q Y R R O I T E O S J O H R H W R S S F
I I Q S F P I D Q R E R K R T I T G L T C Z H I S G F
P V F P Y G L R M Q O S V O I D H Q N V H K R O K S T
I Q A G E L L M D Q V X S P O S M J S O K A W C B H N
L F I V D N O A B H F O I I N F U N D I B U L U M F M
W R M X S X X O N A J L Y N N Q S Q H U N D A A O P B
D X R P H Y J M A D U C T L E S S D A H O S O T M C L
V X Y C E J O U B R F Y F E U G G T F T T B I Y R U W
W B L D G G H L Q E E M G O N Y E R X D F L Y X A Q S
V C H Q T B Q D X N F Q B Q P X Y U S X G L O L Z Q X
T W Q D W L H Q E A J Q J U J X S E C P N V H R N G F
P Q J N X I U A L L B Y W U C R J X T X B X R T H J F
```

Can you find the 20 words hidden in this puzzle? All hidden words puzzles have words running from top to bottom, left to right, and diagonally downward.

HYPOTHALAMUS	ESTROGEN	GLAND
VASOPRESSIN	ISTHMUS	SOMATOTROPIN
DUCTLESS	MASTER	THYROXINE
COLLOID	PARATHYROIDS	ADRENAL
GONADS	SECRETION	THYROID
INFUNDIBULUM	PANCREAS	LOBE
HYPOPHYSIS	OVARIES	

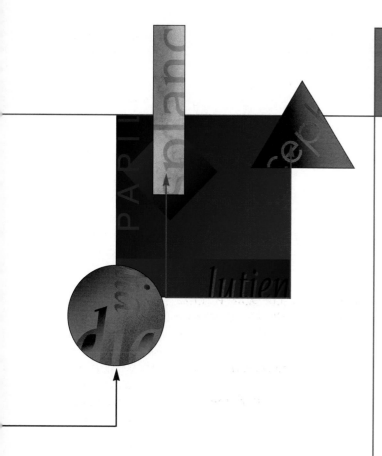

The Nervous System

the central processing unit

This chapter explores the structure and functions of both divisions of the nervous system, central and peripheral, including the brain, spinal cord, nerves, and fluids.

CHARACTERISTICS OF THE NERVOUS SYSTEM

The nervous system has been compared to a computer system, with the brain acting as the central processing unit, relaying messages by way of the spinal cord, through nerve fibers that radiate to every structure in the body, to provide connections for input and output data. Sensory nerves bring impulses, or information, from the various systems of the body, whereas motor nerves carry impulses from the central coordinating point to muscles or glands that need to respond for appropriate adjustment of the body.

The nervous system is divided into the *central nervous system (CNS)*, which includes the *brain* and *spinal cord*, and the *peripheral nervous system (PNS)*, composed of the *craniospinal nerves* and the *autonomic nervous system (ANS)*, which controls and coordinates the functioning of the vital organs. Nervous tissue is composed of many types of cells and fibers, working together in one central mass, with many peripheral strands.

Its a **FACT**

Brain cells are the only cells of the body that cannot reproduce themselves.

Nerve Structure and Function

Nervous system cells are called *neurons.* All neurons are similar in that they have one *axon,* one or more *dendrites,* and a grayish *cell body* in between, containing a nucleus responsible for maintaining the life of the whole cell. The dendrites are numerous short branches that conduct nerve impulses toward the cell body. The axons are longer branches that carry impulses away from the cell body, either to other neurons, through contact with their dendrites, to the cell body itself, or directly to other organs or tissues (see Figure 5.5). It is estimated that each neuron interconnects with about 1000 other neurons.

Neurons are divided into *sensory* (or *afferent*), *motor* (or *efferent*), and *connector* (or *interneuron*) neurons. In sensory neurons, the dendrites are connected to receptors (eyes, ears, and other sense organs), and the axons are connected to other neurons. The receptors change information from external sources, such as light waves or sound vibrations, into electrical impulses. In motor neurons, the dendrites are connected to other neurons, and the axons to effectors (muscles and glands). In connector neurons, the dendrites and axons are both connected to other neurons.

Normally, impulses pass in only one direction. Sensory neurons conduct impulses from the sense organs to the spinal cord and brain. Motor neurons conduct impulses from the brain and spinal cord to muscles and glands. Sensory or afferent impulses are transmitted to the brain through the ascending tracts of the spinal cord, whereas motor or efferent impulses are carried from the brain through the descending tracts of the spinal cord.

The impulses are essentially the same in all types of neurons and may be compared to the wavelike action of peristalsis. The initiating stimulus of the impulse in one section of a nerve fiber causes a similar reaction in the next connecting section, and this chain reaction continues until the impulse reaches the end of the nerve fiber. Nerve impulses differ only in terms of the body part affected: an impulse caused by light rays entering the eye may result in vision; an impulse received in the ear may result in hearing; other impulses may result in muscle movement; and still others may result in glandular secretions.

The threadlike dendrites and axons are also called nerve *fibers.* Bundles of these fibers bound together are called *nerves.* Groups of neuron cell bodies within the brain and spinal cord are called *nuclei,* whereas those outside are called *ganglia* (singular—*ganglion*). A side branch of the axon is called a *collateral,* which ends in a fine, spreading branch called a *terminal twig,* deriving its name from its resemblance to a twig or branch of a tree.

The point at which an impulse is transmitted from the axon of one neuron to the dendrite of another is a microscopic space called a *synapse.* The electrical impulses carried by the neuron do not directly jump the synapse, but instead produce a *neurotransmitter* chemical, which activates other electrical impulses in the dendrites of the connecting neuron.

Nerve fibers are of different types. Some are myelinated, with a coat of white fatty material called a *myelin sheath* surrounding them, found mainly in the central nervous system. Nonmyelinated fibers have a tubelike membrane covering called the *neurilemma* or *sheath of Schwann* and are found especially in the autonomic nervous system. A myelin sheath and a neurilemma are found in peripheral somatic fibers. There are axon fibers that have no sheath, found in the central nervous system and within organs (Figure 15.1).

The nerve cells and their gossamer filaments are held together and supported by a specialized type of tissue called *neuroglia.* Neuroglial cells have many processes, or branches, that form a dense network between neurons. They are divided into four main types: *astrocytes* (*astro*—star), *microglia, oligodendroglia,* and *Schwann cells.* Astrocytes cover the surfaces of

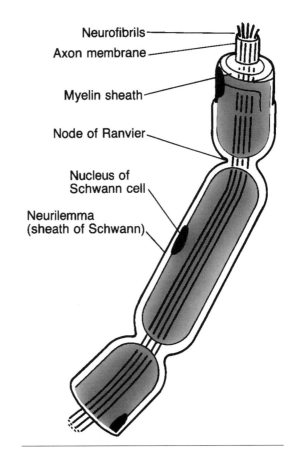

Neurofibrils
Axon membrane
Myelin sheath
Node of Ranvier
Nucleus of Schwann cell
Neurilemma (sheath of Schwann)

Figure 15.1 Diagram of a nerve and its coverings.

the capillaries of the brain. Together with the walls of the capillaries they form the blood-brain barrier, which regulates the passage of nutritive and chemical molecules to the brain neurons. Microglia are phagocytic cells that fight infection and help in healing. Oligodendroglia aid in holding nerve fibers together and in forming the myelin sheath within the central nervous system. Schwann cells, which are found only outside the central nervous system, form the neurilemma and a thin layer of myelin around nerve fibers.

The central nervous system contains both white and gray matter. The white color is created by the myelinated fibers of the bundles of axons and dendrites, and the gray color is due to the masses of nerve cell bodies.

The cell body is vital to the neuron. If the cell body dies, the neuron also dies and can never be replaced. Neurons are so specialized that they have lost their power to reproduce new cells. When an axon is severed, that part distal to the cell body dies, with both the fiber and its surrounding myelinated sheath degenerating. A new axon may gradually grow and restore the nerve, but such regeneration occurs only in the peripheral nervous system. Once a connection is broken within the central nervous system, it is broken forever, although other nerve structures may take over the functions of the injured nerves.

REVIEW 15.A

Complete the following:

1. The nervous system is divided into the __Central__ and __peripheral__ nervous systems.

2. All neurons have one __axon__ and one or more __dendrites__, with a grayish __Cell body__ in between.

3. The three types of neurons are __Sensory__, __motor__, and __connector__.

4. Threadlike dendrites and axons are also called __(nerve) fibers__.

5. Groups of neuron cell bodies within the brain and spinal cord are called __nuclei__.

6. The microscopic space over which an impulse is transmitted is called a __Synapse__.

7. The sheath of Schwann is also called the __neurilemma__.

8. The nerve cells and their filaments are held together and supported by a type of tissue called __neuroglia__.

9. Receptors change information from external sources such as light waves into electrical __impulses__.

10. Groups of neuron cell bodies outside the brain and spinal cord are called __ganglia__.

THE CENTRAL NERVOUS SYSTEM

The central nervous system (CNS) includes the brain and the spinal cord. This system is also referred to as the *cerebrospinal* system. The brain lies in the cranial cavity, and the spinal cord, continuous with the lower end of the brain, passes through the *foramen magnum,* an opening in the occipital bone of the head, and continues down through the vertebral column. The brain and spinal cord are both protected from injury by the skeletal system, the brain by the bones of the skull, and the spinal cord by the vertebrae.

The Meninges

The *meninges* (plural of *meninx*—meaning membrane) are three membranes that envelop the central nervous system, separating the brain and spinal cord from the body cavities in which they lie, and aiding in their support and protection (Figure 15.2). The meninges are composed predominantly of white fibrous connective tissue.

The *dura mater*—the outermost layer, is the hardest, toughest, and most fibrous of the three.
The *arachnoid (arachno* means spider)—the middle membrane is much less dense, and is weblike in appearance.
The *pia mater*—the innermost, thin, compact membrane that is closely adapted to the surface of the brain and spinal cord, is very vascular and supplies the blood for the central nervous system tissues.

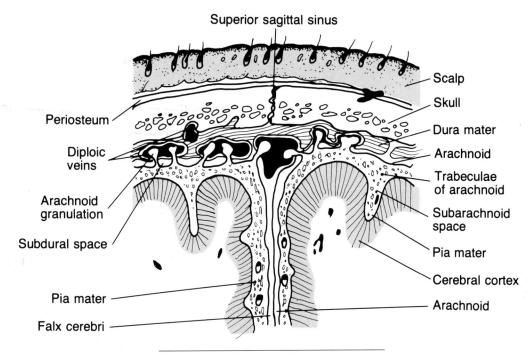

Figure 15.2 Coronal section through skull.

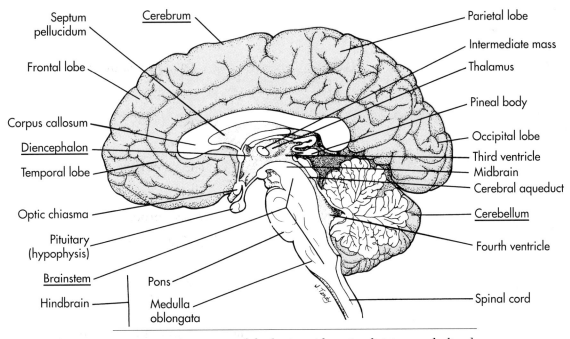

Figure 15.3 Structures of the brain, with major divisions underlined.

The pia mater and arachnoid are often viewed as one membrane, the *pia-arachnoid* (also called the *leptomeninges*). The space between the pia mater and the arachnoid is known as the *subarachnoid space,* and that between the arachnoid and the dura mater as the *subdural space.*

The Brain

The brain is the greatly enlarged part of the central nervous system, weighing about 40 to 60 oz (1.1 to 1.7 kg) in the average adult. In proportion to the size of the body, it is much larger in the neonate than in the adult. The size of the cranium (skull) furnishes only a general index as to the size of the brain, for the shape and thickness of the skull and the subarachnoid space vary in individuals. It is estimated that the average brain contains about 100 to 200 billion neurons at birth, and of these 50 to 100 thousand neurons die each day.

The divisions of the brain are the *brainstem,* the *cerebellum,* the *diencephalon,* and the *cerebrum* (Figure 15.3).

The brainstem. The brainstem is divided into the *medulla oblongata,* the *pons,* and the *midbrain,* with the pons and medulla together commonly referred to as the *hindbrain* (see Figure 15.3).

The medulla oblongata. The medulla oblongata, the lowest and most posterior part of the brain, about 1 inch (2.5 cm) in length, is an extension of the spinal cord at the point where the central canal of the spinal cord enlarges to form the fourth ventricle, extending to the pons. The fourth ventricle, a large kite-shaped cavity that secretes some of the cerebrospinal fluid, contains openings that connect the cavity with the subarachnoid space and with the lateral ventricles in the cerebral hemispheres.

The medulla oblongata is composed of white matter, and a reticular formation, or network, composed of gray and white matter. This network has a *reticular activating system,* connecting with all the sensory systems and the cortex, controlling and regulating the degree of cortical arousal and alertness. The reticular formation also contains groups of nuclei, some of which are highly specialized structures, called nerve centers, that regulate heart action, respiration, and blood pressure.

Nerve fibers (the white matter) in the medulla oblongata establish communication between the cerebrum and the spinal cord. As these nerve fibers pass through the medulla, about 75% cross from one side to the other. This is the basis for the right side of the brain controlling the left side of the body, and the left side of the brain controlling the right side of the body.

The pons. The pons, about 1½ inches (3.8 cm) long and made up of reticular formation and white matter, is the portion of the brain that serves as a bridge (*pons* means bridge) connecting the medulla oblongata, cerebellum, and cerebrum. A portion of the reticular formation, which figures significantly in respiration, extends into the pons. The pons is also associated with the fifth, sixth, seventh, and eighth cranial nerves. These nerves provide sensory input from face, head, muscles, and other internal tissues and the senses of taste, hearing, and balance. They also provide motor control of facial muscles, including the muscles of mastication, and salivary secretion.

The midbrain. The midbrain, or *mesencephalon,* is the uppermost part of the brainstem, above the pons, and, like the hindbrain, is also composed of reticular formation and white matter. It contains auditory, visual, and muscle control centers and is also involved in body posture and equilibrium.

The third and fourth cranial nerves originate in the midbrain, which also contains a small central canal called the *cerebral aqueduct (aqueduct of Sylvius),* that connects the third ventricle of the brain, located

---

R E V I E W   1 5 . B

Complete the following:

1. Another name for the central nervous system is the ___Cerebrospinal___ system.

2. The three meningeal membranes are the
   ___dura mater___,
   ___arachnoid___, and
   ___pia mater___.

3. The four divisions of the brain are the
   ___brain stem___,
   ___diencephalon___,
   ___cerebellum___, and
   ___cerebrum___.

4. The brainstem consists of the
   ___medulla oblongata___, ___pons___,
   and ___midbrain___.

5. The hindbrain is made up of the
   ___medulla oblongata___ and the ___pons___.

in the diencephalon, with the fourth ventricle, located between the cerebellum and the hindbrain.

The cerebellum. The cerebellum is the second largest division of the brain, situated just above the medulla and beneath the rear portion of the cerebrum. It resembles a partially opened shell in appearance and comprises about 10% of the weight of the entire brain. The cerebellum consists of a central portion, called the *vermis,* and two larger sections, one on each side, called the right and left *cerebellar hemispheres* (see Figure 15.3).

The chief functions of the cerebellum are to balance, harmonize, and coordinate muscular activity initiated by the cerebrum. The cerebellum, through its vestibular portion, is connected with the semicircular canals of the ear, which, together with the movements of the eyes, react to gravity and sudden changes or movement of the head. These are further integrated and correlated, by the cerebellum, with nerve impulses from the muscles, tendons, and joints. Through these functions, the cerebellum fine-tunes motor activity and muscle tone, which is essential for precise and complicated voluntary movement, and the maintenance of posture. It also enables the various muscle groups to act harmoniously, or as a cooperative whole, at a given moment. Many motor activities, originally initiated by the cerebrum and coordinated by the cerebellum, such as walking, running, and other skilled movements, eventually become automatic and are not consciously initiated or coordinated.

The diencephalon. The diencephalon is the part of the brain between the midbrain and the cerebrum, containing the *thalamus,* the *epithalamus,* and the *hypothalamus* (*thalamus* means chamber). The diencephalon also contains the third ventricle, a narrow chamber between the right and left halves of the thalamus (see Figure 15.3).

The *thalamus* is a large, gray, oval mass that acts as a center to receive sensory impulses and transmit them on to the cerebral cortex. The thalamus has been referred to as the great integrating center of the brain. It plays a role in integrating visual, auditory, tactile, temperature, pain, and taste sensations with pleasant and unpleasant emotions and with memory storage.

The *epithalamus* contains the pineal body (Chapter 14) and olfactory centers.

The *hypothalamus* is located beneath the thalamus. It connects the endocrine and nervous systems, which coordinate the maintenance functions of the body (Chapter 14). The hypothalamus also regulates the autonomic nervous system and contains centers for control of body temperature, carbohydrate and fat metabolism, appetite, and emotions. It is a key center for the interaction of emotional and bodily functioning and plays a crucial role in psychosomatic illness. The hypothalamus contains the posterior lobe of the pituitary gland, the infundibulum (previously discussed in Chapter 14), and the *optic chiasma.* The optic chiasma, which is also a part of the cerebral hemispheres, is formed chiefly of nerve fibers, and beyond the chiasma these fibers continue as the optic tract.

The cerebrum. The cerebrum, the largest part of the brain, is divided into two hemispheres called the *cerebral hemispheres,* which occupy most of the brain cavity (see Figure 15.3).

The outer surface, or *cortex,* is made up of gray matter, beneath which is white matter that forms the central portion of the brain. As the brain develops, the cerebral hemispheres increase greatly in size in relation to the rest of the brain. As the gray matter of the cortex increases in amount, the surface of each cerebral hemisphere is thrown into folds called *gyri* (singular—*gyrus*), or *convolutions.* These folds are separated from each other by furrows called *sulci* (singular—*sulcus*), with the deeper furrows called *fissures.*

Each cerebral hemisphere contains a *lateral ventricle* separated by a medial wall, the *septum pellucidum.* Each ventricle projects an anterior horn into the frontal lobe, a posterior horn into the occipital lobe, and an inferior horn into the temporal lobe. These horns are also called *cornua* (*cornu* means horn). The lateral ventricles, in conjunction with the third and fourth ventricles, produce the cerebrospinal fluid.

Connecting the structures of one cerebral hemisphere with the other are three groups of *commissural tracts* (connections between corresponding anatomic parts):

> *corpus callosum*—the largest, consisting of dense masses of white matter that transversely unite the two hemispheres.
>
> *anterior commissure*—contains fibers that connect different parts of the temporal lobes with one another.
>
> *posterior commissure*—formed by a thin sheet of fibers that cross transversely under the posterior part of the corpus callosum and connect to the olfactory centers.

The Functional Areas of the Cerebral Cortex

The cerebral cortex is divided into lobes: *frontal, temporal, parietal,* and *occipital,* corresponding with the bones in the region in which they are located (see Figure 15.3). Some anatomists consider a fifth area, the *insula* or *island of Reil*, hidden below the frontal lobe, to be an additional lobe.

Frontal lobe. The frontal lobe, the most anterior of all the lobes, is the center for voluntary movement and is often referred to as the motor area. It contains areas for the control of gross, fine, and complicated muscle movements. One of these areas, the *premotor*, is viewed as the highest level of motor control because it is concerned with learned motor activity of a highly complicated nature, such as playing a musical instrument, dancing, and athletic skills. The most anterior portion of the frontal lobe, the *prefrontal* area, is also the seat of the highest of human functions, including intelligence, creativity, memory, and association of ideas.

Parietal lobe. The parietal lobe collects, recognizes, and organizes sensations of pain, temperature, touch, position and movement. From these sensations we perceive the size, shape, and weight of external objects and of our own physical being.

Temporal lobe. The temporal lobe contains the centers for awareness and correlation of auditory stimuli; it functions in storage of auditory and visual memory and language development. One area, *Broca's speech area*, is especially concerned with speech.

Occipital lobe. The occipital lobe forms the posterior extremity of each cerebral hemisphere. It involves visual perception and visual memory and associations and plays a role in eye movements.

Hemispheric Differences in Function

As previously noted, the left hemisphere of the cerebrum controls the right side of the body, and the right hemisphere controls the left side of the body, because the descending nerve fibers cross over in the medulla and spinal cord, with fibers from the left crossing to the right, and fibers from the right crossing to the left.

General differences in hemispheric function appear to exist, with the left, which is usually dominant, being involved in language, logic, analytic thinking, and ordering of events and symbols, whereas the right hemisphere has been linked to imagination, creativity in art and music, and spatial and depth perception.

Limbic System

The limbic system appears to be a center for emotional experience, emotional behavior, and memory and has been referred to as "the emotional brain." Emotions that have been identified with the limbic system include sadness, pleasure, fear, anger, and sexual arousal, which are subject to moderation by the cerebral cortex.

The limbic system involves areas of the diencephalon and the cerebrum, including the *cingulate gyrus, isthmus, hippocampal gyrus, uncus, hippocampus, septum, amygdala*, and the *hypothalamus*. The hippocampus has been called the "gatekeeper for memory," and has been related to learning and memory problems in diseases like Alzheimer's disease.

Cerebrospinal Fluid

Cerebrospinal fluid is a thin, transparent, watery fluid found within the ventricles of the brain, the central canal of the spinal cord, and the subarachnoid space. It is produced by a network of capillaries that filter plasmalike fluids from blood into the ventricles, with the lateral ventricles producing the major part.

Cerebrospinal fluid drains from the lateral ventricles into the third ventricle, through the cerebral aqueduct (aqueduct of Sylvius) into the fourth ventricle, from which it passes into the subarachnoid space. The cerebrospinal fluid surrounds the brain, providing support for its weight and serving as a protective cushion. The spinal cord is also surrounded and cushioned by the fluid. In addition to the protection provided by the cerebrospinal fluid, it also supplies some nutrients.

Spinal Cord

The spinal cord is an essential extension of the central processing unit, the brain. Sensations received by the sensory nerves are relayed to the spinal cord, where they are transferred either to the brain or to motor nerves. If the sensation is transferred to a motor nerve, it travels out to a muscle or gland and produces an action.

The spinal cord resembles a flattened cylinder and is about the thickness of a pencil. It extends from the medulla oblongata to the level of the first lumbar vertebra.

The spinal cord, constituting about 2% of all the central nervous system, is enclosed in the vertebral column, which protects it from injury. Like the brain, it has three membranous coverings, the pia mater, arachnoid, and dura mater, which have been described in the section on the meninges. Like the brain, it is bathed in cerebrospinal fluid. The spinal cord is made up of an inner core of gray matter and an outer core of white matter, which, in cross section, resembles a butterfly, with its wings divided into two dorsal and two ventral parts called *horns.*

Both ascending and descending tracts are contained in the spinal cord. These tracts are white fibers made up of axons and dendrites. The ascending tracts conduct the afferent (sensory) nerve impulses to the brain, and the descending tracts conduct the efferent (motor) nerve impulses from the brain. Centers for connections between the afferent and the efferent nerve impulses are provided by the gray matter (see Figure 15.7).

It is through the spinal cord, and the attachment of 31 pairs of spinal nerves along its sides, that the brain maintains intimate association with all the organs of the body (see Figures 15.4 and 15.5). Each of the 31 pairs of spinal nerves is attached to the spinal cord by one posterior afferent root and one anterior efferent root, at approximately equal distances throughout the entire length of the cord.

The spinal cord is divided into sections, with 8 pairs of cervical nerves, 12 pairs of thoracic nerves, 5 pairs of lumbar nerves, 5 pairs of sacral nerves, and 1 pair of coccygeal nerves. The functions of these nerves are discussed in the section on the peripheral nervous system.

Injury of the spinal cord in any segment can imperil any or all of its functions. When the spinal cord is injured, the part above the injury functions normally, but there is paralysis of the part below the injury, and the brain receives no impulses from that area.

REVIEW 15.D

Complete the following:

1. The limbic system is referred to as the _____emotional_____ brain.

2. The cerebrospinal fluid is found within the __ventricles of brain__ the __centalcanal of spinal cord__ and the __subarachnoid space__.

3. The spinal cord has ___3___ membranous coverings.

4. The spinal cord has both __ascending__ and __descending__ tracts.

5. There are ___31___ pairs of spinal nerves along the spinal cord.

THE PERIPHERAL NERVOUS SYSTEM

The peripheral nervous system (PNS) includes all the nerves and ganglia located outside of the brain and spinal cord, including the autonomic nervous system (Figures 15.4 and 15.5). Because of the closeness of the connections, the peripheral nervous system overlaps the central nervous system, the spinal cord, and their functions.

Cranial Nerves

The first segment of the peripheral nervous system is the 12 pairs of cranial nerves arising from the brain, especially the brainstem (Figure 15.6).

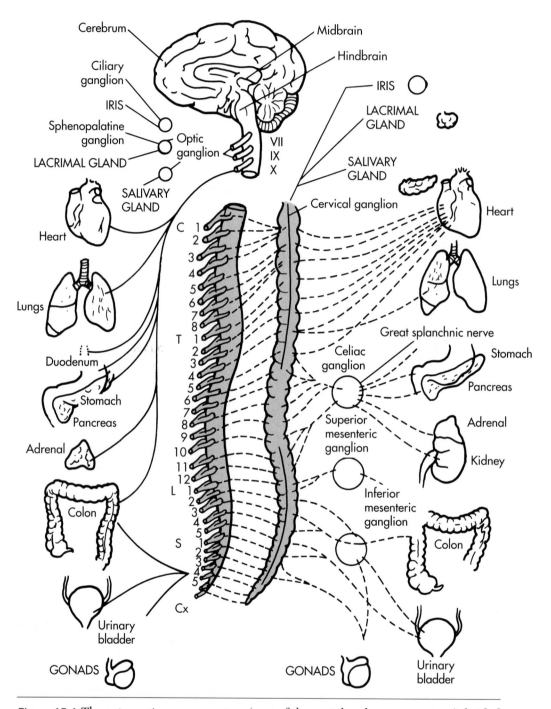

Figure 15.4 The autonomic nervous system (part of the peripheral nervous system) divided into the sympathetic and parasympathetic nervous systems. The sympathetic system is represented by broken lines and the parasympathetic by solid lines. The spinal cord (part of the central nervous system) is also shown.

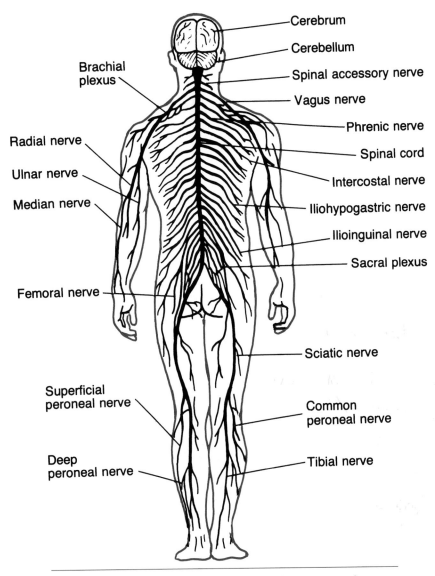

Figure 15.5 Peripheral nervous system, with some cranial nerves.

The first cranial nerve, the *olfactory,* is for the sense of smell.

The second cranial nerve, the *optic,* extends from the retina of the eye to the optic chiasma and is for vision.

The third cranial nerve, the *oculomotor,* functions in movement of the eye, focus, pupil changes, and eye muscle sense.

The fourth cranial nerve, the *trochlear,* functions in movement of the eye.

The fifth cranial nerve, the *trigeminal,* is the largest of the cranial nerves, with both sensory and motor functions. It is divided into three parts, the *ophthalmic,* the *maxillary,* and the *mandibular.* The trigeminal receives sensa-tions from the head and face and innervates the chewing muscles.

The sixth cranial nerve, the *abducens,* innervates the muscles of the eye.

The seventh cranial nerve, the *facial,* is both a sensory and a motor nerve. It controls muscles of the face, ears, and scalp and functions in facial expression, salivary gland secretion, and in taste sensation.

The eighth cranial nerve, the *acoustic* or *auditory* nerve, is divided into two parts, the *cochlear* nerve, which functions in hearing, and the *vestibular* nerve, which functions in maintaining balance and equilibrium.

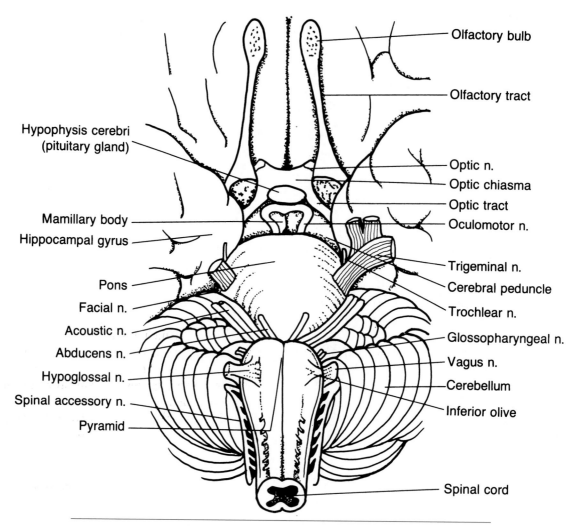

Figure 15.6 Attachment of the cranial nerves to the underside (ventral surface) of the brain.

The ninth cranial nerve, the *glossopharyngeal*, is both a motor and a sensory nerve, which functions in taste sensations, swallowing, and salivary secretion.

The tenth cranial nerve, the *vagus*, is the longest of the cranial nerves and is both a motor and a sensory nerve. It is extensive in distribution, with many branches to the pharynx, larynx, trachea, esophagus, and the thoracic and abdominopelvic viscera, receiving sensations from, and activating, these organs.

The eleventh cranial nerve, the *spinal accessory*, is a motor nerve divided into two parts, *cranial* and *spinal*, and functions in swallowing, head and shoulder movements, visceral movements, and voice production.

The twelfth cranial nerve, the *hypoglossal*, is a motor nerve that controls the muscles of the tongue and functions in speech and swallowing.

Spinal Nerves

As noted previously, 12 pairs of cranial nerves arise from the brain, and 31 pairs of spinal nerves stem from the spinal cord. Both voluntary and involuntary impulses are carried by these nerves. In general, the cranial nerves are voluntary, except for those serving the heart, the smooth muscles of the lungs, the salivary glands, and the stomach and eye muscles. The spinal nerves send fibers to all the muscles of the trunk and extremities, with involuntary fibers going to smooth muscles and glands of the gastrointestinal, urinary, reproductive, and cardiovascular systems.

The spinal nerves are attached to the spinal cord by anterior (efferent) and posterior (afferent) roots. After leaving the spinal cord, the nerves are named after their corresponding vertebra. The first pair of cervical nerves emerge between the first cervical vertebra and the occipital bone, thus providing for 8 pairs of cervical nerves, although there are only seven cervical vertebrae. The next 12 pairs are the thoracic spinal nerves, followed by 5 pairs of lumbar, 5 pairs of sacral, and 1 pair of coccygeal spinal nerves. The lower spinal nerves supply the lower extremities and extend below the level of the spinal cord in parallel strands, resembling a horse's tail, the *cauda equina* (*cauda* means tail, and *equina* means horse). Through openings in the sacrum they extend down the thigh.

Spinal nerves are composed of sensory and motor fibers of both the autonomic and the voluntary nervous systems. In some areas of the body they merge to form an interlacing network called a *plexus.* These plexuses are the *cervical plexus* in the neck, the *brachial plexus* in the shoulder, and the *lumbosacral plexus* in the lumbar, sacral, and coccygeal areas of the back. The names and areas served by a number of the peripheral nerves, many of which are named for bones, organs, or body regions, are shown in Figures 15.4 and 15.5.

The cervical plexus is formed by the first four cervical nerves and supplies the skin and muscles of the shoulders, neck, and head, with phrenic branches going to the diaphragm.

The lower cervical and first thoracic nerves supply the upper limbs through the brachial plexus, which lies in the shoulder area, serving the skin and the arm and hand muscles.

The lumbosacral plexus supplies the skin and muscles of the back, abdomen, buttocks, lower limbs, perineum, and external genitalia. The sciatic nerve is a part of the lumbosacral plexus and is the largest nerve in the body.

Nerve Pathways

Somatic (*soma* means body) motor pathways involve the conduction of impulses from the central nervous system to skeletal muscles. These pathways are classified into *pyramidal (corticospinal)* and *extrapyramidal* tracts. The pyramidal tracts conduct impulses that facilitate conscious, voluntary actions of the muscles. Impulses from the extrapyramidal tracts produce larger, more automatic movements by contracting groups of muscles in sequence, such as those involved in walking, running, and swimming.

Reflex Action

The arrangement of sensory, connector, and motor nerves is referred to as a *reflex arc,* and the action produced is a *reflex action.* An example of a reflex action is that which occurs when a hand touches a hot stove, and the instantaneous pain sensation causes quick withdrawal of the hand. The sensation, in this instance, is relayed to the spinal cord level, because there is not enough time to think of removing the hand, which would be a brain function. When consciousness is involved in an action, it is under the control of the brain. A reflex action occurs below the brain level, within the spinal cord, and is not conscious or voluntary (Figure 15.7).

We have many reflex actions that are automatic, such as walking, dancing, skating, typing, or even driving an automobile, which are first learned by experience or education. When a child is learning to walk, every step taken requires concentration, but in time, experience establishes reflexes, which allow the child the freedom of walking without concentrating. Some reflexes, such as sucking, chewing, swallowing, urination, and defecation, appear to be inherited, because they are present at birth.

Among the most common reflexes are:

knee jerk reflex—the leg extends in response to tapping of the patellar ligament.
Babinski reflex—dorsiflexion of the big toe in response to stroking the sole of the foot.
biceps reflex—contraction of the biceps muscles in response to tapping of the tendon.
Achilles tendon reflex—the foot extends in response to tapping the Achilles tendon.
pupillary reflex—the pupil of the eye contracts in response to exposure of the retina to a bright light.

THE AUTONOMIC NERVOUS SYSTEM

Although a part of the peripheral nervous system, the autonomic nervous system is an integral part of the entire nervous system. It functions automatically and is divided into the *sympathetic* (or *thoracolumbar*) and *parasympathetic* (or *craniosacral*) systems, which act upon the involuntary, smooth, and cardiac muscles and glands (see Figure 15.4). The autonomic

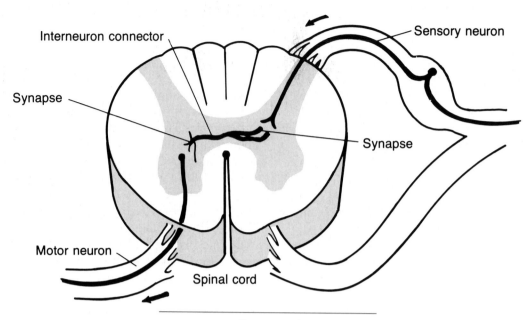

Figure 15.7 Reflex arc in the spinal cord.

nervous system also serves the vital systems that function automatically, such as the digestive, circulatory, respiratory, urinary, and endocrine systems.

Sympathetic System Structure

The sympathetic trunk lies close to the vertebrae and is composed of a series of ganglia (nerve cell clusters) on each side, forming a nodular cord resembling a string of beads (see Figure 15.4). These ganglia extend from the base of the skull to the front of the coccyx and are the basis of the sympathetic system. These ganglia are connected with the thoracic and lumbar spinal cord and with the muscles, organs, and glands they affect through spinal nerves.

Parasympathetic System Structure

The parasympathetic system centers are located in the brainstem and the sacral regions (see Figure 15.4). The centers in the brainstem send out impulses through the oculomotor, facial, glossopharyngeal, and vagus cranial nerves, and the second, third, and fourth sacral nerves make up the sacral group.

Functions

The sympathetic and parasympathetic divisions oppose each other in function and maintain balance in the body mechanisms they serve. They are under the control of the hypothalamus, cerebral cortex, and medulla oblongata in the brain, which coordinates

their actions and keeps the body in **homeostasis** (normal stability of the internal environment). In general, the parasympathetic system maintains the routine functioning of the body, whereas the sympathetic system is called upon to respond under additional stress or emergency conditions.

The following are some examples of opposition of the sympathetic and parasympathetic systems. The sympathetic system dilates the pupils, and the parasympathetic system contracts them. The sympathetic relaxes ciliary muscles so that the eyes are accommodated to distant objects, and the parasympathetic contracts these muscles to accommodate the eyes to near objects. The sympathetic dilates the bronchial tubes, and the parasympathetic contracts them. The action of the heart is quickened or strengthened by the symphathetic system, whereas the parasympathetic system slows its action. The blood vessels of the skin and viscera are contracted by the sympathetic system so that more blood goes to the muscles where it is needed for "fight or flight" under stress, and the parasympathetic system dilates the blood vessels when the need has passed. The gastrointestinal tract and bladder are relaxed by the sympathetic system and contracted by the parasympathetic. The sympathetic system causes contractions of the sphincters to prevent leakage from the anus or urethra, and the parasympathetic system relaxes these sphincters so that waste matter can be expelled. In similar fashion they regulate the body temperature, salivary digestive secretions, and the endocrine glands.

REVIEW 15.E

Complete the following:

1. The peripheral nervous system includes the _____autonomic_____ system, the _____cranial_____ nerves, and the _____spinal_____ nerves.

2. There are __12__ pairs of cranial nerves.

3. The spinal nerves are named for the corresponding _____vertebrae_____.

4. Somatic motor pathways are classified into _pyramidal_ and _extra pyramidal_ tracts.

5. An unconscious, involuntary action occurring below the brain level is a _reflex_ action.

6. The autonomic nervous system has two divisions: _sympathetic_ and _parasympathetic_

7. The two (above named divisions) work in _opposition_ to each other.

8. The first cranial nerve, for the sense of smell, is the _olfactory_ nerve.

9. The second cranial nerve, the _optic_, is the nerve of vision.

10. In the _knee jerk_ reflex, the leg extends in response to tapping of the patellar ligament.

RELATED TERMS THE NERVOUS SYSTEM THE CENTRAL PROCESSING UNIT

DIVISIONS OF THE NERVOUS SYSTEM

autonomic part of the peripheral nervous system that serves the vital systems that function automatically and normally cannot be controlled voluntarily.

central division of the nervous system that includes the brain and spinal cord (also called the *cerebrospinal system*).

parasympathetic one of two divisions of the autonomic system, arising from the central nervous system by preganglionic neurons, with cell bodies located in the brain or in the second, third, and fourth sacral segments of the spinal cord (also called the *craniosacral system*).

peripheral division of the nervous system that consists of nerves and ganglia outside (peripheral) the spinal cord and brain, including the cranial and spinal nerves and the autonomic nervous system.

sympathetic one of two divisions of the autonomic system, arising from the central nervous system by preganglionic neurons, with cell bodies located in the thoracic and first three lumbar segments of the spinal cord, and with ganglia extending from the base of the skull to the coccyx (also called the *thoracolumbar system*).

ANATOMY

Brain, Spinal Cord, and Related Terms

anterior commissure band of white fibers that connects the temporal lobes of the two cerebral hemispheres.

aqueduct of Sylvius see *cerebral aqueduct.*

arachnoid (ah-rak'noid) middle meningeal membrane resembling a spider's web (*arachnoid* means resembling spider's web).

ascending tracts tracts located in the spinal cord, carrying afferent (sensory) nerve fibers that conduct nerve impulses to the brain.

brain central mass of nerve tissue within the cranium, including the cerebrum, cerebellum, diencephalon, midbrain, pons, medulla oblongata, and other structures.

cerebellum (ser"e-bel'um) second largest division of the brain, situated above the medulla oblongata and beneath the rear portion of the cerebrum, commonly referred to as the little, or small, brain.

cerebral aqueduct (ak'we-dukt) canal for the passage of cerebrospinal fluid between the third and fourth ventricles (also called the *aqueduct of Sylvius*).

cerebral cortex outer portion of the cerebrum containing the gray matter or cell bodies of the neurons.

cerebrospinal fluid (ser″e-bro-spi′nal) thin, transparent, watery fluid found around the spinal cord and in the ventricles of the brain, central canal of the spinal cord, and subarachnoid space, providing support for the weight of the brain, and serving as a protective cushion and source of nutrients for the brain and spinal cord.

cerebrum (ser′e-brum) largest part of the brain, occupying most of the cranial cavity, and divided into two cerebral hemispheres.

commissure (kom′i-shur) band of white fibers that joins the two halves of the cerebral hemispheres.

convolution fold in the surface of the cerebral hemisphere (also called *gyrus*).

cornu (kor′nu) hornlike projection, used to describe various projections in the nervous system (plural—*cornua*).

corpus callosum (kor′pus kah-lo′sum) largest commissure of the brain that connects one cerebral hemisphere with another.

descending tracts tracts located in the spinal cord, carrying nerve fibers that conduct efferent (motor), impulses from the brain.

diencephalon (di″en-sef′ah-lon) part of the brain between the midbrain and the cerebrum (*dia* means through, across, or between; *cephalon* refers to brain).

dura mater (du′rah ma′ter) outermost membrane of the brain and spinal cord.

endorphins natural, opiate-like substances, produced in both the brain and pituitary gland, that have narcotic action upon receptor sites in the brain and are believed to play a role in pain experience, emotions, and problems of substance addiction.

ependyma (e-pen′di-mah) membrane lining the ventricles of the brain and the central canal of the spinal cord, producing cerebrospinal fluid.

epithalamus (ep″i-thal′ah-mus) portion of the diencephalon that includes the pineal body and olfactory (smell) centers.

fissure deep groove, or furrow, of the brain on the cortical surface of the cerebrum.

foramen magnum passage for the spinal cord through the occipital bone of the cranium.

fourth ventricle kite-shaped cavity in the hindbrain that produces some of the cerebrospinal fluid.

gyrus surface fold (convolution) of a cerebral hemisphere (plural—*gyri*).

hemisphere (hem′i-sfer) either lateral half of the cerebrum or cerebellum.

hippocampus (hip′o-kam′pus) part of the limbic system often called the "gatekeeper for memory," in which damage or defect has been linked to learning and memory problems such as those in Alzheimer's disease.

hypothalamus (hi″po-thal′ah-mus) portion of the diencephalon located below and between the lobes of the thalamus, containing the optic chiasma, the posterior lobe of the pituitary gland, and the infundibulum.

lateral ventricle space in each hemisphere that projects an anterior cornu (horn) into the frontal lobe, a posterior cornu into the occipital lobe, and an inferior cornu into the temporal lobe and produces most of the cerebrospinal fluid.

leptomeninges (lep″to-me-nin′jez) pia mater and arachnoid membranes of the brain together (singular—*leptomeninx*).

limbic system structures of the cerebrum that lie on the medial surface close to the corpus callosum, and together are described as the "emotional brain" because of their importance in experiencing a wide range of emotions from pleasure and sexual feelings to anger, fear, and sorrow. The hippocampal portion has been related to memory problems.

lobes of cerebrum the cerebral cortex is divided into four lobes named for the cranial bones above them: *occipital, frontal, temporal,* and *parietal.*

medulla oblongata (me-dul′ah ob″long-ga′tah) posterior part of the brain, continuous with the spinal cord.

meninges (me-nin′jez) three membranes enveloping the central nervous system, the dura mater, pia mater, and arachnoid (singular—*meninx*).

midbrain upper part of the brainstem, above the pons.

nucleus mass or cluster of nerve cells in the brain or spinal cord with a common function (see *ganglion* under Nerve Structures and Related Terms).

optic chiasma (op′tic ki′azm-ah) crossing of the optic nerves on the ventral surface of the brain (*chiasm* means crossing).

pia-arachnoid (pi″ah-ah-rak′noid) both the pia mater and arachnoid membranes when considered as one membrane (*pia* means tender).

pia mater innermost, thin, compact membrane closely adapted to the surface of the spinal cord and brain.

pons portion of the brain that serves as a bridge to connect the cerebellum, cerebrum, and medulla oblongata (*pons* means bridge).

posterior commissure thin sheet of fibers that cross transversely under the posterior part of the corpus callosum, connecting the olfactory centers in the cerebral hemispheres.

spinal cord lowest part of the central nervous system, extending from the medulla oblongata to the coccyx, and containing the ascending and descending nerve tracts.

subarachnoid space between the pia mater and arachnoid.

subarachnoid cisterns subarachnoid reservoirs containing cerebrospinal fluid (*cisterna* means closed place).

subdural space space between the dura mater and the arachnoid.

subthalamus portion of the diencephalon that lies between the thalamus and the midbrain.

sulcus (sul′kus) a furrow (groove), separating the gyri from each other (plural—*sulci*).

thalamus (thal′ah-mus) middle portion of the diencephalon that forms part of the lateral wall of the third ventricle and lies between the epithalamus and the hypothalamus (plural—*thalami*).

third ventricle cavity, located below and between the cerebral central hemispheres, producing cerebrospinal fluid.

vermis central body of the cerebellum, shaped something like a worm (*vermis* means worm).

Nerve Structures and Related Terms

afferent neurons neurons that conduct impulses from the sense organs to the spinal cord and brain.

astrocyte (as′tro-site) star-shaped cell of the neuroglia (*astro* means star).

axon long nerve cell process carrying impulses from the cell body.

collaterals side branches of the axon.

connectors neurons in which the dendrites and axons are connected to other neurons.

dendrites numerous short nerve cell processes that conduct nerve impulses toward the cell body.

efferent neurons motor neurons that convey impulses from the brain and spinal cord to the muscles and glands.

ganglion (gang′gle-on) mass of nerve cells, located outside the brain and spinal cord, that serves as a center for nerve impulses (plural—*ganglia*).

microglia (mi-krog′le-ah) phagocytic cells of the nervous system.

motor neurons see *efferent neurons.*

myelinated nerves (mi′-eli-nat″ed) nerves covered with a sheath of white fatty material called myelin (also called *medullated nerves*).

myelin sheath white, fatty coat surrounding nerve fibers, found mainly in the central nervous system.

nerve trunk white, glistening, cordlike bundle formed by nerve fibers running together.

neurilemma (nu″ri-lem′mah) tubelike membrane covering nerve fibers, which may or may not be myelinated (also called *nucleated membrane* and *sheath of Schwann;* also spelled *neurolemma*).

neuroglia (nu-rog′le-ah) specialized type of nervous tissue that holds nerve cells and their gossamer filaments together.

neuron single nerve cell, the structural unit of the nervous system, with a cell body, axon, and dendrites.

neurotransmitters numerous types of chemical substances, including acetylcholine, norepinephrine (adrenaline), dopamine, and serotonin, that act at the synapse to stimulate or inhibit the transmission of impulses.

oligodendroglia (ol″i-go-den-drog′le-ah) cells that aid in holding nerve fibers together and forming the myelin sheath of nerves.

plexus (plek′sus) interlacing network of spinal nerves, in several areas of the body.

Ranvier's node (rahn-ve-ay′s) interruption or constriction in the myelin sheath, at regular intervals.

receptors organs of sensation.

reflex action arrangement of sensory, connector, and motor nerves forming the reflex arc, acting together to produce a reflex action.

sensory neurons peripheral nerves that conduct afferent impulses from the sense organs to the spinal cord.

synapse (sin′aps) microscopic space between an axon of one neuron and the dendrites of another, across which an impulse is transmitted (*synapse* means connection).

terminal twigs peripheral nerve endings, identified according to their action, as vascular, articular, muscular, and cutaneous.

Cranial Nerves

The following list includes the 12 cranial nerves and some of their branches.

abducens (ab-du'senz) sixth cranial nerve; motor nerve that supplies the lateral rectus muscle of the eye.

acoustic eighth cranial nerve, having two sensory divisions, the *cochlear*, which supplies the cochlea of the ear, and the *vestibular*, which supplies the vestibule and semicircular canals of the ear (also called *auditory nerve*).

alveolar two branches of the maxillary division of the trigeminal nerve, *superior* and *inferior*, which receive sensations from the head and innervate the chewing muscles.

auricular, posterior sensory and motor branch of the facial nerve that supplies the ear muscles and the occipitofrontal muscle.

auriculotemporal sensory branch of the mandibular division of the trigeminal nerve, which supplies the skin of the scalp and temple, the superior part of the ear, the external acoustic meatus, and the tympanic membrane.

buccinator sensory branch of the mandibular division of the trigeminal nerve, which supplies the skin of the cheek and gums and mucous membranes of the cheek (also called *buccal*).

cranial nerves twelve pairs of cranial nerves, originating in the brain, with their branches and ganglia.

facial seventh cranial nerve, a sensory and motor nerve, which originates in the pons and supplies facial muscles and some taste buds.

glossopharyngeal ninth cranial nerve, both sensory and motor, which originates in the medulla oblongata and supplies the tongue, pharynx, and eardrum.

hypoglossal twelfth cranial nerve, a motor nerve that originates in the medulla oblongata and innervates the muscles of the tongue.

infraorbital sensory branch of the maxillary division of the trigeminal nerve, supplying part of the nose, lip, skin and conjunctiva of the lower eyelid, and some of the upper teeth and gums.

intermediate nerve sensory root of the facial nerve, supplying salivary glands, palate, tonsils, and tongue.

lacrimal sensory branch of the ophthalmic division of the trigeminal nerve, supplying the lacrimal gland, conjunctiva, and upper eyelid.

laryngeal branches of the vagus nerve, both sensory and motor, that supply the laryngeal, pharyngeal, and tracheal structures.

lingual sensory branch of the mandibular division of the trigeminal nerve that supplies parts of the tongue and mouth.

mandibular sensory and motor division of the trigeminal nerve, with a posterior and anterior division, that gives rise to the lingual, inferior alveolar, and auriculotemporal nerves.

maxillary sensory division of the trigeminal nerve that supplies the mucous membranes of the maxillary sinus and nasal cavity, skin of face and scalp, and some teeth, through its branches, the zygomatic, alveolar, and infraorbital nerves.

oculomotor third cranial nerve, both sensory and motor, which supplies eye muscles, pupillary sphincter, and ciliary processes.

olfactory first cranial nerve, a sensory nerve that supplies the sense of smell.

ophthalmic sensory division of the trigeminal nerve that supplies the skin of the forehead, upper eyelid, external nose, frontal sinus, and the eye, through its branches, the lacrimal, nasal, and frontal nerves.

optic second cranial nerve, a sensory nerve supplying the retina of the eye.

palatine two sensory branches of the maxillary division of the trigeminal nerve that supply the soft and hard palates, uvula, and tonsils.

spinal accessory eleventh cranial nerve, a motor nerve that supplies the sternocleidomastoid and trapezius muscles, cervical lymph glands, pharynx, larynx, and thoracic viscera.

trigeminal fifth cranial nerve, both sensory and motor, with three divisions: ophthalmic, maxillary, and mandibular.

trochlear fourth cranial nerve, a motor nerve that supplies the superior oblique muscles of the eye.

tympanic sensory branch of the glossopharyngeal nerve, supplying the tympanic cavity membranes, mastoid air cells, and parotid gland.

vagus tenth cranial nerve, with meningeal, auricular, pharyngeal, superior laryngeal, superior and inferior cardiac, recurrent laryngeal, bronchial, esophageal, gastric, pyloric, hepatic, and celiac branches that serve the structures for which they are named.

zygomatic sensory branch of the maxillary division of the trigeminal nerve, supplying the skin over the cheekbone and temple.

Spinal Nerves

The following list includes only a portion of the many spinal nerves. Spinal nerve origins are identified using letters to show their anatomic locations and numbers to indicate positions in the spinal column. C refers to cervical, T to thoracic, L to lumbar, and S to sacral. The number following the letter indicates the corresponding vertebra (e.g., C1 indicates the first cervical vertebra).

cauda equina nerves that supply the lower extremities, extending below the level of the spinal cord, deriving their name from the arrangement of their strands, which resembles a horse's tail.

dorsal scapular motor nerve that originates in the spinal cord (C5 to C7) and supplies muscles of the upper back.

femoral sensory and motor nerve that originates in the spinal cord (L2 to L4) and supplies the muscles of the hip, thigh, and leg.

genitofemoral sensory and motor nerve that originates in the spinal cord (L1 to L2) and serves the genitalia and lumboinguinal regions.

gluteal sensory and motor nerve, with inferior and superior branches, originating in the spinal cord (L4 to S2), supplying the gluteal muscles and hip joint.

hypogastric branches of the superior hypogastric plexus that supply the pelvic and ureter areas.

iliohypogastric sensory and motor nerve that originates in the spinal cord (L1) and supplies the abdominal muscles and the skin above the pubis and lateral gluteal region.

iloinguinal sensory nerve that originates in the spinal cord (L1) and supplies the skin of the upper thigh, scrotum, and labia majora.

intercostobrachial sensory nerve that originates in the spinal cord (T2 to T3) and supplies the skin of the axilla and medial side of the arm.

interosseus group of sensory and motor nerves supplying muscles and membranes of the upper and lower extremities.

long thoracic motor nerve that originates in the spinal cord (C5 to C7) and supplies muscles that move the scapula.

median sensory nerve that originates in the spinal cord (C6 to T1) and supplies the muscles of the forearm and muscles and skin of the hand.

musculocutaneous sensory and motor nerve that originates in the spinal cord (C5 to C7) and supplies the brachial and biceps muscles and skin of the radial side of the forearm.

obturator sensory and motor nerve that originates in the spinal cord (L2 to L4) and supplies muscles of the thigh, and skin of the hip, thigh, and knee joint.

peroneal sensory and motor, deep and superficial nerves that originate in the sciatic nerve and supply the muscles of the lower leg and skin of the foot and toes.

phrenic sensory and motor nerve that originates in the spinal cord (C4 to C5) and supplies the diaphragm, lungs, pericardium, and peritoneum.

pudendal sensory and motor nerve that originates in the spinal cord (S2 to S4) and supplies skin, erectile tissue, and muscles of the perineal area.

radial sensory and motor nerve that originates in the spinal cord (C5 to T1, and C6 to C8) and supplies the skin and muscles of the arm and hand.

saphenous sensory branch of the femoral nerve that supplies the skin of the leg and foot.

sciatic sensory and motor nerve, the largest in the body, originates from the sacral plexus (L4 to S3) and supplies the lower limbs.

tibial sensory and motor division of the sciatic nerve that supplies the hamstring muscles and the muscles and skin of the back of the leg and the sole of the foot.

ulnar sensory and motor nerve that originates in the spinal cord (C7 to T1) and supplies muscles of the forearm and hand, and skin of the hand.

PATHOLOGIC CONDITIONS

Inflammations and Infections

arachnoiditis (ah-rak″noid-i′tis) inflammation of the arachnoid membrane (also called *arachnitis*).

cerebrospinal syphilis syphilitic infection of the brain and spinal cord, or syphilis of the central nervous system (also called *Erb's paralysis*). See *syphilis*—Chapter 18.

choriomeningitis (ko″re-o-men″in-ji′tis) inflammation of the cerebral meninges (meningitis), with infiltration by lymphocytes of the choroid plexuses of the ventricles.

Creutzfeldt-Jakob disease (kroits′felt-yak′ob) encephalopathy believed to be caused by a pathologic protein called a *prion* that attaches to normal proteins and converts them to prions that then form a long pathologic chain indestructible by stomach acid, heat, and radiation. The disease produces holes and sponginess in the brain. Transmission is believed to be transmitted by eating infected meat (especially brain and spinal cord tissue). The incubation period may be up to 30 years. *BSE—bovine spongiform encephalopathy* affects cattle (also called *mad cow disease*). The sheep disease is called *scrapie*.

encephalitis (en″sef-ah-li′tis) inflammation of the brain, with a variety of types. One virulent type is *Eastern equine encephalitis,* a rare but usually fatal virus, transmitted by the Asian tiger mosquito.

encephalomyelitis (en-sef″ah-lo-mi″e-li′tis) inflammation of the brain and spinal cord, with a variety of types.

ependymitis (ep″en-di-mi′tis) inflammation of the ependymal lining of the ventricles of the brain and the central canal of the spinal cord.

ganglionitis (gang″gle-on-i′tis) inflammation of a nerve ganglion.

Guillain-Barré syndrome (ge-yan′bar-ray) a postinfectious neurologic condition with symptoms of fever, pain, tenderness, weakness or paralysis of muscles, with suspected viral or immune response causes (also called *Landry's paralysis, polyradiculitis, acute polyneuropathy, infectious polyneuritis,* and *acute idiopathic polyneuritis*).

herpes zoster (her′pez zos′ter) infection caused by a herpes virus (*varicella-zoster* or **VZV**) that follows nerve pathways, characterized by small blisters or vesicles on the skin (also called *shingles*).

leptomeningitis (lep″to-men″in-ji′tis) inflammation of the leptomeninges (pia-arachnoid membrane) of the brain and spinal cord.

meningitis (men″in-ji′tis) inflammation of the meninges of the brain or spinal cord, caused by viral or bacterial infection. (In children, the most common bacterial cause is *Haemophilus influenzae* type B).

meningoencephalitis (me-ning″go-en-sef″ah-li′tis) inflammation of the brain and meninges (also called *cerebromeningitis* and *encephalomeningitis*).

meningoencephalomyelitis (me-ning″go-en-sef″ah-lo-mi″e-li′tis) inflammation that involves the brain, meninges, and spinal cord.

meningomyelitis (me-ning″go-mi″e-li′tis) inflammation of the spinal cord and its membranes.

meningomyeloradiculitis (me-ning″go-mi″e-lo-rah-dik″u-li′tis) inflammation of the meninges, spinal cord, and spinal cord roots (*radiculo* refers to root).

meningoradiculitis (me-ning″go-rah-dik″u-li′tis) inflammation of the meninges and the nerve roots.

myelitis (mi″e-li′tis) inflammation of the spinal cord (*myel* refers to both spinal cord and bone marrow and the context in which it is used will determine which tissue is involved).

myeloradiculitis (mi″e-lo-rah-dik″u-li′tis) inflammation of the spinal cord and nerve roots.

myelosyphilis syphilis of the spinal cord.

neuritis inflammation of a nerve or nerves, caused by infection, toxicity, or trauma.

neuroamebiasis (nu″ro-am″e-bi′ah-sis) neuritis that results from infection by amebae.

neurochorioretinitis (nu″ro-ko″re-o-ret″i-ni′tis) inflammation of the optic nerve, retina, and choroid of the eye.

neuromyelitis (nu″ro-mi″e-li′tis) spinal cord inflammation with neuritis (also called *myeloneuritis*).

neuromyositis (nu″ro-mi″o-si′tis) neuritis with inflammation of corresponding muscles.

pachyleptomeningitis (pak″e-lep″to-men″in-ji′tis) inflammation of all three membranes of the brain or spinal cord.

pachymeningitis (pak″e-men″in-ji′tis) inflammation of the dura mater (also called *perimeningitis*).

polioencephalitis (po″le-o-en-sef′ah-li′tis) inflammation of the gray matter of the brain, caused by polio virus (*polio* refers to the gray matter of the nervous system).

polioencephalomeningomyelitis (po″le-o-en-sef″ah-lo-me-nin″go-mi″e-li′tis) inflammation of gray matter of the brain and spinal cord and their covering membranes.

poliomyelitis (po″le-o-mi″e-li′tis) acute viral infection and inflammation of the gray matter of the spinal cord, caused by one of three polio viruses, resulting in asymptomatic, paralytic, or mild types (relatively uncommon since the development of preventive vaccines such as the Salk and Sabin vaccines).

poliomyeloencephalitis (pol″e-o-mi″el-o-en-sef′a-li′tis) inflammation of the gray matter of the brain and spinal cord caused by the polio virus (also called *poliomyelencephalitis*).

polyneuritis inflammation of a large number of spinal nerves at the same time.

polyneuroradiculitis (pol″e-nu″ro-rah-dik″uli′tis) inflammation of the spinal ganglia, nerve roots, and peripheral nerves.

polyradiculitis (pol″e-rah-dik″u-li′tis) inflammation of nerve roots.

rabies (ra′bez) a once fatal viral disease infecting the central nervous system and salivary glands, transmitted by an infected animal's bite or a wound contacting infected saliva (also called *hydrophobia* because of the painful glottal and throat spasms produced by drinking water).

rachiomyelitis (ra"ke-o-mi"e-li'tis) inflammation of the spinal cord.

radiculitis (rah-dik"u-li'tis) inflammation of a spinal nerve root.

radiculomeningomyelitis (rah-dik"u-lo-me-ning"go-mi"e-li'tis) inflammation of the nerve roots, the spinal cord, and its covering (also called *rhizomeningomyelitis*).

Reye's syndrome (riz) encephalopathy associated with fatty degeneration of the liver occurring in children as a rare sequela to influenza and other viral infections, with late stages showing intracranial pressure and cerebral edema (Chapter 18).

tetanus (tet'ah-nus) acute, bacterial infectious disease caused by *Clostridium tetani* whose source is in soil, street dust, or animal and human feces. It is transmitted by spores at the site of an injury, burn, or wound, primarily affecting the nervous system and involving the peripheral nerves and anterior horn cells (also called *lockjaw*, which is a symptom along with generalized muscle spasms and seizures).

Hereditary, Congenital, and Developmental Disorders

adrenoleukodystrophy (ALD) rare, fatal disease caused by a sex-linked X chromosome defect, affecting males, resulting in myelin sheath deterioration, and degeneration of brain tissue, with symptoms of muscular spasticity, optic neuritis, deafness, and mental and emotional deterioration (also called *Siemerling-Creutzfeldt disease*).

amyelencephalia (a-mi"el-en-seh-fa'le-ah) absence of both brain and spinal cord.

amyelia (a"mi-e'le-ah) absence of the spinal cord.

anencephaly (an"en-se-fa'le) congenital defective development of cranial bones, with failure of brain and spinal cord to develop (also called *anencephalia*).

Arnold-Chiari syndrome (ke-ar'e) malformation, with downward displacement of the cerebellum into the fourth ventricle and underdevelopment of hindbrain, and internal hydrocephalus, usually associated with an opening in the spinal column (also called *cerebellomedullary malformation syndrome*).

ataxia-telangiectasia (AT) (tel-an'gie-ek-tas"e-ah) hereditary, progressive disorder of immunoglobulin metabolism that appears when a child begins walking, with symptoms of lack of coordination, dilation of the ends of blood vessels in ears, eyes, and face, and susceptibility to respiratory infection, which usually causes death in early adulthood (also called *Louis-Bar's syndrome*).

atelencephalia (a-tell'en-se-fa'le-ah) incomplete or imperfect development of the brain (*atel* means incomplete).

atelomyelia (at"e-lo-mi-e'le-ah) incomplete development of the spinal cord.

atelorachidia (at"e-lo-rah-kid'e-ah) incomplete development of the spinal column.

cephalocele (se-fal'o-sel) protrusion of a part of the cranial contents through a defect in the skull (also called *encephalocele* and *craniocele*).

cerebral sphingolipidosis (sfing'go-lip'i-do'sis) group of inherited diseases characterized by excessive muscle tone, underdevelopment, spastic paralysis, blindness, convulsions, and mental deterioration, associated with abnormal retention of lipids in the brain (includes *Tay-Sachs disease*, an infantile form formerly called *amaurotic familial idiocy; Jansky-Bielschowsky disease*, an early juvenile type; *Spielmeyer-Vogt disease*, a late juvenile form; and *Kufs' disease*, an adult form).

Charcot-Marie-Tooth disease (shar'ko) inherited neuromuscular disease, characterized by atrophy of peroneal muscles of the fibula, producing footdrop, clubfoot, and ataxia.

craniomeningocele (kra"ne-o-me-nin'go-sel) herniation of the cerebral membranes through a defect in the skull.

craniorachischisis (kra"ne-o-rah-kis'ki-sis) congenital incomplete closure of the skull and spinal column.

diastematomyelia (di"ah-stem"ah-to-mi-e'le-ah) separation of the lateral halves of the spinal cord by a septum of bone or cartilage (also called *diastomyelia; diastasis* means separation).

encephalomyelocele (en-sef"ah-lo-mi-el'o-sel) herniation of the spinal cord, meninges, and medulla caused by abnormality of the foramen magnum.

epilepsy (ep'i-lep"se) hereditary or idiopathic nervous system disorder, with or without convulsions, that may also develop following infection or trauma. Characterized by a temporary disturbance of brain impulses, with several types: *grand mal*, loss of consciousness with convulsions; *petit mal*, temporary loss of awareness and suspension of activity; *psychomotor*, brief clouding of consciousness accompanied by meaningless repetition of movement, such as handclapping; and *focal*, in which the seizures are one-sided or affect limited body areas (*epilepsy* means a condition of seizure).

Friedreich's ataxia (fred'riks) progressive spinocerebellar degeneration with an early onset characterized by kyphoscoliosis, cardiac abnormalities, nystagmus, and ataxia.

heterotopia (het″er-o-to′pe-ah) displacement of gray matter into the white matter of the brain and spinal cord.

Huntington's chorea rare, progressive, hereditary disease, usually beginning after age 30, associated with degenerative changes of the basal ganglia and cerebral cortex, producing personality change, with irritability, poor judgment, indifference, and memory loss, progressing to total incapacitation and eventual death within 10 to 20 years. There is a 50:50 chance of inheriting the disease if either parent has the defective gene (also called *chronic chorea* and *degenerative chorea*).

hydrencephalocele (hi″dren-sef′ah-lo-sel) hernial protrusion of the brain substance through a cranial defect, with an accumulation of cerebrospinal fluid in the sac (also called *hydrocephalocele*).

hydrencephalomeningocele (hi″dren-sef′ah-lo-me-nin′go-sel) hernial protrusion of the meninges through a cranial defect, with accumulations of cerebrospinal fluid and brain substance in the sac.

hydrocephalus (hi-dro-sef′ah-lus) abnormal accumulation of fluid in the cerebral ventricles, with thinning of the cortex and enlargement of the head caused by separation of the cranial bones.

hydromeningocele (hi″dro-me-nin′go-sel) protrusion of the meninges through a defect in the skull or spine, with an accumulation of cerebrospinal fluid in the sac.

hydromyelia (hi″dro-mi-e′le-ah) accumulation of fluid in the spinal cord, resulting in an enlarged central canal.

hydromyelocele protrusion, through a spina bifida (see entry), of membranes and tissue of the spinal cord, forming a sac containing cerebrospinal fluid (also called *hydromyelomeningocele*).

Krabbe's disease (krab′ez) rare, infantile, familial cerebral sclerosis, with death usually occurring in 1 to 2 years (also called *globoid cell leukodystrophy*).

Lesch-Nyhan cerebral palsy an X-linked, inherited disorder of males, associated with an enzyme formation defect, and characterized by spastic cerebral palsy and mental retardation.

macrocephaly (mak″ro-se-fa′le) excessively large size of head (also called *macrocephalia* and *megacephaly*).

Marie's sclerosis hereditary form of sclerosis of the cerebellum.

meningocele (me-ning′go-sel) herniation of the meninges through a cranial or spinal column defect.

meningoencephalocele (me-ning″go-en-sef′ah-lo-sel) herniation of the meninges and brain substance through a defect in the skull.

meningomyelocele (me-ning″go-mi-el′o-sel) herniation of a part of the spinal cord and meninges through a defect in the spinal column.

Menkes' syndrome rare, congenital, genetically determined, fatal nerve disorder involving inability to metabolize copper, affecting only males, producing a characteristic kinky hair, failure to thrive, seizures, and brain deterioration (also called *kinky hair disease*).

microcephalus (mi″kro-sef′ah-lus) person with an excessively small head.

microcephaly condition of excessive smallness of the head (also called *microcephalia*).

microgyrus (mi″kro-ji′rus) abnormally small, narrow convolution of the brain.

micromyelia (mi″kro-mi-e′le-ah) abnormally short or small spinal cord.

Möbius syndrome (me″be-us) rare, congenital, developmental facial palsy, often accompanied by oculomotor disorders (inability to control facial and eye muscles).

myelocele (mi′e-lo-sel) herniation of the substance of the spinal cord through a defect in the vertebral column (also called *myelocystocele, myelocystomeningocele,* and *myelomeningocele*).

myelodysplasia (mi″e-lo-dis-pla′ze-ah) defective development of the spinal cord.

myeloradiculodysplasia (mi″e-lo-rah-dik″u-lo-dis-pla′ze-ah) developmental abnormality of the spinal cord and spinal nerve roots.

myeloschisis (mi″e-los′ki-sis) developmental anomaly in which there is a cleft spinal cord.

neurofibromatosis hereditary disorder that affects not only the nervous system but other systems as well (Chapter 18).

porencephaly (po″ren-se-fa′le) abnormal presence of cavities in the brain substance usually opening into the lateral ventricles (also called *porencephalia* and *spelencephaly; spel* means cavity).

spina bifida (spi′nah bif′i-dah) developmental anomaly characterized by a defective formation of the bony spinal canal through which spinal membranes and/or cord may protrude.

spina bifida occulta (ok-kul′tah) spina bifida without associated protrusion of the spinal cord or meninges.

syringobulbia (si-ring″go-bul′be-ah) presence of a cavity filled with fluid in the brainstem.

syringoencephalomyelia (si-ring″go-en-sef″ah-lo-mi-e′le-ah) presence of a tubular cavity in the substance of the brain and spinal cord.

syringomyelia (si-ring″go-mi-e′le-ah) cavities, lined with dense tissue, within the spinal cord, producing deterioration of sensation, paralysis, and scoliosis of the spine.

syringomyelocele (si-ring″go-mi′e-lo-sel) protrusion of the spinal cord through the bony defect in spina bifida, in which the cavity of the herniated sac is connected with the central canal of the spinal cord (also called *syringocele*).

Tay-Sachs disease a form of inherited cerebral sphingolipidosis (occurring largely in families of Eastern European Jewish background), with destruction of ganglion cells, myelin degeneration, and glial proliferation that results in blindness, dementia, and psychomotor retardation, with death within 4 years of age.

tuberous sclerosis congenital familial disease, producing tumors on the surfaces of the lateral ventricles, and sclerotic patches on the surface of the brain, resulting in marked mental deterioration and epilepsy (also called *Bourneville's disease*).

Circulatory Disturbances

cerebral hemorrhage bleeding into the structure of the cerebrum, usually caused by rupture of an artery or a congenital aneurysm, that may be followed by destruction of brain tissue, with ensuing paralyses, sensory losses, and cognitive confusion and losses.

cerebrovascular accident (CVA) commonly called *stroke* or *apoplexy,* includes rupture (hemorrhagic stroke) or obstruction (ischemic stroke) of an artery of the brain, with symptoms of severe headache, nausea, vomiting, and confusion. This may be accompanied by localized and widespread neurologic deterioration, with possible coma, paralysis, and aphasia. Outcome may be fatal, with survival often leaving some residual damage and reduced functioning (see also *transient ischemic attack*).

encephalomalacia softening of brain tissue caused by reduced blood supply.

epidural hematoma collection of blood outside the dura mater.

intracranial hemorrhage cranial blood vessel leakage leading to escape of blood within the cranium and development of hematomas.

subarachnoid hemorrhage escape of blood into the subarachnoid space, usually caused by rupture of an aneurysm.

subdural hemorrhage escape of blood between dura mater and arachnoid membranes (also called *subdural hematoma* and *hemorrhagic pachymeningitis*).

transient ischemic attack (TIA) condition that may precede an ischemic stroke, producing symptoms of double vision, or loss of vision, numbness in upper extremities, dizziness and falling, usually lasting about 24 hours.

Other Organic Abnormalities

Alzheimer's disease (altz′hi-merz) a brain degenerative disorder classified as a *primary degenerative dementia, senile dementia Alzheimer's type (SDAT)* is a progressive brain atrophy disease characterized by neuronal degeneration, neurofibrillary tangles, and senile plaques in the brain, usually occurring in persons older than 65, with rare cases in persons younger than 50 classified as *presenile dementia,* with prognosis of death within 10 years. Possible factors implicated in the disease include impairment of the proteins that make up the structure of cells, viral infection, and low neurotransmitter activity.

amyotrophic lateral sclerosis (ALS) chronic progressive disease of the nervous system, occurring in middle age, in which there is atrophy of muscles and sclerosis (hardening) of the lateral columns of the spinal cord, characterized by disturbance in motility, weakness and wasting of afflicted muscles, and irregular twitching (also called *Lou Gehrig's disease* and *Charcot's disease*).

aphasia loss of oral or written language caused by brain damage, of various types, mainly receptive and expressive.

ataxia muscular incoordination.

athetosis (ath′e-to-sis) recurring series of purposeless motions of the extremities, due to brain lesion or drug toxicity (*athetos* means not fixed).

aura experience that precedes and marks the onset of a paroxysmal attack such as an epileptic seizure, that may take the form of visual, auditory, olfactory, or tactile sensations.

Bell's palsy palsy characterized by peripheral facial weakness with retraction of the angle of the mouth and impaired closure of the eye on the affected side.

bradylalia abnormally slow speech, caused by a brain lesion (*lalia* means talking).

Brown-Séquard's syndrome paralysis of motion on one side of the body and of sensation on the other caused by a lesion on one side of the spinal cord.

cephalalgia headache (also called *cephalodynia* and *cerebralgia*).

cerebral ataxia lack of muscular coordination caused by cerebral disease (*ataxia* means lack of order).

cerebral palsy group of conditions with a variety of symptoms caused by brain damage, affecting muscular control and coordination, described by symptoms as *spastic, athetoid, rigid, ataxic,* and *tremor.*

chorea (ko-re'ah) a convulsive nervous disease with involuntary jerky movements (*chorea* means to dance).

coma stuporous condition of depressed responsiveness, with absence of response to strong stimuli.

decerebration loss of higher mental functions because of brain damage.

delirium mental disturbance marked by hallucinations, excitement, physical restlessness, and incoherence, that may occur as a result of fever, disease (especially alcoholic psychosis), or injury (*delirium* means off the track).

dementia mental deterioration of the brain because of organic disease.

diplegia paralysis of like parts on both sides of the body.

dysbasia difficulty in walking, because of central nervous system lesion (*basia* means step).

dyskinesia impaired voluntary movement resulting in fragmentary, incomplete, or involuntary movements, because of brain damage or disorder.

dysphasia speech impairment caused by central nervous system lesion.

dyspraxia partial loss of ability to perform coordinated motions.

Erb-Duchenne paralysis paralysis of the upper arm, with the absence of involvement of the small hand muscles (also called *Erb's paralysis*).

hemiplegia paralysis of one side of the body, of several types.

Horner's syndrome paralysis of the cervical sympathetic fibers, causing inward sinking of the eyeball, ptosis of the upper eyelid, constriction of the pupil, and narrowing of the opening between the eyelids.

hyperpathia exaggerated response to stimuli, marked by severe pain or discomfort in response to light stimulation of the skin, caused by damage to the thalamus.

jacksonian seizure focal seizure or convulsion, beginning with distal twitching of a group of muscles such as the fingers, and progressing proximally in "marchlike" fashion, reflecting cortical activity in a particular form of epilepsy.

monoplegia paralysis of one part.

multiinfarct dementia one of the dementias of aging caused by a series of small strokes that cause brain cell damage, giving rise to mental function decline (previously called *senile dementia*).

multiple sclerosis (MS) an immune system disorder, the most common demyelinating disorder of the brain and spinal cord (CNS), usually appearing in early adulthood. There are four types: *relapsing-remitting; primary progressive; secondary progressive;* and *progressive-relapsing.* All are characterized by sporadic sclerotic patches on the myelin sheath, which form scars so that nerve impulses are interrupted, lost, or misrouted, resulting in a variety of symptoms including paralysis, nystagmus, lack of coordination, ataxia, tremor, paresthesia, visual and speech disturbances (also known as *insular, disseminated,* or *focal sclerosis*).

myeloplegia spinal paralysis.

narcolepsy uncontrollable urge to sleep or sudden attacks of sleep (*narco* refers to sleep).

neuralgia pain in a nerve or nerves (also called *neurodynia*).

opisthotonos (o"pis-thot'o-nos) tetanic spasm with head and heels bent backward and body bowed forward (*opistho* means backward).

palsy (pawl'ze) paralysis (see entries under individual types).

panplegia total or complete paralysis (also called *pamplegia*).

paralysis loss or impairment of motor function in a part as the result of disease or a lesion of the neural or muscular mechanism.

paraparesis partial paralysis.

paraphasia partial aphasia in which wrong words with senseless meaning are used (also called *paraphrasia*).

paraplegia (par"ah-ple'je-ah) paralysis of the lower torso and extremities.

paresis a form of paralysis.

Parkinson's disease disease primarily of late life, usually caused by deterioration of cerebral nuclei neurons that fail to produce sufficient dopamine to counter the excitatory action of acetylcholine, resulting in a masklike expression, rigidity, tremor of the resting muscles, and a drooping posture (also called *paralysis agitans* and *parkinsonism*).

Pick's disease one of the primary degenerative dementia disorders classified as a presenile dementia, with insidious onset occurring around ages 45 to 50. It produces vascular and degenerative changes in the brain, with symptoms including thinking and memory difficulties, fatigue, and personality changes. As the disease progresses, increasing disorientation, apathy, and impairment of thought and judgment are noted, with death within 8 years.

pragmatagnosia inability to recognize formerly known objects.

progressive bulbar paralysis progressive paralysis of the muscles, as well as atrophy of the lips, tongue, mouth, and throat (also called *Duchenne's paralysis*).

retrograde amnesia loss of memory for events preceding the event causing brain damage.

senility deterioration, both physical and mental, related to aging.

shaken infant syndrome (SIS) brain damage in infants and young children, caused by severe shaking, exuberant play, or physical abuse, that produces intracranial hemorrhage and pressure on brain tissue.

syncope (sin'ko-pe) transient loss of consciousness resulting from a decrease in cerebral blood flow, usually accompanied by a fall in blood pressure, and commonly referred to as fainting.

tabes dorsalis degeneration of the dorsal columns of the spinal cord and sensory nerve trunks as a result of tertiary syphilis.

torpor no response to normal stimuli.

Tourette's disease or syndrome onset in childhood, characterized by facial and vocal tics, progressing to generalized lack of coordination and coprolalia (uncontrollable urge to say obscenities). It is believed to be caused by a defect in the basal ganglia of the brain, with resulting excess of the neurotransmitter dopamine, treatable with dopamine-blocking tranquilizers (named for French physician, Gilles de la Tourette).

Wernicke's syndrome (ver'ni-kez) a degenerative encephalopathy attributed to thiamine deficiency associated with chronic alcoholism. It is characterized by ataxia, mental dullness, impaired retentive memory, diplopia, and nystagmus (also called *Wernicke's encephalopathy*).

Oncology*

astroblastoma (as"tro-blas-to'mah) tumor composed of immature astrocytes (preastrocyte cells).

astrocytoma (as"tro-si-to'mah) tumor made up of adult astrocytes (star-shaped cells).

ependymoblastoma (ep-en"di-mo-blas-to'mah) tumor derived from embyronic ependymal cells.

ependymoma (ep-en"di-mo'mah) tumor derived from adult ependymal cells.

gangliocytoma (gang"gle-o-si-to'mah) tumor derived from mature ganglion cells (also called *ganglioneuroma*).

glioblastoma multiforme* (gli"o-blas-to'mah) malignant cystic tumor of the cerebrum or spinal cord (also called *glioma multiforme*).

glioma (gli-o'mah) any tumor composed of any of the various cells forming the interstitial tissue of the brain, spinal cord, pineal body, posterior pituitary, and the retina.

glioneuroma (gli"o-nu-ro'mah) tumor composed of gliomatous and neural elements.

medulloblastoma* (me-dul"o-blas-to'mah) malignant tumor of the cerebellum.

meningematoma (me-nin"jem-ah-to'mah) hematoma of the dura mater of the meninges (also called *meninghematoma*).

meningioma (me-nin"je-o'mah) benign, encapsulated tumor originating in the arachnoid

meningofibroblastoma (me-ning'go-fi"bro-blas-to'mah) type of meningioma.

neurilemoma (nu"ri-le-mo'mah) tumor of the peripheral nerve sheath of Schwann (also called *neurolemmoma, neurinoma,* and *Schwannoma*).

neuroblastoma* (nu"ro-blas-to'mah) malignant tumor of the nervous system composed mainly of neuroblasts.

neurocytoma (nu"ro-si-to'mah) brain tumor composed of undifferentiated ganglionic nerve cells (also called *medulloepithelioma*).

neuroepithelioma (nu"ro-ep"i-the"le-o'mah) rare type of glioma usually occurring in the retina.

neurofibroma (nu"ro-fi-bro'mah) tumor of peripheral nerve cells resulting from abnormal proliferation of Schwann cells.

*Indicates a malignant condition.

neurogliocytoma   (nu-rog"le-o-si-to'mah) tumor made up of neuroglial cells.

neuroglioma (nu"ro-gli-o"mah) tumor made up of neuroglial tissue.

oligodendroblastoma (ol"i-go-den"dro-blas-to'mah) tumor composed of young oligodendroglial cells.

oligodendroglioma (ol"i-go-den"dro-gli-o'mah) tumor composed of oligodendroglia.

paraganglioma (par"ah-gang"gle-o'mah) tumor that contains chromaffin cells and occurs in the sympathetic nervous system (also called *chromaffinoma*).

spongioblastoma   (spon"je-o-blas-to'mah) tumor composed of spongioblasts (also called *spongiocytoma*).

sympathicoblastoma* (sim-path"i-ko-blas-to'mah) malignant tumor that contains embryonic sympathetic nerve cells (also called *sympathoblastoma* and *sympathogonioma*).

SURGICAL PROCEDURES

chordotomy (ko-dot'o-me) any operation on the spinal cord.

craniectomy (kra"ne-ek'to-me) excision of a part of the skull.

cranioplasty (kra'ne-o-plas"te) repair of defects of the skull.

craniotomy (kra"ne-ot'o-me) surgical opening of skull to remove a tumor, or relieve intracranial pressure.

duraplasty plastic repair of the dura mater.

gangliectomy (gang"gle-ek'to-me) excision of a ganglion (also called *ganglionectomy*).

hemicraniectomy (hem"e-kra"ne-ek'to-me) procedure for exposing part of the brain in preparation for surgery (also called *hemicraniotomy*).

hemidecortication   (hem"e-de-kor"ti-ka'shun) removal of half of the cerebral cortex.

hemispherectomy (hem"i-sfer-ek'to-me) removal of a cerebral hemisphere.

leukotomy (lu-kot'o-me) cutting of the white matter in the frontal lobe of the brain (also spelled *leucotomy*).

lobectomy (lo-bek'to-me) excision of a lobe of the brain.

lobotomy (lo-bot'o-me) incision into the frontal lobe of the brain through drilled holes in the skull.

meningeorrhaphy (me-nin"je-or'ah-fe) suture of the meninges, especially those of the spinal cord.

neurectomy (nu-rek'to-me) excision of a part of a nerve.

neuroanastomosis (nu"ro-ah-nas"to-mo'sis) anastomosis, or connection, between nerves.

neurolysis (nu-rol'i-sis) surgical freeing of perineural adhesions.

neuroplasty plastic repair of a nerve.

neurorrhaphy suturing of a nerve.

neurotomy dissection of a nerve.

neurotripsy (nu"ro-trip'se) surgical crushing of a nerve.

pallidotomy surgical destruction of the subcortical tract *globus pallidus* to relieve involuntary muscle movement.

phrenemphraxis (fren"em-frak'sis) surgical crushing of the phrenic nerve (also called *phreniclasia* and *phrenicotripsy*).

phrenicectomy (fren"i-sek'to-me) excision or resection of part of the phrenic nerve (also called *phreniconeurectomy* and *phrenectomy*).

phrenicotomy surgical division of the phrenic nerve.

rachicentesis (ra"ke-sen-te'sis) lumbar puncture (also called *rachiocentesis*).

radicotomy (rad"i-kot'o-me) sectioning of nerve roots of the spine to relieve pain or spastic paralysis (also called *radiculectomy* and *rhizotomy*).

sympathectomy resection of a sympathetic nerve or ganglion (also called *sympathetectomy* and *sympathicectomy*).

sympathicotripsy   (sim-path"i-ko-trip'se) surgical crushing of a sympathetic ganglion.

tractotomy (trak-tot'o-me) surgical interruption of a nerve tract.

vagotomy sectioning of a vagus nerve.

ventriculocisternostomy (ven-trik"u-lo-sis"ter-nos'to-me) surgical creation of an opening or shunt between the ventricles and the cisterna magna (enlarged subarachnoid space) to relieve cerebrospinal fluid pressure (also called *ventriculostomy*).

volumetric interstitial brachytherapy (VIB) the use of radiation implants through catheters inserted into small holes drilled in the skull and left in place for 3 to 4 days, delivering radiation directly to a tumor and preserving surrounding tissue, after which catheters are removed, producing comparatively long remission.

°Indicates a malignant condition.

LABORATORY TESTS

amyloid beta-protein precurser (APP) test antibody assay test of cerebrospinal fluid to measure the level of a substance that produces the protein plaques in the brains of Alzheimer's victims.

brain electrical activity map (BEAM) computer-generated map of the brain emitting electrical activity evoked by flashes of light, with the patterns of wavelike electrical activity revealing the presence of tumors or other lesions.

brain scan a scanner is used, in conjunction with intravenous injection of radioactive substance, which circulates to the brain, concentrating in areas of abnormality, to diagnose lesions, tumors, and areas of necrosis.

cerebral angiography using a contrast medium injected into the carotid, brachial, subclavian, or femoral arteries, a series of x-rays is taken to visualize the blood vessels of the brain.

cerebrospinal fluid scan injection of radioactive material into the spinal canal in conjunction with a brain scan to detect abnormalities of the skull or spinal fluid leaks.

cerebrospinal fluid tests series of tests to detect the presence of blood, infection, and other abnormalities. It includes a cell count to detect infection in the brain or spinal canal, abnormal levels of calcium present in tuberculous meningitis, and culture to detect disease-causing microorganisms.

coccidioidomycosis antibodies blood test to identify a fungal infection that affects the central nervous system and other body parts.

computerized tomography (CT) use of a thin beam of x-rays to derive cross-sectional images (tomograms) of the head that are put together and analyzed to form a picture on a computer screen that shows tumors, tissue atrophy, and other anatomic abnormalities; a more effective tool for diagnosis than ordinary x-ray and pneumoencephalography (also called *computerized axial tomograph—CAT*).

diffusion-weighted magnetic resonance imaging imaging method to detect the flow of fluid through the brain after trauma; for early detection of ischemic and infarct problems.

echoencephalogram scan of the brain using ultrasound to detect abnormalities.

echo-planar imaging (EPI) a type of functional MRI (fMRI) that reduces imaging time from minutes to fractions of a second, using changes in blood oxygenation to highlight active areas of the brain.

electroencephalograph (EEG) a machine used to reveal patterns of electrical activity of the brain in the form of brain waves that aids in diagnosing epilepsy, tumors, and other abnormalities reflected in electrical activity. With advanced computer technology used with the EEG in what is called the "evoked potential" or neurometrics technique, it shows promise in diagnosing even more difficult conditions including senility, learning disorders, stroke, and traumatic injury disorders.

magnetic resonance imaging (MRI) noninvasive method of scanning the body by use of an electromagnetic field and radio waves that provides visual images on a computer screen and magnetic tape recordings; used to examine soft tissue, and especially useful for diagnosis of multiple sclerosis and tumors (also called *nuclear magnetic resonance— NMR*).

magnetoencephalography (MEG) measure of the magnetic fields produced by electrical activity of the brain. Used to detect neural activity too rapid for MRI or PET methods.

multiplane imager brain scanning device using injected radioactive isotopes in the bloodflow of the brain, to study brain function.

myelography x-ray of the spinal cord and subarachnoid space, using a contrast medium, to identify spinal lesions caused by disease or trauma.

perfusion magnetic resonance imaging rapid method of MRI scanning, using a contrast agent in the blood to detect brain damage at the capillary level. (Together with diffusion-weighted MRI, provides a complete picture of an acute ischemic attack.)

pneumoencephalography injection of gas such as air or oxygen into cerebral ventricles and subarachnoid spaces to allow x-ray visualization (pneumoencephalogram) of the cranium and contents for diagnosis of tumors, atrophy of tissue, and similar abnormalities.

positron emission transaxial tomography (PET) A further refinement of CT scan technology, PET uses a thin beam of x-ray scans to take computer-assisted, cross-sectional images of the brain after injection of a radioactive substance, to visualize the metabolism of this substance, and, consequently, the biochemical activity within the cells of the brain.

serum ammonia blood test to detect elevated levels of ammonia; helps in diagnosing Reye's syndrome.

single photon emission computed tomography (SPECT) imaging method to reveal abnormal metabolic action of the brain; for diagnosis of cancer, stroke, Alzheimer's disease, some mental illnesses, localization of seizures in epilepsy; and for monitoring the treatment of tumors. A solution of radioactive sugar is injected into the patient, and as the sugar is metabolized by the brain, the imaging device rotates around the head, scanning, analyzing, and recording by computer.

stereotaxic neuroradiography x-ray procedure frequently used during neurosurgery to guide a needle into a specific area of the brain.

vitamin B tests group of tests done for vitamin B_2 on blood and urine, and for vitamin B_6 on urine, to detect a vitamin deficiency that relates to nervous system problems.

PSYCHIATRIC DISORDERS

DSM-IV Sampling

The following disorders, which are largely nonorganic or functional in origin, are named and described according to the most recent manual of mental disorders *(DSM-IV)* of the American Psychiatric Association.* This list is a sampling, and not intended to describe all disorders listed in the manual.

alcohol-related disorders disorders listed under substance-related disorders, including: *alcoholic intoxication,* a confused, disoriented state, with subsequent amnesia, following consumption of even moderate quantities of alcohol; *delirium tremens,* an acute mental disturbance characterized by delirium with trembling and great excitement, anxiety, disorientation, mental distress, hallucinations, restlessness, and convulsions, seen in alcoholic psychosis or following withdrawal of heavy alcohol or narcotic ingestion; *acute alcoholic hallucinosis,* a severe psychotic reaction with terrifying auditory hallucinations as the major symptom; and *Korsakoff's psychosis,* a psychosis characterized by memory defect, disorientation, delirium, hallucinations, and falsification of memory, symptoms believed to be caused by nutritional inadequacies, especially vitamin B deficiency, in chronic alcoholism.

anorexia nervosa an *eating disorder* with potential for death from starvation, in which severe weight reduction is produced by voluntarily refusing food or vomiting ingested food, with onset in adolescent or young adult years, primarily seen in females (20:1 ratio) who have histories of unusual eating habits and tendencies to conscientiousness in school work and social behavior (both psychosocial and neurologic factors are believed to be involved in various stages of progression of the disorder).

antisocial personality disorder a *personality disorder* with characteristic antisocial, unconventional, or criminal behavior (also called *sociopathic personality* and *psychopathic personality*).

anxiety disorders a general category of disorders, including *phobic disorders, panic disorder, generalized anxiety disorder, posttraumatic stress disorder,* and *obsessive-compulsive disorder,* all of which involve anxiety (generalized apprehension) and defensive mechanisms that block anxiety to varying degrees, but, unlike psychoses, include continued contact with reality.

attention deficit/hyperactivity disorder (ADHD) a disorder of children and adolescents with symptoms of school underachievement, short attention span, restlessness, disorganization, and excessive physical activity.

bulimia (bu-lim'e-ah) abnormal appetite or hunger (*limia* refers to hunger), in which large amounts of food are consumed, and also referring to one variety of *eating disorder* in which food is vomited after eating large quantities, thus producing severe weight loss to the point of starvation and death (also called *phagomania* and *sitomania*).

conversion disorder term for a disorder classified under *somatoform disorders* in which there is sensory or motor impairment in the absence of organic cause.

depression see *mood disorders.*

dissociative disorder mental disorder including amnesia, fugue, multiple personality, and depersonalization, in which stress is avoided by or escaped from (dissociated) the true self by varying degrees of memory or identity changes.

Down syndrome a form of mental retardation with multiple-system involvement (Chapter 18).

factitious disorders disorders that are characterized by physical or psychologic symptoms that are produced voluntarily by the individual to gain attention (the chronic form is also called *Munchausen syndrome*). This category includes *factitious disorder by proxy,* in which the individual (usually a parent) induces symptoms in another (usually the individual's child) to gain attention for himself or herself, without regard for the hazards to the other (also called *Munchausen by proxy disorder*).

*American Psychiatric Association: *Diagnostic and statistical manual of mental disorders,* ed 4, Washington, DC, 1994, The Association.

fragile X syndrome a form of X-linked moderate to severe mental retardation (Chapter 18).

Hurler's syndrome a form of mental retardation with multiple-system involvement (Chapter 18).

mania abnormal mental state characterized by extreme excitement.

manic-depressive obsolete term for the mood disorder called *bipolar affective disorder.*

mental retardation condition of significantly below average general intellectual functioning, classified by level of function as mild, moderate, and severe.

mood disorders a group of disorders ranging from mild to psychotic, including melancholia, despondency, hopelessness, sadness, and loss of interest in outside activities, classified as follows: *bipolar disorder,* involving both depression and elation (mania); *major depressive disorder,* a severe depressive condition; *cyclothymic disorder,* a persistent pattern of mood swings without severe disruption of functioning; and *dysthymic disorder,* neurotic depression with mild rather than severe disruption of functioning.

paranoia (par″ah-noi′ah) chronic form of psychosis characterized by delusions of persecution or grandeur.

paraphilias (par″ah-fil′ee-yuhs) group of sexual disorders involving abnormal objects and types of sexual gratification.

personality disorders group of disorders in which interpersonal problems are blamed on others, leading to lifetime histories of repetitive, irresponsible, manipulative, and disturbed relationships, classified according to the most prominent characteristic pattern: *paranoid, schizoid, schizotypal, histrionic, narcissistic, antisocial, borderline, avoidant, dependent, passive-aggressive,* and *obsessive-compulsive.*

phobia (fo′be-ah) morbid fear, currently classified under *anxiety disorders,* referring to the generalized, unreasonable fear or anxiety that underlies the disorders, commonly referred to by their roots. (A simplified, limited list follows.)

acrophobia heights.

agoraphobia (ag″o-rah-fo′be-ah) open spaces, crowded or public places.

algophobia (al″go-fo′be-ah) pain.

aquaphobia water.

astraphobia lightning, thunder, and storms.

claustrophobia (klaws″tro-fo′be-ah) closed spaces.

cynophobia or **kynophobia** dogs.

entomophobia insects.

erotophobia sexual love.

gynephobia women.

microbiophobia germs.

mysophobia (mi″so-fo′be-ah) contamination or dirt.

musophobia mice.

necrophobia corpses.

noctiphobia or **nyctophobia** night or darkness.

ophidiophobia (o-fid″e-o-fo′be-ah) snakes.

thanatophobia (than″ah-to-fo′be-ah) death.

xenophobia strangers.

zoophobia animals or some particular animal.

posttraumatic stress disorder classified as an *anxiety disorder,* the symptoms follow a traumatic event and involve reexperiencing the event, and/or symptoms of depression, autonomic arousal, dissociative states, and a variety of emotional problems (commonly seen in war veterans, rape and crime victims).

psychotic disorder mental disorders in which there is a loss of contact with reality, as well as personality disintegration.

schizophrenia (skiz″o-fre′ne-ah) this term, which literally means "split personality," covers a group of psychotic conditions in which there is a profound tendency to withdraw from reality, disorientation, and thought disorder, with subtypes including: *undifferentiated,* mixed-symptom type with delusions, hallucinations, thought disorder, and bizarre behavior; *paranoid,* illogical, changeable delusions and hallucinations with confused ideas of reference (object of others' interest) and grandiosity, that lead to unpredictable and sometimes dangerous behavior; *catatonic,* state of either excited or stuporous motor activity, sometimes changing abruptly to the opposite, with potential for dangerous behavior; *disorganized,* a more severe form than the others, with greater personality breakdown, usually occurring at an earlier age, with silliness, peculiar mannerisms, bizarre behavior, and changeable and often fantastic hallucinations and delusions; and *residual,* involving individuals who have recovered from one of the other subtypes but who still manifest some mild schizophrenic thinking and behavior.

somatization disorder disorder pertaining to mind-body relationship, as in psychosomatic reactions, classified as a *somatoform disorder,* in which the person is severely limited in effectively coping with stress and attaining goals, and defensive and self-defeating strategies are repeatedly used without success, leading to frustration and constant emotional arousal of the autonomic nervous system, which produces internal bodily changes, leading to breakdown of some organ systems.

substance-related disorders this classification covers substance dependence and maladaptive behavior associated with the regular use of alcohol and/or drugs (barbiturates, sedatives, opioids, cocaine, amphetamines, hallucinogens, marijuana, tobacco, etc.), including interference with social or occupational functioning.

Other Psychiatric Terms

agraphia (ah-graf'e-ah) inability to express thoughts in writing; may be functional or the result of brain pathology.

alexia inability to read, sometimes associated with cerebral dysfunction (*lexia* refers to word).

amentia (ah-men'she-ah) mental deficiency.

amnesia (am-ne'se-ah) loss of memory.

analgesia (an"al-je'ze-ah) insensibility to pain.

anepia (an-e'pe-ah) inability to talk (*epia* refers to speech).

anergic (an-er'jik) characterized by abnormal inactivity, with lack of energy (*ergic* means work).

anesthesia loss of sensation.

anomia (ah-no'me-ah) loss of ability to recognize or name objects (*nomia* refers to name).

anosognosia (an-ah"sog-no'ze-ah) loss of ability to recognize that one has a disease or bodily defect (*noso* means disease; *gnosia* means knowledge).

apathy absence of emotion, or indifference to the environment or other people, with attention directed inward rather than outward.

aphonia loss of voice.

apraxia (ah-prak'se-ah) loss of ability to perform intricate skilled acts that had been previously mastered.

asthenia (as-the'ne-ah) weakness or lack of strength and energy.

autism (aw'tizm) condition of being dominated by subjective, introspective thinking, and a symptom of schizophrenia, that may affect some children who show schizophrenic-like conditions in a disorder referred to as *infantile autism* or *Kanner's syndrome.*

autoeroticism (aw"to-e-rot'i-sizm) sexual gratification of self by various means without participation of another (*auto* means self).

automatism (aw-tom'ah-tizm) performance of undirected actions without evident conscious volition.

bestiality (bes-te-al'i-te) sexual relations between humans and animals, classified as a *paraphilia.*

bradykinesia (brad"e-ki-ne'se-ah) slow movement (*kinesis* means movement).

bradyphrenia slowness of thinking (*phrenia* refers to mind).

bradypragia (brad"e-pra'je-ah) slowness of action.

bradypsychia (brad"e-si'ke-ah) slowness in mental reactions.

catalepsy (kat'ah-lep"se) waxy rigidity of the muscles, with limbs tending to remain in any position in which placed, observed in catatonic schizophrenia and other conditions.

cataphasia (kat"ah-fa'ze-ah) speech disorder involving constant repetition of the same word or phrase.

catatonia (kat"ah-to'ne-ah) form of schizophrenia (see *schizophrenia*).

cathexis (kah-thek'sis) concentration of mental or emotional energy that may be abnormal in intensity, on a person or object.

confabulation (kon-fab"u-la'shun) act of making up answers and concocting experiences without regard to truth.

coprolalia (kop"ro-la'le-ah) use of vulgar, or obscene language (*copro* refers to dung or feces).

cyclothymia (si"klo-thim'e-ah) cyclic alternation of moods between elation and depression (see *mood disorders*).

deja entendu (day"zhah on-ton-doo') impression, in a new situation, that one has heard the same thing previously.

deja vu (voo') impression, in a new situation, that one has seen the same thing previously.

delusion false belief or idea, a major symptom of psychosis.

dereism irrational thinking or fantasy that is not in accord with logic, experience, and reality.

dipsomania (dip'so-ma'ne-ah) uncontrollable desire for alcohol.

disorientation loss of proper bearings for time, place, and/or identity during mental confusion.

drug dependency drug addiction or habituation.

dysarthria (dis-ar′thre-ah) imperfect articulation in speech, such as stuttering or stammering.

dysgraphia (dis-gra′fe-ah) inability to write properly.

dyslexia impaired reading ability.

dyslogia (dis-lo′je-ah) impaired logical thinking.

dysphonia difficulty in speaking, or any impairment of voice.

dysphoria (dis-fo′re-ah) sadness and depression.

dysthymia (dis-thim′e-ah) disorder of mood (*thymia* refers to mind or emotion).

echolalia (ek″o-la′le-ah) meaningless repetition of words.

echopathy (ek-op′ah-the) senseless repetition of words or actions.

egocentric self-centered.

empathy process of imaginative projection of one's own consciousness into other persons in order to understand their feelings and emotions.

erotic relating to or producing sexual excitement or love.

erotomania (e-rot″to-ma′ne-ah) exaggerated sexual interest or behavior.

euphoria (u-fo′re-ah) exaggerated sense of well-being, the opposite of dysphoria.

euthymia (u-thi′me-ah) pleasant feeling, and state of well-being.

exhibitionism exposing the genitals to public view or to members of the opposite sex, popularly referred to as "flashing" in lay terminology, classified as a *paraphilia.*

extrovert one whose interests are centered in external objects and actions.

fetishism practice of attaching unusual or magical qualities to an object, or the investment of sexual feeling in an inanimate object, classified as a *paraphilia.*

flagellantism getting pleasure from whipping someone or being whipped, psychoanalytically viewed as sexual pleasure, related to sadism and masochism, classified as a *paraphilia.*

folie a deux (foal-ee ah duh) disorder in which two closely associated people share the same deluded or distorted ideas (popularly called a "gruesome twosome").

fugue (fug) dissociated state in which a person seems rational and conscious and may perform purposeful acts, but later is unable to recall the occasion or events.

gay popular term for homosexual; used more commonly for males.

glossolalia speaking in an unknown or imaginary language.

hallucination (hah-lu″si-na′shun) sense perception not based upon objective reality.

haplology omissions of syllables in speaking, found in manic speech.

hedonia (he-do′ne-ah) excessive interest in pleasure.

heterolalia use of inappropriate or meaningless words in place of those intended (also called *heterophasia*).

homosexuality (ho″mo-seks″u-al′i-te) sexual attraction to persons of the same sex (commonly called *gay* for males and *lesbian* for females), no longer considered an abnormal disorder unless it is ego-dystonic (unacceptable to the person's deeper self).

hyperpragia (hi″per′a′je-ah) pronounced increase in mental activity (also called *hyperphrenia*).

hypnosis (hip-no′sis) induced state of altered awareness or trance.

hypoalgesia decreased sensitivity to pain (also called *hypalgesia*).

hypochondria term used to describe excessive somatic complaints without evident organic cause.

hypoesthesia (hi″po-es-the′ze-ah) decreased sensibility to pain.

hypokinesia decrease of motor function.

hypomania excitement, with increased activity and speech, but not as extreme as in mania.

hypophrasia slow speech associated with psychosis.

id Freudian term for the self-preservative and sexual instincts.

incest sexual relations between close relatives (between parent and child, brother and sister, uncle and niece, etc.).

inertia (in-er′she-ah) inactivity.

insomnia (in-som′ni-a) sleeplessness.

introverted thoughts and activities centered on self instead of toward others, with the person becoming isolated, introspective, and relatively uncommunicative, the opposite of extroverted.

inversion turning inward.

kleptomania impulse to steal (*klepto* means steal).

lesbian female homosexual.

lethargy lack of energy.

libido (li-be'do) Freudian collective term for energy, motive, force, or striving, especially with reference to sexual drive.

logographia (log"o-graf'e-ah) inability to express ideas in writing.

malingering simulating or feigning illness for purposes other than getting attention.

masochism (mas'o-kism) deriving gratification or pleasure by the recipient of cruel treatment or pain, classified as a *paraphilia.*

misogyny (mis-oj'i-ne) aversion to women (*gyn* refers to women).

misopedia (mis"o-pe'de-ah) hatred of children (*pedia* refers to children).

mogilalia (moj-e-la'le-ah) stuttering, also called *molilalia* (*mogi* means with difficulty).

narcissism (nar'si-sizm) excessive self-interest or self-love, and inability to love another.

necromania (nek"ro-ma'ne-ah) morbid preoccupation with death or the dead (*necro* means death).

necrophilia (nek"ro-fil'e-ah) morbid attraction to a corpse or sexual intercourse with a dead person, classified as a *paraphilia.*

necrosadism (nek"ro-sa'dizm) gratification of sexual needs through mutilation of a corpse, classified as a *paraphilia.*

negativism (ne'ah-tiv-izm) abnormal opposition to suggestions or advice.

neurosis obsolete term used to describe a less serious psychiatric problem than psychosis, and now referred to as a *disorder.*

nosophilia abnormal desire to be ill (*noso* refers to disease).

nymphomania (nim"fo-ma'ne-ah) abnormally intense sexual desire in a female.

oligophrenia mental deficiency.

onychophagy (on"i-kof'ah-je) habitual biting of nails.

palilalia (pal"i-la'le-ah) pathologic repetition of words (*pali* means again).

paragraphia (par"ah-gra'fe-ah) disorder in which one word is written in place of another.

paralalia speech disturbance.

paralgesia (par"al-je'se-ah) abnormally painful sensation.

paralogia (par"ah-lo'je-ah) impaired reasoning.

paraphilia (par"ah-fil'e-ah) aberrant sexual activity; sexual deviations.

pavor diurnus attack similar to nightmare, but occurring during the daytime (*pavor* means terror; *diurnus* means day).

pavor nocturnus nightmare, night terror (*nocturnus* means night).

phantom limb phenomenon vivid feeling of still having an amputated limb, usually associated with subjective feelings of pain, perceived as originating in the lost limb.

pica (pi'ka) craving for ingestion of unnatural substances such as ashes, lead, hair, or dirt, usually seen in severely disturbed persons, although it may occur in pregnant women and in malnourished children.

poriomania (po"re-o-ma'ne-ah) tendency to wander from home.

pornographomania morbid desire to collect pornographic or erotic literature, art, etc., as opposed to casual collection by relatively normal persons.

premenstrual syndrome (PMS) emotional counterpart of physiologic endocrine distress that precedes the onset of the menstrual period in females of reproductive age, with symptoms of fatigue, irritability, tension, anxiety, and depression.

pseudocyesis (su"do-si-e'sis) false pregnancy, classified as a *somatoform disorder* (*cyesis* means pregnancy).

pseudographia (su"do-graf'e-ah) writing of meaningless symbols.

pseudologia (su"do-lo'je-ah) pathologic oral or written lying.

pseudomania pretended mental disorder

psychalia (si"ka'le-ah) hearing of voices or seeing images in mental disorders.

psyche (si'ke) term meaning soul or mind, including both conscious and unconscious processes.

psychogenic originating from psychologic mechanisms and not from organic disease or disorder; for example, phobias are considered to be psychogenic in origin, but senile psychosis is regarded as organic.

psycholepsy (si-ko-lep'se) condition characterized by sudden changes in mood, tending toward depression.

psychosis term for severe mental disorder with loss of reality contact, unlike neurotic disorder in which reality contact is retained.

pyromania excessive preoccupation with fires and gaining pleasure from setting fires.

rationalization one of many unconscious defense mechanisms, by which a plausible explanation is concocted to justify one's beliefs, behavior, needs, feelings, or motives, with the real motivation remaining hidden.

sadism (sad′izm) gratification through cruelty inflicted on others, classified as a *paraphilia.*

sadomasochism (sad″o-maz′o-kizm) characterized by both sadism and masochism, classified as a *paraphilia.*

sodomy (sod′o-me) sexual practices including fellatio and anal intercourse between humans and coitus between humans and animals (bestiality).

somnambulism sleepwalking.

sophomania (sof″o-ma′ne-ah) exaggerated belief in one's own brilliance.

stress term referring to physical or psychosocial adjustment demands placed on people, who differ in capacity to adapt, producing reactions that may be oriented either toward coping or toward protecting oneself from harm and damage.

theomania obsession with religion or with God, or belief that one is God (*theo* means God).

transvestism sexual deviation, most common in males, classified as a *paraphilia,* in which the individual gets sexual gratification from wearing clothes of the opposite sex, and may extend to wanting to be accepted as a member of the sex they are emulating, in which case they may even have sex change surgery to anatomically resemble the preferred sex identity, thereby becoming *transsexual.*

trichophagia (tri-kof′ah-je-ah) practice of eating hair.

trichotillomania uncontrollable urge to pull out one's own hair.

voyeurism (voi′yer-izm) sexual deviation in which sexual excitation or gratification is derived from looking at sexual organs or watching sexual activity by others, classified under *paraphilias* (also called *scopophilia*).

zoosadism deriving pleasure from cruelty to animals, classified as a *paraphilia.*

Tests for Psychiatric and Neurologic Conditions

The following is a listing of a few of the many psychologic and psychiatric tests used to evaluate mental functioning and brain disorders.

Beck Depression Inventory (BDI) self-report measure of feelings, attitudes, and behaviors that are diagnostic of depression.

Brief Psychiatric Rating Scale (BPRS) method of analyzing the clinical symptoms of patients with a standardized method of rating more than 18 separate scales that cover a wide range of psychiatric conditions.

Minnesota Multiphasic Personality Inventory (MMPI and MMPI-2) extensive self-report by patient, using true-false inventory, that assesses psychiatric pathology.

Millon Clinical Multiaxial Inventory (MCMI and MCMI-II) extensive self-report by patient, using true-false inventory, that assesses personality traits, symptoms, and disorders.

neuropsychologic tests tests that assist in the diagnosis of brain damage or disorder and assess the extent of change from normal functioning. Some of the widely used tests for these purposes include:

Bender Visual Motor Gestalt Test drawing a set of geometric figures to assess perceptual impairment.

Benton Test of Visual Retention-Revised drawing, by memory, a set of complex geometric figures.

Halstead-Reitan Neuropsychologic Battery a comprehensive battery of 11 basic tests of perception, cognition, and motor functioning, plus the use of the *WAIS-III* and *MMPI,* for diagnosing and assisting in localization of brain damage.

Neurosurgery Center Comprehensive Examination of Aphasia battery of 24 tests evaluating visual, auditory, tactile, sensory, and motor aphasia problems.

sorting tests tests of abstract categorical function, using objects, colors, and shapes.

Rorschach Test a set of 10 standardized ink blots used to analyze thought processes, motives, characteristic defenses, and effectiveness of coping, based on the "projective hypothesis" that, in trying to identify vague and unstructured materials, people will "project" their own feelings, motives, and problems into the materials.

Thematic Apperception Test (TAT) ambiguous and unstructured set of pictures about which patients make up stories by projecting their own conflicts into the pictures, revealing needs and motives, perception of reality, and characteristic coping or defensive strategies.

Wechsler Adult Intelligence Scale-III (WAIS-III) this measure of intelligence, which has a variety of different types of verbal and performance tests, is used to analyze cognitive competence, bizarre ideas, anxiety problems, and other structural components of psychiatric functioning.

Treatment Methods for Psychiatric Conditions

electroconvulsive therapy (ECT) form of shock therapy used in mental disorders (depression), in which electrical currents are conveyed to the brain by electrodes applied to the scalp, resulting in loss of consciousness and muscle tonic and clonic contractions, followed by amnesia and confusion for varying periods after waking.

insulin coma therapy rarely used method of treating schizophrenics, involving administration of increasing amounts of insulin until the patient experiences hypoglycemic coma, which is terminated by providing glucose.

pharmacologic methods of treatment drugs are extensively used in treatment of psychiatric conditions, and the following represent some of the chemical types and/or generic (nontrade name) drugs that have been used during a long period of time. New drugs are constantly being developed for use in this area, and some of the currently listed drugs may become obsolete.

   antianxiety drugs group of minor tranquilizers that include *propranolol* and the *benzodiazepines.*

   antidepressant drugs two major groups are used to treat severe depressive symptoms, especially of the unipolar type: *tricyclics* and *monoamine oxidase (MAO) inhibitors.*

   antimanic drugs primary drug used for manic states and bipolar disorders is *lithium carbonate.*

   antipsychotic drugs three major groups of antipsychotic drugs, or major tranquilizers, that are used to treat extreme agitation, delusions, hallucinations, and violent behavior, include the *phenothiazines, butyrophenones,* and *thioxanthenes.*

   neurotransmitter reuptake inhibitors these drugs act by preventing absorption of the neurotransmitters serotonin and norepinephrine, and are used primarily to reduce depression and produce feelings of well-being (one popular drug is *Prozac*).

   stimulant drugs these drugs, used primarily for hyperactivity in children, include *amphetamines* and *methylphenidate.*

prefrontal lobotomy surgical procedure in which the frontal lobes are separated from the deeper centers in the diencephalon, producing significant personality changes, primarily used as a method for psychoses that do not respond to other methods, severe and debilitating obsessive-compulsive disorders, and for severe pain in terminal illness.

psychotherapies this group of therapies involve the application of psychologic theory and knowledge to treatment of psychiatric disorders, with the following the best known of a large group.

   behavior modification the use of scientific principles of *contingency management* (rewarding desired behavior) to modify the symptoms and effect some personality change in a wide range of psychiatric disorders, including psychoses and personality disorders.

   behavior therapy this approach uses conditioning principles in the application of methods like *systematic desensitization, aversion therapy,* and *flooding* in the treatment of paraphilias, panic disorders, and phobias in particular.

   client-centered therapy this approach uses the overall relationship between the patient and therapist, and the therapist's positive attitudes, to open the patient to a "growth potential" that encourages increased openness for the development of behavior change and insight.

   cognitive therapy assists patients to examine beliefs and attitudes that produce and maintain their emotional disorders and has been found especially effective with depression.

   psychoanalytic therapy this approach uses principles and methods of various psychoanalytic schools to produce insight in the patient about the origins of the pathology and the defensive tactics that the patient uses to maintain it.

EXERCISES **THE NERVOUS SYSTEM** THE CENTRAL PROCESSING UNIT

Exercise 15.1 *Complete the following:*

1. The brain and spinal cord are located in the _____Central nervous_____ system.
2. The craniospinal nerves are located in the _____peripheral nervous_____ system.
3. The sympathetic and parasympathic systems are located in the _____autonomic nervous_____ system.
4. The groups of neuron cell bodies outside the central nervous system are called _____ganglia_____.
5. The membranes that envelop the central nervous system are called _____meninges_____.
6. The three membranes that envelop the nervous system are the _____dura mater_____, the _____arachoid_____, and the _____pia mater_____.
7. The portion of the brain that is referred to as a bridge is the _____pon_____.
8. The part of the brain in which the thalamus, epithalamus, and hypothalamus are located is the _____ _____diencephalon_____.
9. The thin, transparent, watery fluid found in the ventricles of the brain, central canal of the spinal cord, and the subarachnoid space is called _____cerebro spinal fluid_____.
10. The passage for the spinal cord through the occipital bone of the cranium is called the _foramen magnum_

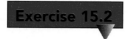**Exercise 15.2**   *Using the list of terms below, identify each part in Figure 15.8 by writing the name in the corresponding blank.*

Cerebrum   Midbrain   Diencephalon

Frontal lobe   Occipital lobe   Medulla oblongata

Corpus callosum   Pons   Third ventricle

Pineal body   Parietal lobe   Optic chiasma

Septum pellucidum   Temporal lobe   Cerebellum

Pituitary (hypophysis)   Cerebral aqueduct   Spinal cord

Fourth ventricle   Intermediate mass   Thalamus

Brainstem

1. _____cerebrum_____
2. _____septum pellucidum_____
3. _____frontal lobe_____
4. _____corpus callosum_____
5. _____diencephalon_____
6. _____temporal lobe_____
7. _____optic chiasmal_____
8. _____pituatory_____
9. _____brainstem_____
10. _____pens_____
11. _____medulla oblogata_____

12. _____parietal lobe_____
13. _____intermediate mass_____
14. _____thalamus_____
15. _____pineal body_____
16. _____occipital lobe_____
17. _____thurd ventricle_____
18. _____midbrain_____
19. _____cerebral aqueduct_____
20. _____cerebellum_____
21. _____fourth ventricle_____
22. _____spinal cord_____

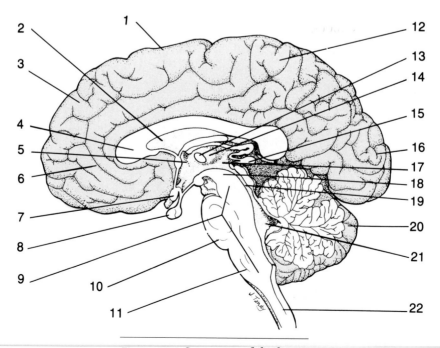

Figure 15.8 Structures of the brain.

Exercise 15.3   *Matching*

H 1. long nerve cell processes that carry impulses from the cell body

F 2. numerous short nerve cell processes that conduct nerve impulses toward the cell body

N 3. neurons concerned with muscle or gland action

K 4. peripheral neurons that conduct afferent impulses from the sense organs to the spinal cord

D 5. the region of connection between processes of two adjacent neurons for transmission of impulses

G 6. peripheral nerve endings

A 7. space between the pia mater and the arachnoid

I 8. space between the dura mater and arachnoid

M 9. central body of the cerebellum, shaped like a worm

C 10. a furrow, or groove, separating folds of the brain

L 11. second cranial nerve, which innervates the retina of the eye

E 12. third cranial nerve, which innervates the eye muscles and the sphincter of the pupil and ciliary processes

J 13. interlacing network of spinal nerves

O 14. nerve that originates in the spinal cord and innervates the diaphragm

B 15. a so-called wandering nerve, both motor and sensory, with an extensive distribution, with some gastric, pyloric, hepatic, and celiac branches

A. subarachnoid
B. vagus
C. sulcus
D. synapse
E. oculomotor
F. dendrites
G. terminal twigs
H. axon
I. subdural
J. plexus
K. sensory neurons
L. optic
M. vermis
N. motor neurons
O. phrenic

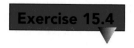

Give the meaning of the components in the following words and then define the word as a whole. Suffixes meaning *pertaining to* or *state* or *condition*, shown following a slash mark (/), are not to be defined separately. Before reaching for your medical dictionary, check the Related Terms list in this chapter.

1. Encephalomyelitis:

   encephalo _brain_

   myel _spinal cord_

   itis _inflammation_

   _____

2. Arachnoiditis:

   arachnoid _arachnoid membrane_

   itis _inflammation_

   _____

3. Meningoencephalitis:

   meningo _meninges_

   encephal _brain_

   itis _inflammation_

   _____

4. Pachymeningitis:

   pachy _dura mater_

   mening _meninges_

   itis _inflammation_

   _____

5. Polioencephalomeningomyelitis:

   polio _gray matter_

   encephalo _brain_

   meningo _meninges_

   myel _spinal cord_

   itis _inflammation_

   _____

6. Rachiomyelitis:

   rachio _____

   myel _spinal cord_

   itis _inflammation_

   _____

7. Anencephalia:

   an _no_

   encephal/ia _brain_

   _____

8. Cephalocele:

   cephalo _brain_

   cele _hernia_

   _____

9. Encephalomyelocele:

   encephalo _brain_

   myelo _spinal cord_

   cele _hernia_

   _____

10. Heterotopia spinalis:

    hetero _other_

    top/ia _place_

    spinal/is _spinal_

    _____

CROSSWORD PUZZLE CHAPTER 15

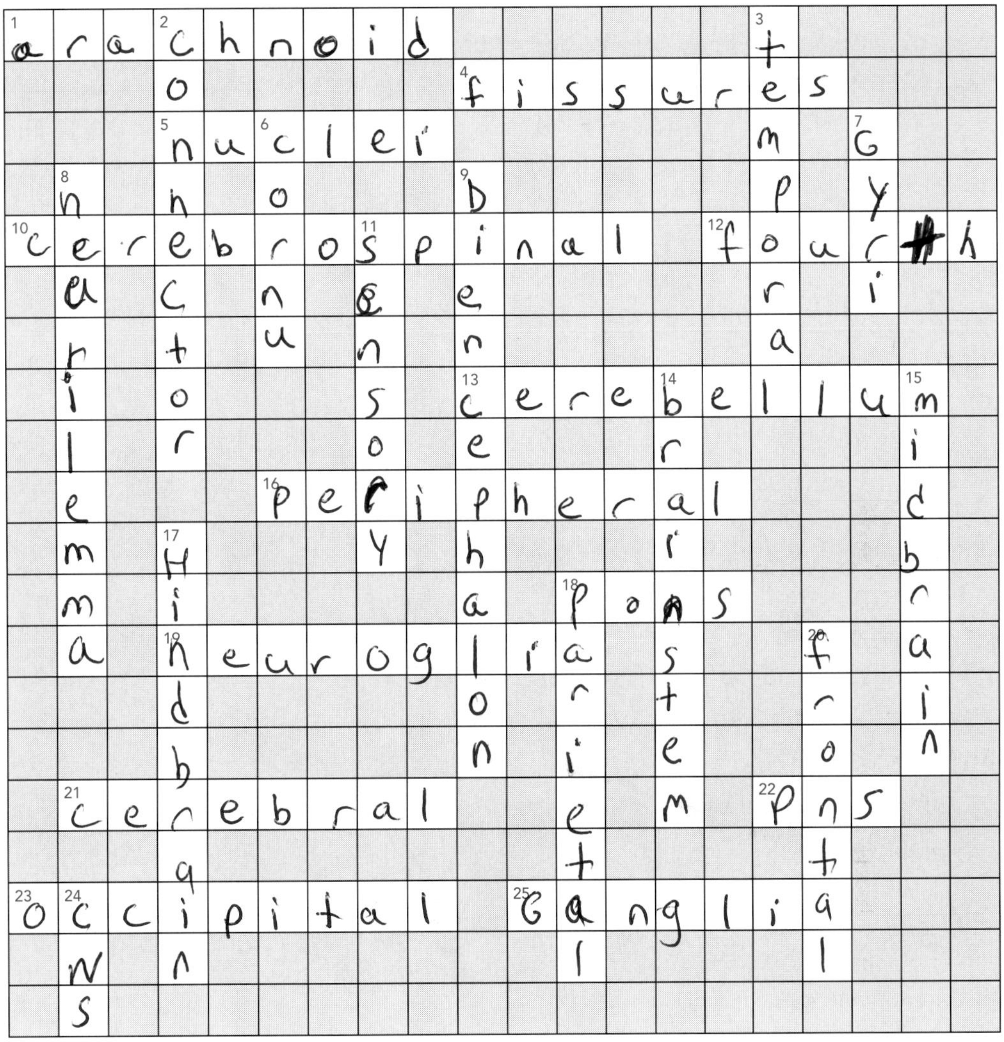

ACROSS

1. Weblike membrane
4. Deeper furrows
5. Neuron cell body groups in central nervous system
10. Fluid of central nervous system
12. Kite-shaped ventricle
13. A division of the brain
16. Craniospinal and autonomic nerves
18. Bridge
19. Hold and support nerve cells
21. Aqueduct (of Sylvius)
22. Peripheral nervous system abbreviation
23. Posterior lobe of cerebral cortex
25. Nerve cell clusters outside central nervous system

DOWN

2. Interneuron neuron
3. A lobe of the cerebral cortex
6. Means horn
7. Cerebral hemisphere convolutions
8. Sheath of Schwann
9. A division of the brain
11. Afferent neurons
14. A division of the brain
15. The mesencephalon
17. Pons and medulla together
18. A lobe of the cerebral cortex
20. Anterior lobe of cerebral cortex
24. Central nervous system abbreviation

HIDDEN WORDS PUZZLE

```
A  G  Y  Z  E  Z  Y  F  B  G  Y  M  S  O  T  U  V  K  D  N  M
I  X  W  R  E  C  E  P  T  O  R  R  T  F  M  P  J  Y  T  F  L
E  Y  O  J  V  L  O  Z  Y  W  J  J  Y  E  N  N  W  N  J  U  U
L  C  E  N  T  R  A  L  P  D  I  Y  V  C  C  J  H  I  C  M  U
L  T  I  V  L  K  U  O  L  I  X  G  Y  C  Y  V  C  I  U  S  K
S  Y  H  N  Q  S  Y  M  P  A  T  H  E  T  I  C  O  M  W  S  H
D  Y  A  F  M  R  U  U  P  D  T  J  H  Z  X  M  R  Y  O  B  D
H  T  N  V  Q  Z  R  B  E  X  D  E  N  D  R  I  T  E  X  U  P
J  H  Y  A  T  G  B  T  A  F  F  E  R  E  N  T  L  L  J  H  G
K  J  U  O  P  K  W  C  U  R  F  F  W  A  E  E  T  I  J  R  X
Q  L  K  H  L  S  P  S  T  J  A  E  D  V  L  H  X  N  U  Y  P
B  O  U  C  B  U  E  Q  O  S  H  C  R  M  U  S  Q  K  D  S  V
F  M  M  E  M  B  R  A  N  E  P  S  H  E  Q  V  X  M  P  G  H
E  Q  M  F  S  D  M  I  O  Y  T  I  T  N  N  O  L  I  B  S  F
O  A  X  K  O  U  U  Y  M  K  J  W  U  I  O  T  P  W  I  S  G
U  K  K  T  T  R  U  H  I  P  B  N  J  N  M  I  M  A  Y  B  Q
E  X  H  D  R  A  A  V  C  I  U  N  D  G  B  U  D  H  G  L  W
W  Q  Y  I  U  L  D  M  V  Y  I  L  O  E  S  W  L  X  B  R  C
K  V  F  B  Y  O  S  R  E  C  S  E  S  S  C  N  E  U  R  O  N
X  F  W  G  M  O  W  J  Y  N  W  C  U  E  C  L  W  D  S  A  I
```

Can you find the 20 words hidden in this puzzle? All hidden words puzzles will have words running from top to bottom; left to right; and diagonally downward.

SUBARACHNOID	RECEPTOR	AXON
AFFERENT	FORAMEN	AUTONOMIC
MENINGES	NEURON	MEMBRANE
CENTRAL	COLLATERAL	SUBDURAL
MYELIN	EFFERENT	SYNAPSE
SYMPATHETIC	STIMULUS	TWIG
DENDRITE	IMPULSE	

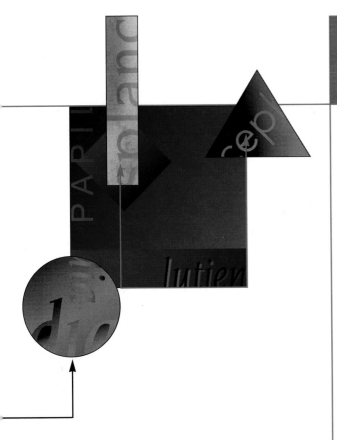

The Special Senses

the sources of information

In this chapter we discuss the five special senses: vision, hearing, smell, taste, and touch, and their unique structures and sensation mechanisms.

THE SENSE OF VISION

The organ of vision is the *eye,* with its various accessory organs, such as the *extrinsic muscles,* the *eyelids,* and the *tear apparatus.* Strictly speaking, the eye includes only the *bulb* of the eye (the *eyeball*) and the *optic nerve,* which connects it with the brain. This constitutes the essential part of the organ of vision. (The term *optic* refers to the eye, as do the combining forms *oculo* and *ophthalmo.*)

The eye is the most important sense organ in the body. It is from the eye that we receive most of our information, not only in what we can see around us or in the near distance, but also in what we learn through the printed word.

The eyeball occupies the front half of the orbital cavity, where it is embedded (cushioned) in fat and connective tissue. The eyeballs lie on either side of the root of the nose and are almost sphere shaped. Attached to the eyeball and contained in its orbital cavity are the *optic nerve, ocular muscles,* and certain other nerves and vessels. A soft mucous membrane, called the *conjunctiva,* covers the anterior (or exposed) third of the eyeball and lines the eyelids. The

---

It's a FACT

Vision is so sensitive that, on a clear moonless night, a person on a mountain can detect the striking of a match 50 miles away.

eyes are protected by the eyelids (referred to as *palpebrae;* combining form is *blepharo*), which are fringed with *cilia* (eyelashes), and, above the eyes another row of hairs, usually arched in appearance, forms the *supercilia* (eyebrows). The eyes are moistened and kept clean by the tears from the *lacrimal glands,* and the eyelids blink frequently to spread the secretions of the lacrimal glands over the external surface of the eye, keeping it moist.

Movement of the eyeball is by six slender *extrinsic* muscles, attached to each eye, that act together. The movement of opening the eyes, however, is confined to the upper lid. The eyes are free to move in any direction, upward, downward, and sideways, or the gaze may be fixed and straight ahead.

The eyeball is like a hollow sphere whose wall is made up of three concentric coats and whose cavity is filled with transparent *refracting media* (tissues and fluid that transmit light). The outer fibrous coat, the *sclera,* has a white, opaque, posterior portion and a transparent anterior portion called the *cornea.* The intermediate coat, the *choroid,* is vascular and pigmented and divided into a posterior portion and a smaller anterior portion, which has three structures, the *ciliary body,* the *suspensory ligament,* and the *iris.* The choroid, the ciliary body, and the iris together are referred to as the *uvea.* The *retina* (internal coat), is the light-sensitive layer that is made up of differentiated nervous receptors continuous with the optic nerve. Three transparent refractive media fill the optic cavity; the *vitreous body* (semigelatinous substance contained in a thin, clear membrane) between the retina and the lens, and two *aqueous humor* (watery fluid) chambers anterior to the lens (Figure 16.1).

The eye is like a camera, with an opening in front, the *pupil,* that lets light in, a *crystalline lens* behind the pupil focusing the rays of light to form an image on the retina, which contains the vision sense organs, the *rods* and *cones.* The optic nerve carries the impulses from the rods and cones to the visual area.

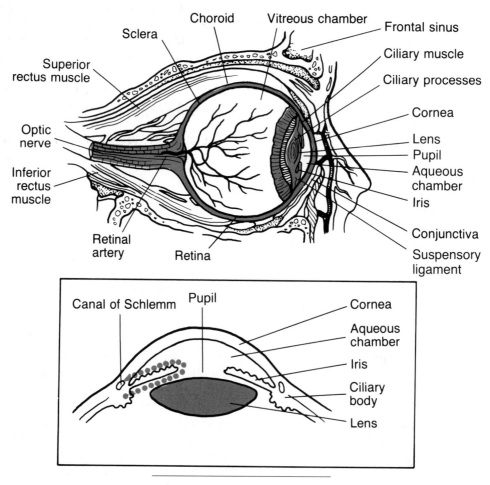

Figure 16.1 Structures of the eye.

Structures of the Eye

Sclera. The *sclera* is the white, opaque portion of the eye, "the white of the eye," and constitutes the posterior five sixths of the eyeball. It is composed of white fibrous tissue and fine elastic fibers, with the front portion covered by a membrane called the *conjunctiva*, through which small, superficial blood vessels can be seen. In children, the sclera is often very thin and allows the underlying choroidal pigment to show through, giving the sclera a bluish cast, and, in the aged, one often sees a yellowish cast. The conjunctival surfaces are lubricated and washed by the tears secreted by the lacrimal glands.

Cornea. The *cornea* is the anterior, transparent portion of the fibrous coat of the eyeball through which light enters the eye. It is nearly circular in shape, and its marked curvature makes it bulge with a domelike protrusion that varies among individuals and diminishes somewhat with age. It is devoid of blood and lymph vessels, except at the extreme periphery, and this lack of vascularity makes the cornea subject to infection after injury.

Choroid. The *choroid* is located between the sclera and retina, and its posterior part is a thin membrane with a rich vascular layer. The cells of the choroid are filled with melanin, a black or dark brown pigment, which gives it a dark brown appearance. Extra light is absorbed by the pigment which helps to prevent blurring of an image by internally reflected light. The chief function of the choroid is to maintain the nutrition of the retina through its capillary plexus and numerous small arteries and veins.

Ciliary body. The *ciliary body,* an extension of the choroid, is a thickened portion of the vascular layer which extends from the visual layer to the iris. The ciliary body is a wedge-shaped, flattened ring, with muscles connected to the *suspensory ligament* that attaches the lens to it and *processes* (ridges) that secrete the *aqueous humor* (fluid). The ciliary processes consist of a rich vascular plexus embedded in pigmented *stroma* (connective tissue). Focusing on far or near objects (called *accommodation*) is accomplished through changing the shape of the lens by action of the *ciliary muscles.*

Suspensory ligament. The *suspensory ligament,* made up of separate fibers, is another structure of the anterior extension of the choroid, continuous with the capsule that encloses the lens, and attaching the lens to the ciliary muscles.

Iris. The *iris,* the most anterior portion of the vascular layer, continuous with the ciliary body, is doughnut shaped, and its central opening, the *pupil,* appears to be black in color. The iris is composed of rings of muscle fibers, some of which are arranged circularly, contracting to reduce the size of the pupil, with others arranged radially, contracting to increase the size of the pupil, regulating the amount of light admitted to the lens. The iris is suspended in the aqueous space between the cornea and lens, dividing it into anterior and posterior chambers. The larger anterior chamber is between the iris and the cornea, and the posterior chamber is between the lens and the iris. These chambers are filled with the lymphlike aqueous humor, which aids in maintaining the shape of the eyeball, and empties into the *canal of Schlemm,* an oval channel circling the anterior chamber. The aqueous humor, which is secreted by the ciliary processes, flows through the pupil into the anterior chamber, and the pressure maintained by the balance between secretion and removal of fluid is known as the *intraocular pressure.*

The reflection of light scattered by pigment substances in the iris results in different colors, with dark eyes having abundant pigment and blue eyes having less pigment. Some neonates have blue eyes because the pigment does not develop in the stroma (connective tissue fibers forming the major part of the iris) until after birth; however, others have brown eyes at birth because the stromal pigment is already developed.

Lens. The transparent crystalline **lens** is directly behind the iris of the eye, enclosed in an elastic capsule supported by the suspensory ligament, and focuses the light rays on the retina. The shape of the lens is altered by the action of the ciliary muscles, which affects the *refraction* (bending) of light rays.

Retina. The innermost of the three coats of the eyeball, the *retina,* is a soft, delicate membrane that is in contact with, and nourished by, the vascular coat. The retina is the nervous tissue layer with special neuroepithelial cells, the *rods* and *cones,* named for their shape, that serve as the photosensitive receptors of light stimuli. The cones are much less numerous than the rods and are adapted to bright light and color perception as well as for the fine details of an object. The rods are much more sensitive for low light vision but are color blind. Near the center of the back of the retina is a small yellow area called the *macula lutea,* with a central depression, the *fovea centralis,* which is the region of clearest vision, in which the cones are most concentrated, and no rods are found. The retina also contains numerous sensory and connector neurons and their processes. At a point in the back of the retina, nearer the nose, there is an *optic disk,* where the nerve fibers from the entire eye converge to form the *optic nerve,* producing a blind spot because there are no rods or cones present. At the point where the optic nerve pierces the sclera, it is accompanied by the optic central artery and vein, which come from the choroid.

Lacrimal glands. The *lacrimal glands,* about the size of an almond kernel, lie under the bones forming the upper, outer orbit, secrete *tears,* which are carried to the conjunctiva by lacrimal ducts. There are several small accessory lacrimal glands lying in folds under the eyelids, which under ordinary circumstances secrete sufficient tears to lubricate and clean the eyes, with the main glands called into play only during crying or in response to irritation of the conjunctiva.

The blinking of the eyes spreads the tears over the conjunctival surfaces and directs the fluid into a lacrimal lake at the nasal corner, the *inner canthus.* The tears are drained from the lake by two small lacrimal ducts that lead into the nose. The opening of the tear ducts into the nose accounts for the "running" of the nose during crying.

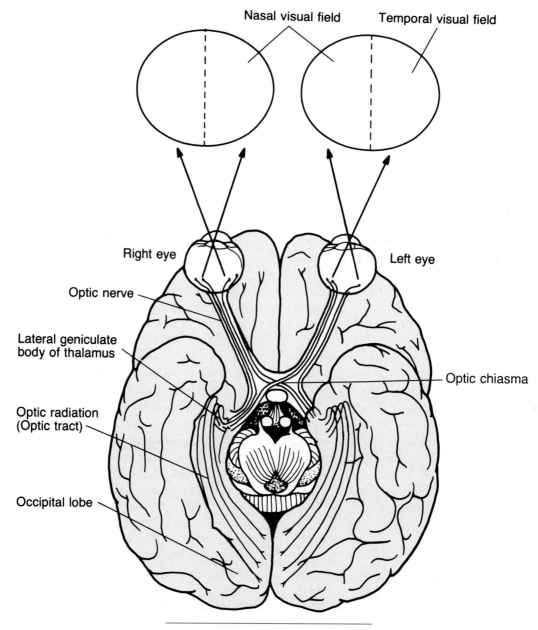

Figure 16.2 Visual fields and pathways.

The Mechanism of Vision

Vision occurs when light rays enter the pupil and are focused upon the retina by the lens, cornea, and aqueous and vitreous humors. This process of focusing is accomplished by all four components, any of which may develop defects. Light rays from objects 20 feet or more away are relatively parallel and are readily focused on the retina by the normal eye. Closer light rays must be bent more sharply to focus them on the retina. This process, called *accommodation,* involves an increase in convex curvature of the lens (which is elastic) by ciliary muscle contraction, along with some constriction of the pupil to restrict stray light that might blur the image.

Since both eyes must focus the light rays from an object on corresponding points on the retina to achieve single rather than double vision, the eyeballs are *converged* (moved together) by six extrinsic muscles that are attached to the outside of the eyeball and to the bones of the orbit. The slight difference in corresponding points of the retina on which the light rays from the same object are focused, caused by the few inches separating the eyes, as well as the individual's history of visual experiences with near and far objects, accounts for depth perception, or three-dimensionality.

Stimulations of the retinal receptors (rods and cones) are transmitted through the optic nerves to the *optic chiasma,* then to midbrain areas and the visual cortex areas of the occipital lobe. In the optic chiasma, the optic nerve fibers from the inner (or nasal) half of each retina crossover and join those from the outer (or temporal) half of the retina of the other eye before continuing on. For example, the fibers from the right half of the left eye link up with those from the right half of the right eye. This accounts for the finding that in conditions producing total loss of nerve transmission in the visual cortex of one hemisphere, there is partial loss of vision in both eyes rather than total loss in either (Figure 16.2).

REVIEW 16.A

Complete the following:

1. The most important sense organ is the
   __eye__ .

2. The mucous membrane covering the exposed third of the eyeball is the
   __conjunctiva__ .

3. Tears are secreted by __lacrimal__ glands.

4. There are __3__ concentric coats making up the wall of the eyeball.

5. The receptors of light stimuli are the
   __rods__ and __cones__ .

6. The "white of the eye" is called the
   __sclera__ .

7. Light enters the eye through the transparent part of the eyeball called the
   __cornea__ .

8. The pigment melanin fills the cells of the
   __choroid__ .

9. The process by which light rays are bent to focus them on the retina is called
   __accommodation__ .

10. Stimulations of the retinal receptors are transmitted through the optic nerves to the
    __optic chiasma__ .

THE SENSE OF HEARING

We usually think of the *ear* as the organ of hearing, which is divided into the *external ear, middle ear,* and *inner ear* (*oto* and *auris* refer to ear; *audi* refers to hearing). However, the ear also contains structures responsible for equilibrium.

Structures of the Ear

External ear. The *external ear* is made up of the *auricle* (or *pinna,* meaning wing), the cartilaginous, cutaneous appendage, and the *external auditory meatus* (*meatus* means opening), which is a short, tortuous passage that leads to, and penetrates, the temporal bone. The external auditory canal is entirely lined by skin containing modified sweat glands that secrete a yellow-brown waxy substance called *cerumen* (earwax). This canal ends blindly at the *tympanic membrane* (eardrum). Sound waves reach the tympanic membrane through this canal, are picked up by the inner bones of the ear, and transmitted by the auditory nerve to the brain (Figure 16.3).

Middle ear. This small, air-filled *tympanic cavity* in the skull is lined by a mucous membrane and situated between the inner ear and the tympanic membrane, communicating through the *eustachian tube* with the pharynx. This tube keeps the air pressure equal on both sides of the tympanic membrane, making the air pressure in the middle ear the same as that of the atmosphere. The pharyngeal orifice of the tube is normally closed but opens during swallowing and yawning or when a high pressure is created in the nasopharynx, as when blowing the nose or making a forced expiration with the nostrils and mouth closed. The tympanic membrane is very sensitive to any difference in pressure on its two surfaces, and during rapid changes in altitude, as in airplane ascents and descents, annoying aural effects may be produced, such as ringing sounds in the ears (tinnitus).

In the middle ear there are three tiny connected bones called the *auditory ossicles* (*ossicle* means little bone), deriving their names from their shape: the *malleus* (hammer), the *incus* (anvil), and the *stapes* (stirrup). These bones are connected by joints, and they bridge the tympanic cavity (middle ear) to transmit sound waves to the inner ear by the mechanical action of the ossicles.

Inner ear. The *inner ear (labyrinth)* begins at the *oval window,* against which the stapes presses, and continues in a labyrinthine *cochlea* (which means spiral or snail-shell shape), which contains three canals that are separated from each other by thin membranes and almost converge at the apex. Two of these canals are bony chambers filled with a *perilymph fluid,* one of which, the *vestibular canal,* is connected to the oval window that leads to the tympanic cavity (middle ear). The second, the *tympanic canal,* is connected to the *round window* opening into the middle ear. The third canal, the *cochlear canal,* a membranous chamber filled with *endolymph,* is situated between the other two canals. The cochlear canal contains the *organ of Corti,* a spiral-shaped organ located on the *basilar membrane* of the canal that is made up of cells with projecting hairs that transmit auditory impulses to the cochlear nerve.

The Mechanism of Hearing

Sound waves enter the external ear and strike the tympanic membrane, causing vibration, which sets into motion the three ossicles, the malleus, the incus, and the stapes, in that order. The stapes is the last to vibrate, and it strikes against the oval window of the vestibular canal, setting into motion the perilymph fluid in the vestibular and tympanic canals of the cochlea. The vibrating perilymph sets into motion the basilar membrane in the cochlear canal, thereby disturbing the endolymph fluid in the membranous area of the cochlea. *Hair cells* of the organ of Corti are stimulated by the movement of the endolymph; and by bending against another membrane (the *tectorial*), the hair cells transmit the impulse to the brain by way of the auditory nerve. The final interpretation of sound is made by the brain.

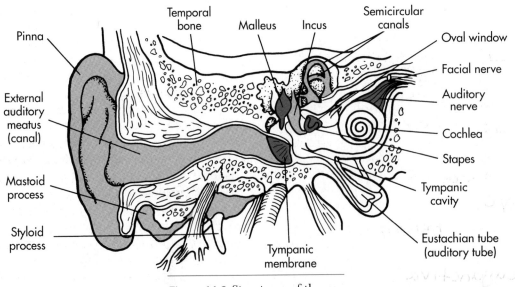

Figure 16.3 Structures of the ear.

The Sense of Equilibrium

In addition to the structures just described, each inner ear has three *semicircular canals* in the labyrinth that lie in planes at right angles to each other, plus a *utricle,* and a *saccule.* These are the structures of equilibrium (see Figure 16.3).

The saccule and utricle are small sacs that are lined with sensitive hairs and contain particles, called *otoliths* (*lith* means stone), that are made up of calcium carbonate. The otoliths press on the hair cells through the pull of gravity and stimulate the initiation of impulses from the hair cells to the brain through their basal sensory nerve fibers. The utricles and saccules, which together are called the *vestibule,* are responsible for the reactions that result from position change and change of *rectilinear* motion (movement in a straight line).

The semicircular canals, which are liquid filled, respond to rotary, or turning, movement. They are positioned at right angles to each other, each corresponding to one of the three spatial planes. Turning the head in any direction stimulates at least one of the canals. Inside each canal are hair cell receptors that bend in response to rotary motion, stimulating nerve fibers that carry impulses to the vestibular branch of the auditory nerve and then to the brain.

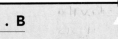

R E V I E W 1 6 . B

Complete the following:

1. The ear has two functions, _hearing_ and _equilibrium_ .

2. The tympanic membrane is also known as the _eardrum_ .

3. The _eustachian tube_ equalizes air pressure on both sides of the tympanic membrane.

4. The inner ear has a labyrinthine cochlea, which contains _3_ canals.

5. The three ossicles are the _malleus_ , _incus_ , and _stapes_ .

6. The external auditory canal is entirely lined by _skin_ .

7. The stapes presses against the _oval window_

8. Hair cells transmit sound stimulation to the brain by way of the _auditory_ nerve.

9. The _Cochlea_ canal lies between the vestibular and tympanic canals.

10. The structures of equilibrium are three _semicircular canals_, plus a _utricle_ and a _saccule_ .

THE SENSE OF SMELL

Smell is one of the most primitive senses. In many animals it is very acute and of paramount importance because it serves to warn the animal of approaching enemies, guides it in its quest for food, and even motivates the sex reflexes. In humans it also serves to warn of danger. Smoke is often smelled before the fire is located; escaping gas from a leaky burner or pipeline can be smelled before a person is overcome or carelessly lights the match that causes an explosion.

The peripheral organ for smell is the *nose* (*naso* and *rhino* refer to nose), with its external parts and nasal cavities. The organ of smell is the *olfactory* (*olfact* refers to smell) *epithelium* of the nose, and odor is perceived through stimulation of its cells. The olfactory receptors are confined to the nasal mucosa over a relatively small area in a narrow niche formed by the *superior nasal concha* (*concha* means shell shaped), the upper part of the *septum* (wall between the two nasal cavities), and the *root* of the nose (Figure 16.4).

The *root* of the nose is the upper, narrow end between the eyes, and the *bridge* of the nose is the part that extends from the root to the *tip (apex).* The *external nares (nostrils)* are the two oval openings separated from one another by the lower part of the *septum,* and the flexible lower portions on each side bordering the nostrils are the *alae* (*ala* is the singular form and means winglike).

The nose is formed by the nasal bones and cartilage. The nasal bones are the *turbinates, superior* (upper), *medial* (middle), and *inferior* (lower) *conchae.* Nasal cartilages are connected to each other and to the bones by fibrous tissue. Just inside the nasal cavities is a lining of skin with a ring of coarse hairs, whose function is to trap dust and foreign particles during inspiration.

The mucous membrane lining the nose is continuous with particular connecting areas, and infections of this membrane are easily spread to them. These con-

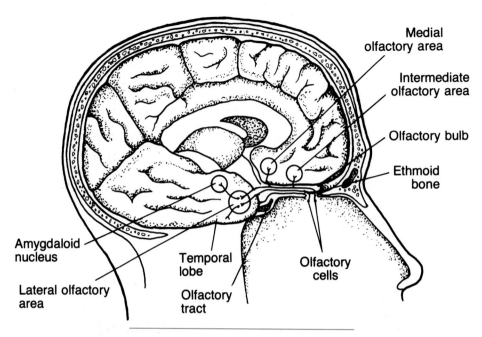

Figure 16.4 Olfactory centers in the brain.

necting areas include the nasopharynx; the eustachian tube (auditory canal); the middle ear cavity; the sphenoidal, ethmoidal, frontal, and maxillary sinuses; and the palatine bones and tear ducts.

The stimulation of the olfactory epithelium is initially transmitted to the *olfactory bulb* and from there continues to the olfactory centers in the brain. Six basic odors have been identified, interacting with each other to produce almost 10,000 odors we can experience: flowery, fruity, spicy, resinous, burned, and putrid. The sense of smell is far more sensitive than the sense of taste, and complements it, as is evident when a respiratory infection blocks the sense of smell, causing food to lose its customary flavors.

THE SENSE OF TASTE

The organs of taste in humans are the *taste buds*, located mainly in the *papillae* (small projections) on the tongue, but a few may be found in the mucous membrane that covers the soft palate, the fauces (opening from the mouth to the pharynx), and the epiglottis.

The sense of taste is limited to four primary, or fundamental, tastes: sweet, sour (acid), salt, and bitter. The various other tastes that we experience are blends of these. For a substance to arouse a sensation of taste, it must be dissolved either in solution or by the saliva, which accounts for the location of the taste buds on a moist surface. Many substances that we think we taste are, in reality, only smelled, and their taste depends upon their odor. For this reason smell is sometimes described as "taste at a distance."

REVIEW 16.C

Complete the following:

1. The five special senses are _Vision_, _hearing_, _smell_, _taste_, and _touch_.

2. The _olfactory epithelium_ of the nose is the organ of smell.

3. Another term for nostrils is _external nares_

4. There are _6_ basic odors.

5. Stimulation of the organ of smell is initially transmitted to the olfactory _bulb_.

6. The organs of taste are located mainly on the _tongue_.

7. The organs of taste are the _taste buds_.

8. There are _4_ fundamental tastes.

9. Taste depends on _odor_.

10. To arouse a sensation of taste a substance must be _dissolved_.

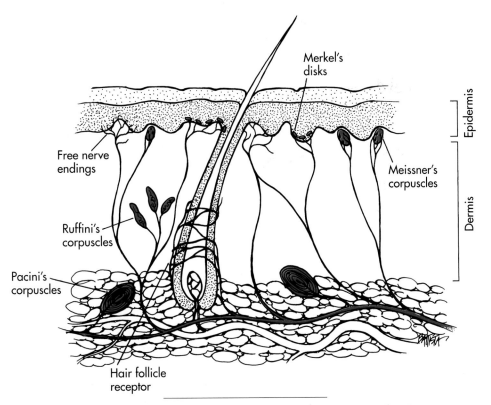

Figure 16.5 Sensory receptors.

TOUCH AND OTHER CUTANEOUS SENSES

The skin is a receptor for the sensations of touch, as well as those of heat, cold, and pain (Chapter 8 and Table 16.1).

Touch (also called light pressure) is experienced as a function of stimulation of *free sensory nerve endings* (*dendrites*) everywhere in the skin but especially around hair follicles. Tactile corpuscles in the epidermis called *Merkel's disks* relay light touch and superficial pressure, and other structures in the corium (layer below the epidermis) called *Meissner's corpuscles* are believed to mediate light pressure sensations. Heavier pressure stimulates the *Pacini's corpuscles,* which are lamellated (layered) bodies of sensory nerve tissue located in the subcutaneous layer.

Thermal sensations of heat and cold are experienced in response to changes of even a few degrees from skin temperature, but the precise mechanisms are not known. Free nerve endings are believed to be the main receptors, along with Ruffini's corpuscles, which are sensory end structures located in the corium. Also considered as mediators of heat and cold are the *capillaries* of the skin (Figure 16.5).

Pain sensations have not been linked to any specific nerve structures but are believed to be transmitted by free sensory nerve endings found just below the surface of the skin.

The skin areas of the body have varying sensitivities to sensation as a function of the distributions of receptors in the differing areas. The most sensitive areas generally are those that are most involved in obtaining information about oneself and the external world, such as the lips and fingers, whereas fewer receptors are found on the back of the hand or the dorsal surfaces generally.

TABLE 16.1 THE SPECIAL SENSES

Sense	Organ	Receptors	Stimulus
sight (vision)	retina of eye	Rods (120 million/eye)* cones (8 million/eye)*	Wavelengths of light
hearing (audition)	basilar membrane of cochlea (inner ear)	Hair cells of the organ of Corti	Sound vibrations
balance (equilibrium)	utricle, saccule, and semicircular canals of inner ear	Hair cells	Mechanical and fluid pressure
smell (olfaction)	mucous membranes of upper nasal cavity	Olfactory epithelium hair cells (60 million)	Chemical gas
taste (gustation)	surface of tongue	Taste buds on papillae (10,000)	Dissolved chemicals
touch pressure	layers of skin	Free nerve endings, Meissner's corpuscles, Pacini's corpuscles Merkel's disks	Mechanical pressure
pain		Free nerve endings	High intensity of stimuli
warmth, cold		Free nerve endings, Ruffini's corpuscles, skin capillaries	Thermal energy

*/means per (each).

REVIEW 16.D

Complete the following:

1. The skin is a receptor for __touch__ , __heat__ , __cold__ , and __pain__ .

2. Stimulation of free sensory nerve endings produces the sense of __touch / pain__ .

3. The most sensitive skin areas are the __lips__ and __fingers__ .

4. The least sensitive skin areas are the __dorsal__ surfaces.

5. Pacini's corpuscles are stimulated by __heavy / heavier__ pressure.

RELATED TERMS **THE SPECIAL SENSES** THE SOURCES OF INFORMATION

SENSE OF VISION

Anatomy

accommodation process by which the lens and pupil adjust to focus light rays on the retina.

aqueous chamber space within the eye that encloses the aqueous humor, divided by the iris into anterior and posterior chambers.

aqueous humor watery fluid within the aqueous chamber between the cornea and vitreous humor.

blepharon eyelid (also called *palpebra*).

canal of Schlemm exit duct for aqueous humor, located in the anterior cavity, which keeps intraocular pressure constant under normal conditions.

canthus (kan'thus) angle at either end of the slit between the eyelids, the outer, temporal canthus, and the inner, nasal canthus (plural—*canthi*).

choroid (ko'roid) coat, located between the sclera and the retina, with cells filled with melanin, whose posterior part is a thin membrane with a rich vascular layer.

cilia eyelashes.

ciliary body (sil'e-er"e) thickened extension of the choroid from the visual layer to the iris, consisting of the ciliary processes and muscles, assisting in accommodation, and secreting aqueous humor.

cones specialized neuroepithelial cells of the retina that serve as the color and fine-detail receptors of vision.

conjunctiva (kon"junk-ti'vah) membrane that lines the eyelid and covers the eyeball.

cornea (kor'ne-ah) transparent structure that forms the anterior part of the external tunic of the eye.

emmetropia (em"e-tro'pe-ah) perfect vision (*emmetros* means in proper measure).

extrinsic muscles six slender muscles attaching the outside of the eyeball to the bones of the orbit, acting together to move the eyeballs.

fovea (fo've-ah) depressed area in the center of the macula of the retina, with no rods and the greatest concentration of cones, producing the area of clearest vision.

intraocular pressure pressure maintained by the balance between secretion and removal of aqueous humor in the anterior chamber.

iris most anterior portion of the vascular layer of the eye, a doughnut-shaped, pigmented ring of muscles that regulates the size of the pupil.

lacrimal glands organs of secretion of tears, which cleanse and lubricate the conjunctiva.

lens transparent part of the eye, directly behind the iris, that focuses light rays on the retina (also called *crystalline lens*).

levator palpebrae muscles muscles that raise upper lid.

macula yellow spot near the center of the back of the retina with a central depression, the fovea (also called *macula lutea*).

optic term referring to the eye.

optic chiasma brain structure receiving transmissions of the optic nerves.

orb eyeball.

orbit bony socket that contains the eye.

palpebra eyelids.

pupil central hole or opening in the iris.

refracting media transparent tissues and fluids in the eye through which light passes, and by which it is refracted (bent) and brought to focus.

retina innermost, nervous tissue or sensory layer, of the three coats of the eyeball; contains the rods and cones.

rods highly specialized, cylindric, neuroepithelial cells of the retina, that react to light but not color, and are most sensitive to low light intensity.

sclera (skle'rah) tough, white, supporting tunic of the eyeball.

supercilia eyebrows.

suspensory ligament ligament attaching the lens to the ciliary body.

uvea term used to include the iris, ciliary body, and choroid.

vitelliform resembling the yoke of an egg.

vitreous humor semigelatinous transparent substance that fills the membrane-enclosed space between the lens and the retina.

Pathologic Conditions

Inflammations and infections of the eye

acute contagious conjunctivitis purulent infection of the conjunctiva (also called *pinkeye*).

blepharitis inflammation of the eyelid.

chorioretinitis (ko"re-o-ret"i-ni'tis) inflammation of the choroid and retina (also called *retinochoroiditis*).

choroiditis inflammation of the choroid.

conjunctivitis inflammation of the conjunctiva.

dacryoadenitis (dak"re-o-ad"e-ni'tis) inflammation of the lacrimal gland (also called *dacryadenitis*).

dacryocystitis inflammation of the lacrimal sac.

episcleritis (ep"i-skle-ri'tis) inflammation of the tissue of the sclera.

hordeolum (hor-de'o-lum) inflammation of an eyelid sebaceous gland, commonly called a sty.

iridocyclitis (ir"i-do-si-kli'tis) inflammation of the iris and ciliary body.

iridocyclochoroiditis (ir"i-do-si"klo-ko"roid-i'tis) inflammation of the iris, the ciliary body, and the choroid coat.

iridokeratitis (ir"i-do-ker"ah-ti'tis) inflammation of the cornea and iris (also called *keratoiritis*).

iritis inflammation of the iris.

keratitis inflammation of the cornea.

keratoconjunctivitis (ker"ah-to-kon-junk"ti-vi'tis) inflammation of the cornea and conjunctiva.

keratoiridocyclitis (ker"ah-to-ir"i-do-sik-li'tis) inflammation of the cornea, iris, and ciliary body.

ophthalmitis inflammation of the deeper structures of the eye (also called *ophthalmia*).

optic neuritis inflammation of the optic nerve.

panophthalmitis inflammation of all structures of the eye.

retinitis inflammation of the retina.

scleritis inflammation of the sclera.

sclerochoroiditis inflammation of the sclera and choroid.

scleroconjunctivitis inflammation of the sclera and conjunctiva.

sclerokeratitis inflammation of the sclera and cornea.

trachoma chronic, granulating, contagious infection of the conjunctiva, caused by the bacterium *Chlamydia.*

uveitis inflammation of the uvea, which includes the iris, ciliary body, and choroid.

Hereditary, congenital, and developmental disorders of the eye

achromatopsia (ah-kro"mah-top'se-ah) total color-blindness (also called *achromatopia*).

albinism absence of pigment in the eye.

aniridia (an"i-rid'e-ah) absence of the iris.

anophthalmos (an"of-thal'mos) absence of, or rudimentary development of, one or both eyes (also called *anophthalmia*).

congenital cataract opacity of lens originating before birth.

corectopia (kor-ek-to'pe-ah) abnormal placement of the pupil (*core* refers to the pupil of the eye).

cyclopia (si-klo'pe-ah) developmental anomaly characterized by a single orbit.

deuteranomaly partial color-blindness, involving subnormal perception of green because of a deficiency of green-sensitive cones.

deuteranopia green color-blindness.

dichromatopsia (di"kro-mah-top'se-ah) partial color blindness, with ability to distinguish only two of the primary colors (red, blue, yellow, green).

ectopia of lens misplacement of the lens.

ectropion uveae eversion or outward turning of the pupillary margin of the eye (also called *iridectropium*).

embryotoxon congenital opacity at the margin of the cornea (*toxon* means a bow or anything arched).

megalocornea developmental anomaly characterized by a large cornea.

megalophthalmos abnormally large size of the eyes.

microcornea abnormally small cornea.

microphakia abnormally small lens.

microphthalmos abnormally small eyes.

polycoria existence of more than one pupil in an eye.

protanomaly (pro"tah-nom"ah-le) form of color blindness, with an imperfect perception of red, caused by deficiency of red-sensitive cones (also called *protanomalopsia*).

protanopia red color blindness, with absence of red-sensitive cones.

retinitis pigmentosa (pig"men-to'sah) group of retinal diseases that may be inherited, with retinal atrophy, weakening of the retinal vascular system, clumping of pigment, and narrowing of the visual field.

tritanomaly partial color blindness, with a deficiency of blue-sensitive pigment in the cones.

tritanopia (tri"tah-no'pe-ah) form of color blindness, with an absence of blue-sensitive pigment in the cones, sometimes associated with drug effects, retinal detachment, or nervous system diseases (also called *tritanopsia*).

Other abnormal conditions of the eye

adhesions of iris fibrous bands or strictures in the iris or adhering the iris to other eye structures.

age-related macular degeneration (AMD) two types of degeneration of the retinal macula appearing in later life: the most common form, a dry type, causing visual dimming or distortion; and a much less common wet, or neovascular, type associated with abnormal growth of new blood vessels that leak into the macula, damaging the retina.

altered pupillary reflexes hyper- (over), or hypo- (under) contraction of the pupil on exposure to light.

amblyopia (am″ble-o′pe-ah) dimness of vision (*ambly* means dimness).

ametropia (am″e-tro′pe-ah) defect in the refractive powers of the eye in which images are not brought into proper focus on the retina (*ametro* means disproportionate).

aniseikonia (an″i-si-ko′ne-ah) image seen by one eye differs in size and shape from that seen by the other eye (*anis* means unequal; *eikon* means image).

anisopia (an″i-so′pe-ah) inequality of vision in the two eyes.

anterior ischemic optic neuropathy (AION) sudden vision loss resulting from reduced blood supply to the optic nerve.

aphakia (ah-fa′ke-ah) absence of lens, usually used to describe the absence of lens after cataract surgery; may also be a congenital anomaly.

arcus senilis (ar-kus se-nil′is) white or gray ring around the cornea, caused by lipoid degeneration of the corneal tissue in the aged (*senilis* refers to old age).

astigmatism defective curvature of the refractive surfaces of the eye, causing light rays to spread over a more or less diffuse area and not sharply focus on the retina (*stigma* means point).

blepharospasm spasm of the eyelid or excessive winking of the eyes.

blindness lack or loss of sight, with a variety of causes and a number of types:

aknephascopia (ak″nef-ah-sko′pe-ah reduced vision with poor lighting such as twilight (also called *twilight blindness—knepha* refers to twilight).

cortical blindness caused by lesion of cortical visual center.

eclipse (solar) blindness caused by viewing a partial eclipse of the sun, resulting in amblyopia as a result of retinal thermal lesion.

hemeralopia day blindness or defective vision in bright light.

niphablepsia dimness of vision, usually temporary, caused by glare of the sun upon the snow (also called *snow blindness—nipha* means snow)

nyctalopia night blindness.

cataract opacity of the crystalline lens or its capsule, with a number of types and varying causes.

corneal opacity opacity of the cornea.

corneal ulcer lesion of the cornea.

diabetic retinopathy (ret″i-nop′ah-the) noninflammatory degeneration of the retina, characterized by retinal ischemia, hemorrhages, and exudation, which tends to develop in persons who have had diabetes for a long period of time.

diplopia double vision (*diplo* means double).

enophthalmos (en-of-thal′mos) abnormal retraction of the eye into the orbit.

floaters small bits formed of clumps of vitreous gel, that appear to float in the visual field.

glaucoma (glaw-ko′mah) disease characterized by excessive intraocular pressure, with hardness of the eye, atrophy of the retina, and possible progression to blindness.

hypermetropia farsightedness, caused by insufficient refracting power to focus parallel rays on the retina (also called *hyperopia*).

hypertensive retinopathy retinal degeneration caused by hypertension.

hypopyon (hi-po′pe-on) accumulation of pus in the anterior chamber of the eye.

lenticular opacity opacity in the lens.

maculopathy (mak-u-lah′path-ee) degeneration of the retinal macula.

myopia nearsightedness, caused by refraction error which focuses parallel rays in front of the retina.

nystagmus (nis-tag′mus) involuntary, rapid, horizontal, vertical, rotary, or mixed movements of the eyeball (*nys* means nod).

ophthalmoplegia paralysis of eye muscles.

pannus abnormal membrane-like corneal vascularization (*pannus* means cloth).

presbyopia farsightedness resulting from normal aging changes in the lens (also called *hyperopia*).

ptosis drooping or falling of the eyelid.

retinal detachment separation of the retina from the choroid causing loss of vision; due to abscesses or hemorrhages in the vitreous body, trauma, complications of intraocular surgery, inflammation or tumors of the choroid, and passage of vitreous and/or aqueous humor through a hole in the retina.

Stargardt's disease juvenile type of macular degeneration.

Stellwag's sign infrequent or incomplete blinking of the eyelid, a sign of Graves' disease.

strabismus (strah-biz′mus) deviation of the eye, with various forms called *tropias* (meaning turning).

    esotropia turning inward (also called *convergent strabismus* or crossed eyes).

    exotropia turning outward (also called *wall-eye*).

    hypertropia upward deviation of one eye.

    hypotropia downward deviation of one eye.

synechia (si-nek′e-ah) adhesion of one part of the eye to another, especially iris to cornea or lens (*synechia* means continuity).

von Graefe's sign (gra′fez) lid lag, a sign of Graves' disease.

xerophthalmus (ze″rof-thal′mus) abnormally dry cornea and conjunctiva caused by vitamin A deficiency (also called *xerophthalmia*).

Oncology of the eye*

Other tumors occur in the structure of the eye, as they do in other parts of the body, but only those peculiar to the eye are listed here.

angiomatosis retinae condition of multiple and bilateral hemangiomas of the retina, which may be associated with hemangiomas of the cerebellum, fourth ventricle, and spinal cord.

retinoblastoma* (ret″i-no-blas-to′mah) malignant tumor that arises from retinal germ cells, usually occurring in children younger than 3 years.

Surgery

blepharectomy (blef′ah-rek′to-me) excision or removal of all or part of an eyelid.

blepharoplasty (blef′ah-ro-plas″te) plastic repair of an eyelid.

blepharorrhaphy suturing together of the eyelid margins (also called *tarsorrhaphy*).

blepharosphincterectomy (blef′ah-ro-sfingk″ter-ek′to-me) excision of some fibers of the eyelid muscle to relieve pressure on the cornea.

blepharotomy incision of eyelid (also called *tarsotomy*).

canthectomy surgical removal of a canthus.

canthoplasty (kan′tho-plas″te) plastic surgery of the palpebral fissure, especially the section of a canthus to lengthen the fissure, and surgical restoration of a defective canthus (also called *cantholysis*).

canthotomy incision of a canthus.

capsulectomy excision of the capsule of the crystalline lens.

capsulotomy incision of the capsule of the crystalline lens.

cataract implant procedure for the implantation of a permanent artificial lens after cataract removal.

conjunctivoplasty plastic repair of the conjunctiva.

corectomedialysis (ko-rek″to-me″di-al′i-sis) formation of an artificial pupil by detachment of the iris from the ciliary body (also called *coretomedialysis* and *iridodialysis*).

coreoplasty plastic repair of the pupil.

cyclodialysis (si″klo-di-al′i-sis) procedure for glaucoma, to form a communication between the anterior chamber of the eye and the suprachoroidal space.

cyclodiathermy (si″klo-di′ah-ther″me) treatment of a portion of the ciliary body by diathermy.

dacryoadenectomy (dak″re-o-ad″e-nek′to-me) excision of a tear gland.

dacryocystectomy excision of a lacrimal (tear) sac.

dacryocystorhinostomy (dak″re-o-sis″to-ri-nos′to-me) anastamosis of the lacrimal sac to the nasal mucosa, through the lacrimal bone.

dacryocystosyringotomy (dak″re-o-sis″to-sir″in-got′o-me) incision of the lacrimal sac and duct.

dacryocystotomy incision of the lacrimal gland or duct (also called *lacrimotomy*).

enucleation excision of the eyeball.

evisceration excision of the contents of eyeball.

goniotomy (gon″ne-ot′o-me) surgical procedure in congenital glaucoma consisting of opening the canal of Schlemm at the angle of the anterior chamber (*gonio* means angle).

intrastromal corneal ring (ICR) small plastic ring implanted in the cornea to correct myopia.

---

* Indicates a malignant condition.

iridectomy excision of part of the iris.

iridencleisis (ir″i-den-kli′sis) procedure used to reduce intraocular pressure, forming a permanent drain for the aqueous humor by strangulation of a slip of the iris in a corneal incision.

iridocyclectomy (ir″i-do-si-klek′to-me) removal of a portion of the iris and the ciliary body.

iridocystectomy (ir″i-do-sis-tek′to-me) plastic surgery on the iris, to establish an artificial pupil.

iridomesodialysis (ir″i-do-me″so-di-al′i-sis) loosening of adhesions around the inner edge of the iris (also called *iridomedialysis*).

iridosclerotomy (ir″i-do-skle-rot′o-me) incision of sclera and edge of iris in treatment of glaucoma.

iridotasis (ir″i-dot′ah-sis) stretching the iris in treatment of glaucoma.

iridotomy formation of artificial pupil by cutting the iris (also called *iritomy*).

iritoectomy (i″ri-to-ek′to-me) removal of a portion of the iris.

keratectomy excision of a portion of the cornea.

keratocentesis puncture of cornea for aspiration of aqueous humor.

keratoplasty corneal transplant or repair of the cornea.

keratotomy incision of the cornea.

lacromotomy incision of the lacrimal gland or duct.

laser surgery use of an instrument that concentrates light energy into a narrow beam, so that treatment of tissue can be done so quickly that the surrounding areas are not affected; used within the eyeball to repair the retina, and also in cataract and glaucoma surgery.

orbitotomy incision of the orbit.

peritectomy excision of a ring of conjunctiva around the cornea, followed by cauterization of the trench made—an operation for pannus (an abnormal membranelike vascularization of the cornea).

photorefractive keratotomy (PRK) use of an excimer laser pulsing into the cornea to correct myopia.

radial keratotomy (RK) microscopic radial incisions on the corneal surface to flatten the cornea to correct myopia.

sclerectomy excision of part of the sclera (also called *scleroticectomy*).

scleriritomy incision of sclera and iris in anterior staphyloma (defect in the eye inside the cornea, with protrusion of the cornea or sclera).

scleroplasty repair of the sclera.

sclerostomy creation of an opening through the sclera for the relief of glaucoma.

sclerotomy incision of the sclera.

vitrectomy repair of a macular hole by peeling away scar tissue and replacing the vitreous body with a bubble of gas, which closes the hole.

Vision Tests

color perception tests designed to reveal defects in color vision by means of standard colors presented to the individual, including:

Bodal's test colored blocks.

Cohn's test colored embroidery.

Holmgren's test skeins of colored yarn.

Mauthner's test bottles of colored liquid.

Nagel's test printed concentric colored circles.

pseudoisochromatic test series of printed plates composed of round dots of varied standard colors and sizes, which are arranged to be read as numbers and letters in normal color perception, which, with subsequent revisions, is the most widely used and best standardized test available (used by the *Ishihara* and *A.O. Hardy-Rand-Rittler* tests).

fluorescent eye stain test to detect abnormalities or injuries in the cornea, and to aid in the fitting of contact lenses.

Hering's test test of binocular vision.

magnetic resonance imaging (MRI) noninvasive method of scanning the eye by use of an electromagnetic field and high-frequency radio waves, which provides visual images on a computer screen, and magnetic tape recordings, used to detect tissue changes and eye cancers (also called *nuclear magnetic resonance—NMR*).

ophthalmodiaphanoscope (of-thal″mo-di-ah-fan′o-skop) instrument for viewing the interior of the eye by transmitted light.

ophthalmodynamometer (of-thal″mo-di″nah-mom′e-ter) instrument for measuring retinal arterial pressure.

ophthalmoleukoscope (of-thal″mo-lu′ko-skop) instrument that uses polarized light to test color perception.

ophthalmoscope (of-thal″mo-skop) instrument that examines the interior of the eye using a light source, a perforated mirror, and a system of lenses.

opthalmotonometer (of-thal"mo-to-nom'e-ter) instrument used to measure intraocular tension or pressure (also called *tonometer*).

refraction determination of type and degree of refractive deviations in the eye structures along with their correction by external lenses.

retinoscopy detection of refractive errors by noting the movement of light shined directly on the retina (also called *shadow test*).

scanning laser ophthalmoscope laser device that produces a picture to diagnose retinal sections that are functioning abnormally.

Snellen eye chart standardized visual acuity measure using block letters in successive lines of decreasing size to be read at a set distance; the most commonly used eye chart for gross screening.

sonogram use of ultrasound to detect diseases of the eye.

visual field test measure of the extent of retinal area within which visual stimuli can be perceived.

SENSE OF HEARING

Anatomy

auricle external projecting part of the ear (also called *pinna*).

auris term that refers to the ear.

cerumen earwax.

cochlea (kok'le-ah) snail-shaped canal in the inner ear.

endolymph fluid that fills the semicircular canals and the membranous labyrinth of the ear.

eustachian tube (u-sta'she-an) tube that leads from the ear to the throat (also called *auditory tube*).

incus anvil-shaped bone in the middle ear (also called *anvil*).

labyrinth (lab'i-rinth) inner ear, consisting of numerous canals and membranes and the organ of Corti, the organ of hearing.

malleus hammer-shaped bone in the middle ear (also called *hammer*).

meatus opening to the ear; both internal and external.

middle ear small, air-filled tympanic cavity in the skull, between the labyrinth and tympanic membrane.

organ of Corti spiral organ of hearing located on the basilar membrane of the cochlear canal.

ossicles little bones of the middle ear, including malleus, incus, and stapes.

otolith stone in the utricle and saccule of the inner ear (*lith* means stone).

oval window opening between the middle ear and the inner ear.

perilymph fluid that fills some chambers of the inner ear.

saccule small hair-lined sac of the inner ear, which, together with the utricle and semicircular canals, is the organ for equilibrium.

semicircular canals three membranous canals (lateral, superior, and posterior) contained within the bony semicircular structures of the labyrinth, involved with equilibrium.

stapes (sta'pez) stirrup-shaped bone in the middle ear (also called *stirrup*).

tympanic membrane membrane *(eardrum)* that separates the middle ear from the external ear, and transmits vibrations to ossicles.

utricle (u'tre-k'l) small hair-lined sac of the inner ear that is concerned with equilibrium.

Pathologic Conditions

Inflammations and infections of the ear

eustachitis (u"sta-ki'tis) inflammation of the eustachian tube.

labyrinthitis inflammation of the inner ear, or labyrinth.

mastoiditis inflammation of the mastoid process behind the ear.

myringitis inflammation of the eardrum.

otitis media, externa, and interna inflammation of the middle ear (also called *tympanitis*), external ear, and inner ear, respectively.

panotitis inflammation of all parts of the ear.

tympanomastoiditis inflammation of the eardrum and mastoid.

Congenital and developmental disorders of the ear

deformity of auricle a variety of abnormal pinna formations, including pointed ear, dog ear, and ridged ear.

macrotia excessively large ears.

microtia excessively small ears.

otosclerosis hereditary disorder, with formation of spongy bone tissue around the stapes and oval window, preventing transmission of vibration to the inner ear, resulting in progressive deafness.

polyotia presence of more than one ear on a side of the head.

Other abnormal conditions and descriptive terms of the ear

deafness complete or partial loss of the sense of hearing, of many different types, including:

central deafness disease or defect in the auditory pathways of the brainstem or cerebral hemispheres.

conductive deafness defective sound-conducting apparatus in the auditory meatus, eardrum, or ossicles.

cortical deafness caused by a lesion of the cerebral cortex.

labyrinthine deafness disease or defect of the labyrinth.

sensorineural deafness caused by lesion or dysfunction of the nerve tracts of the cochlea and nerve centers.

diplacusis (dip″lah-ku′sis) hearing of one sound as two, caused by a difference in perception between the two ears, usually related to cochlear pathology.

Meniere's syndrome condition in which there is dizziness, nausea, tinnitus, and progressive deafness, caused by nonsuppurative disease of the labyrinth (also called *labyrinthine syndrome*).

otalgia earache (also called *otodynia*).

otoneuralgia neuralgia of the ear.

otopyorrhea (o″to-pi″o-re′ah) discharge of pus from the ear.

otorrhagia (ot″to-ra′je-ah) hemorrhage from the ear.

otorrhea (o″to-re′ah) discharge from the ear.

presbycusis progressive late-life hearing loss caused by inner ear and/or nerve deterioration.

tinnitus (ti-ni′tus) ringing in the ears.

tympanophonia (tim″pah-no-fo′ne-ah) condition of increased resonance in which the voice sounds unnatural to oneself, found in diseases of the middle ear or nasal fossae (also called *autophony*).

tympanosclerosis (tim″pah-no-skle-ro′sis) hardening of tympanic membrane.

vertigo dizziness.

Oncology of the ear

Other tumors occur in the structures of the ear, as they do in other parts of the body, but only one peculiar to the ear is given here.

acoustic neuroma usually arising from the acoustic nerve, this tumor grows within the internal auditory meatus, encroaching upon the brainstem, and may adhere to and displace the facial nerve, and involve the trigeminal nerve.

Surgical Procedures

fenestration (fen″es-tra′shun) formation of an opening into the labyrinth of the ear for the restoration of hearing in cases of otosclerosis.

incudectomy removal of the incus.

labyrinthectomy (lab″i-rin-thek′to-me) excision of the labyrinth of the ear.

labyrinthotomy (lab″i-rin-thot′o-me) incision into the labyrinth.

malleotomy (mal″e-ot′o-me) dividing the malleus in cases of ankylosis of the ossicles of the middle ear.

myringectomy excision of the tympanic membrane (also called *myringodectomy*).

myringoplasty plastic repair of the eardrum.

myringotomy incision of the tympanic membrane.

ossiculectomy (os″i-ku-lek′to-me) excision of ossicles, or small bones of the ear, incus, malleus, and stapes.

ossiculotomy incision of the small bones of the ear.

stapedectomy (sta″pe-dek′to-me) excision of the stapes.

tympanectomy (tim″pan-ek-to-me) excision of the tympanic membrane.

tympanolabyrinthopexy (tim″pah-no-lab″i-rin′tho-pek″se) surgical procedure to cure progressive deafness caused by otosclerosis.

tympanosympathectomy (tim″pah-no-sim″pah-thek′to-me) excising of the tympanic plexus for the relief of tinnitus.

tympanotomy surgical puncture of the tympanic membrane.

Hearing Tests

audiometer instrument for measuring hearing acuity by testing the thresholds for electrically or electronically generated pure tones of varying frequency and amplitude.

audiometry measurement of hearing by audiometer.

Bekesy audiometry (bay-kay-se) semiautomatic method in which the examinee responds by signal (button press) to indicate perception of monaural tones that cover the audiometric scale.

caloric test test of the functioning of the inner ear by instilling hot or ice water into the ear and watching the eye movements, which normally move toward the hot and away from the cold, used for patients with ear disease, trauma, or symptoms of syncope or vertigo.

computerized tomography (CT) imaging device using x-rays at multiple angles through specific sections, analyzed by computer to provide a total picture of the part being examined (also called *computerized axial tomography—CAT*).

conduction deafness tests tests designed to determine the location of defect in the sound-conducting apparatus, including:

bone conduction test a vibrating tuning fork handle is placed against the skull to determine middle ear conduction loss.

Kabaschnik's test transfer of below-threshold vibration of a tuning fork to the nail of the examiner's finger, which closes the external auditory meatus, in which the normal ear will detect sound.

Rinne test compares air and bone conduction by alternate placement of a vibrating tuning fork on the mastoid process and just outside the external auditory meatus.

Schwabach test comparison of bone conduction efficiency of examinee with that of the examiner.

Weber's test bone conduction test placing vibrating tuning fork on the forehead or vertex midline and noting sound perception on right, left, or midline.

electrocochleography test that measures the electrical current generated in the inner ear by sound stimulation.

electrodermal audiometry the use of a mild electric shock to condition the patient to a pure tone, which then elicits an electrodermal response to measure hearing threshold.

magnetic resonance imaging (MRI) non-invasive method of scanning the tissues of the ear by means of an electromagnetic field and high frequency radio waves, which provide visual images on a computer screen, and magnetic tape recordings, to detect and locate tumors (also called *nuclear magnetic resonance—NMR*).

SENSE OF SMELL

Anatomy

concha (kong'kah) shell-shaped turbinate bones of the nose.

external nares nostrils.

olfactory center center for smell located in the brain.

olfactory epithelium organ of odor reception located in a small area in the nasal mucosa.

septum wall between the two nasal cavities.

vomeronasal organs minute pits located just inside the nostrils, containing nerve cells that are directly connected to the olfactory bulb that are sensitive to pheremones (sex chemicals).

Pathologic Conditions and Associated Terms

anosmia absence of the sense of smell.

dysosmia (dis-oz'me-ah) defect or impairment of the sense of smell.

hyperosmia abnormally marked sensitivity to odors (also called *hyperosphresia*).

hyposmia (hi-poz'me-ah) impairment or defect of the sense of smell.

osmesis (oz-me'sis) act of smelling.

osmesthesia (oz"mes-the'ze-ah) olfactory sensibility involving inability to perceive and distinguish odors.

osmodysphoria (oz"mo-dis-fo're-ah) abnormal dislike of certain odors.

Laboratory Test

Proetz test test for acuity of smell, using different concentrations of substances with recognizable odors to the lowest concentration at which recognition occurs, which is called the *olfactory coefficient* or *minimal identifiable odor*.

SENSE OF TASTE

Anatomy

papillae tiny projections on the mucous membrane of the tongue that contain the taste buds.

primary tastes the four fundamental tastes are sweet, sour, salt, and bitter.

taste buds organs of taste located mainly on the tongue.

Pathologic Conditions and Associated Terms

ageusia (ah-gu'ze-ah) lack or impairment of the sense of taste (also called *ageustia; geusia* refers to taste).

dysgeusia (dis-gu'ze-ah) abnormal or perverted sense of taste (also called *parageusia*).

hypergeusia (hi"per-gus"e-ah) excessive or abnormal acuteness of the sense of taste (also called *oxygeusia*).

hypogeusia (hi"po-gus"e-ah) impairment of the sense of taste.

TOUCH AND OTHER CUTANEOUS SENSES

esthesiometer (es-the"ze-om'e-ter) instrument for measuring or mapping tactile and other cutaneous sensitivity, using both a fixed and a movable point of touch to determine how closely the points may come before they are perceived as a single stimulus, called two-point discrimination (also called *tactometer*).

free nerve ending sensory dendritic nerve endings located close to the surface of the skin and around hair follicles.

Meissner's (tactile) corpuscle small, oval body in the corium (layer of skin below the epidermis) with interlaced sensory fibrils and epitheloid cells believed to be receptors for light touch, along with free nerve endings.

Merkel's (tactile) disks flattened, domelike expansions of nerve endings in the epidermis, believed to be receptors for light touch and superficial pressure.

Pacini's corpuscle oval sensory body located deep in the subcutaneous layer, which appears to be the receptor for heavy pressure (also called *lamellated corpuscle*).

Ruffini's corpuscle oval sensory end structure in the corium that is believed to be a receptor for warmth, which also seems to be a function of free nerve endings and capillary responses.

EXERCISES THE SPECIAL SENSES THE SOURCES OF INFORMATION

Exercise 16.1   *Complete the following:*

1. The peripheral organ for smell is the ____nose____ .
2. The upper narrow end of the nose between the eyes is called the ____root____ .
3. The structures that constitute the essential part of the eye are the ___eyeball___ and the ___optic nerve___ .
4. The movement of opening the eye is a function of the ____upper____ eyelid.
5. The anterior, transparent portion of the fibrous coat of the eyeball, through which light enters the eye, is the ____cornea____ .
6. The part between the sclera and retina whose posterior part is a thin membrane with a rich vascular layer is the ____choroid____ .
7. The innermost of the three coats of the eyeball, constituting the nervous layer on which light rays are focused, is the ____retina____ .
8. The divisions of the ear are the ____external____ , ____middle____ , and ____inner____ .
9. The malleus, incus, and stapes perform the important function of ___transmission of sound waves to inner ear___ .
10. The structures of equilibrium are the ___semicircular canals___ , ___utricle___ , and ___saccule___ .

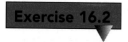**Exercise 16.2**   *Using the list of terms below, identify each part in Figure 16.6 by writing the name in the corresponding blank.*

Vitreous chamber

Conjunctiva

Lens

Retina

Iris

Sclera

Aqueous chamber

Optic nerve

Cornea

Ciliary processes

Choroid

Pupil

Ciliary muscle

Suspensory ligament

1. _Vitreous chamber_

2. _Choroid_

3. _sclera_

4. _optic nerve_

5. _retina_

6. _Ciliary muscle_

7. _Ciliary process_

8. _Cornea_

9. _lens_

10. _pupil_

11. _aqueous chamber_

12. _iris_

13. _conjunctiva_

14. _Suspensory ligament_

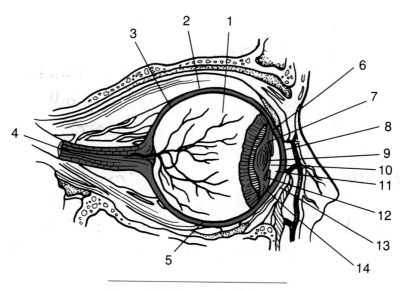

Figure 16.6 Structures of the eye.

Exercise 16.3 *Using the list of terms below, identify each part in Figure 16.7 by writing the name in the corresponding blank.*

Temporal bone

Tympanic cavity

Auditory nerve

Pinna

Cochlea

Incus

Mastoid process

Eustachian tube

Tympanic membrane

External auditory meatus or canal

Malleus

Stapes

Semicircular canals

Styloid process

1. _pinna_
2. _external auditory meatus or canal_
3. _mastoid process_
4. _temporal bone_
5. _malleus_
6. _incus_
7. _semicircular canals_
8. _auditory nerve_
9. _cochlea_
10. _stapes_
11. _tympanic cavity_
12. _eustachian tube_
13. _tympanic membrane_
14. _styloid process_

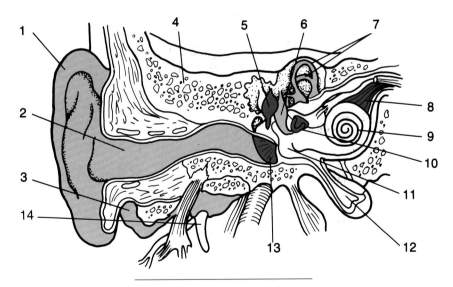

Figure 16.7 Structures of the ear.

Exercise 16.4   *Matching*

___H___   1. the depressed area in the center of the back of the retina; the area of clearest vision.

___B___   2. angles at the ends of the slits between the eyelids.

___E___   3. specialized outer ends of the visual cells in the retina that are adapted to bright light, acute vision, and color perception.

___C___   4. special cylindrical neuroepithelial cells in the retina, highly sensitive to low light.

___G___   5. the partition separating the external nares.

___J___   6. special organ of hearing located on basilar membrane of the cochlea.

___I___   7. the projecting posterior part of the ear that lies outside the head.

___D___   8. structures for equilibrium in the labyrinth.

___A___   9. structure leading from the ear to the throat.

___F___   10. structure that separates the middle ear from the external ear.

A. eustachian tube
B. canthi
C. rods
D. semicircular canals
E. cones
F. tympanic membrane
G. septum
H. fovea
I. pinna
J. organ of Corti

Exercise 16.5   *In the blank following each pair of words, indicate whether their meaning is the same or different.*

1. inner ear
   labyrinth   ___Same___

2. auricle
   external nares   ___different___

3. tympanic membrane
   eardrum   ___Same___

4. eyelid
   palpebra   ___Same___

5. earwax
   cerumen   ___Same___

Give the meaning of the components of the following words and then define the word as a whole. Suffixes meaning pertaining to or state or condition, shown following a slash mark (/), are not to be defined separately. Before reaching for your medical dictionary, check the Related Terms list in this chapter.

1. Blepharitis:

   blephar _eyelid_

   itis _inflammation_

   _____

2. Diplopia:

   Dipl _double_

   op/ia _vision_

   _____

3. Nyctalopia:

   nyct _night_

   al _blind_

   op/ia _vision_

   _____

4. Retinoblastoma:

   retino _retina_

   blast _germ cell_

   oma _tumor_

   _____

5. Dacryoadenectomy:

   dacryo _tear_

   aden _gland_

   ectomy _removal_

   _____

6. Eustachitis:

   eustach _eustachian tube_

   itis _inflammation_

   _____

7. Myringitis:

   myring _eardrum_

   itis _inflammation_

   _____

8. Tympanomastoiditis:

   tympano _tympanic membrane_

mastoid _mastoid_

itis _inflammation_

9. Xerophthalmus:

   xer _dry_

   ophthalm/us _eye_

   _____

10. Otalgia:

    ot _ear_

    algia _pain_

    _____

11. Dacryocystitis:

    dacryo _tear_

    cyst _sac_

    itis _inflammation_

    _____

12. Ageusia:

    a _not_

    geus/ia _taste_

    _____

13. Otorrhea:

    oto _ear_

    rrhea _discharge_

    _____

14. Optic neuritis:

    op/tic _eye_

    neur _nerve_

    itis _inflammation_

    _____

15. Retinitis:

    retin _retina_

    itis _inflammation_

CROSSWORD PUZZLE

The completed crossword grid contains the following answers:

Across: 1. IRIS, 6. CONJUNCTIVA, 7. TOUCH, 9. DENDRITES, 12. STAPES, 14. VESTIBULE, 17. LACRIMAL, 18. NOSE, 20. EARDRUM, 22. RODS, 24. OLFACTORY, 27. INCUS, 28. SEPTUM, 29. EYE, 30. TASTE

Down: 2. RETINA, 3. FOUR, 4. SUPERCILIA, 5. CILIA, 8. OTIS, 10. MALLEUS, 11. VISION, 13. MALLEUS, 15. LABYRINTH, 16. EYELIDS, 19. OTIS, 21. CORNEA, 23. SCLERA, 25. CONES, 26. SENSE

ACROSS

1. Colored portion of eye
6. Membrane covering exposed eyeball
7. One of the special senses
9. Free sensory nerve endings
12. Stirrup (auditory ossicle)
14. Utricles and saccules together
17. Glands forming tears
18. Organ of smell
20. Tympanic membrane
22. Visual sense receptors
24. Sense of smell
27. Anvil (auditory ossicle)
28. Wall between nasal cavities
29. Organ of vision
30. One of the special senses

DOWN

2. Light-sensitive layer of eye
3. Number of primary tastes
4. Eyebrows
5. Eyelashes
8. Little bones
10. One of the special senses
11. One of the special senses
13. Hammer (auditory ossicle)
15. Inner ear
16. Eyelids
19. Combining form meaning ear
21. Transparent portion of eyeball
23. White portion of eye
25. Visual receptors for color
26. One of the special senses

HIDDEN WORDS PUZZLE   CHAPTER 16

```
H  V  L  T  V  T  H  V  T  N  M  U  H  E  J  C  C
E  H  S  A  W  Y  A  S  V  Y  N  S  I  F  Y  D  D
B  F  P  N  N  M  S  C  D  X  S  K  S  O  T  K  J
V  R  O  F  N  P  V  E  T  U  B  P  L  X  B  W  X
P  Q  K  Q  T  A  I  S  S  I  N  U  S  T  X  X  E
R  T  E  N  V  N  T  X  X  V  L  G  P  K  D  L  G
C  N  E  P  L  I  R  E  I  F  Z  E  D  A  P  M  P
B  Q  P  R  O  C  E  S  S  E  S  O  I  K  D  J  H
A  C  C  E  S  S  O  R  Y  L  K  R  U  C  P  X  E
N  G  X  X  R  U  B  X  Q  R  P  L  H  M  P  E  E
N  F  C  T  X  I  S  P  B  G  O  I  L  O  L  W  N
L  C  W  R  T  C  P  F  W  K  U  N  R  R  X  X  M
B  R  D  I  C  O  C  H  L  E  A  N  I  O  D  U  E
R  G  H  N  O  R  F  S  E  N  S  A  T  I  O  N  P
M  B  L  S  A  E  A  R  D  R  U  M  G  D  E  K  Q
A  E  Q  I  G  C  R  Y  S  T  A  L  L  I  N  E  O
P  I  O  C  V  E  A  U  R  I  C  L  E  R  N  U  W
X  I  F  B  M  P  Z  O  K  H  C  A  Y  I  T  N  Z
A  H  L  J  U  T  O  V  K  Y  O  I  P  S  D  E  I
N  R  I  P  V  O  R  L  V  N  M  Y  H  S  R  B  A
G  R  S  N  K  R  M  U  Y  J  M  Z  I  M  U  T  D
C  B  U  D  U  B  F  P  T  O  L  D  P  S  L  V
I  C  I  J  F  L  L  J  N  Y  D  W  K  H  D  I  E
S  S  V  H  R  N  P  R  R  N  A  R  E  S  K  W  J
D  T  W  C  W  W  M  P  U  C  T  K  A  O  C  Q  M
R  E  H  E  Y  T  L  E  Y  A  I  H  E  V  E  R  U
O  H  V  V  Y  L  G  E  R  V  O  X  B  Q  H  S  C
I  F  I  T  D  I  U  Y  T  E  N  G  Y  G  N  V  I
```

Can you find the 20 words hidden in this puzzle? All hidden word puzzles will have words running from top to bottom, left to right, and diagonally downward.

ACCOMMODATION	VITREOUS	SINUS
EXTRINSIC	COCHLEA	ACCESSORY
TYMPANIC	PINNA	RECEPTOR
CHOROID	PERIPHERAL	CAPSULE
NARES	SENSATION	TACTILE
CRYSTALLINE	AURICLE	IRIS
PROCESSES	EARDRUM	

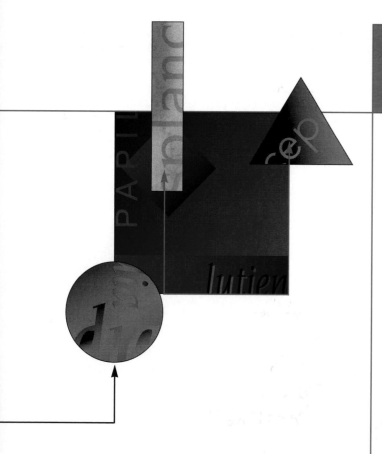

The Lymphatic and Immune Systems

the defenders of the body

In this chapter we describe the lymphatic and immune systems and their component parts and mechanisms.

THE LYMPHATIC SYSTEM

The lymphatic system includes the *lymph nodes, spleen, tonsils,* and *thymus,* and has roles in the cardiovascular and immune systems. It interacts with the cardiovascular system by way of the *lymphatic vessels,* which carry the fluid, called *lymph,* back to the circulation. Lymph is made up of tissue fluids, almost colorless, rich in white blood cells, and similar to blood plasma in appearance and composition. It is circulated throughout the body by the lymphatic vessels. The lymphatic system also has a crucial role in the immune system, because of its production and circulation of white blood cells.

The Lymphatic Vessels

The lymphatic vessels begin as lymphatic capillaries and form a vast network distributed throughout the body. These capillaries join to form slightly larger lymphatic vessels, which progressively repeat the process, forming larger and larger vessels. These vessels collect proteins and water, which continually filter out of the blood into the tissue fluid, and return them to the circulation. The lymphatic structure resembles that of

FACT

It's a

Although few American doctors believed in vaccination in 1777, George Washington's order to vaccinate the entire continental army may have helped ensure victory in the war of independence.

veins, but with a beaded appearance resulting from sinus spaces associated with the numerous valves which prevent backflow. The lymphatic vessels collect the lymph and carry it to either the *thoracic duct* or the *right lymphatic duct,* which in turn empty into the left and right subclavian veins, respectively. In the abdominal area, the thoracic duct has a saclike expansion, the *cisterna chyli* (*cisterna* means storage tank;

chyli refers to liquid contents), which collects and stores lymph on its way back to the venous system.

The Lymph Nodes

Along the course of the lymph vessels are numerous *lymph nodes,* enclosed in fibrous capsules (Figure 17.1). These nodes vary in size from mere dots to

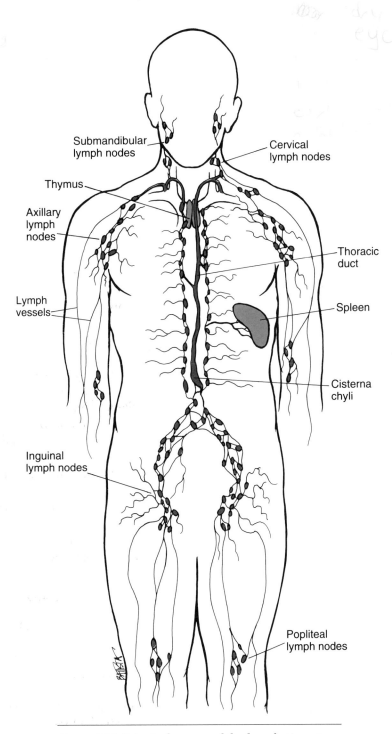

Figure 17.1 • Principal organs of the lymphatic system.

larger, bean-sized and bean-shaped bodies, identified by their location. Some examples are:

submandibular—lower jaw
cervical—neck
axillary—axilla
inguinal—groin
popliteal—knee

The lymph nodes act as filters to remove bacteria and other foreign bodies or particles, including malignant cells. They may be felt, or even seen, when they are inflamed or swollen by ingested bacteria and their toxins. Another important function of the lymph nodes is the manufacture of white blood cells (lymphocytes and monocytes), making the nodes an extremely important part of the body's defense against infection.

The Spleen

The spleen is a large, flattened, oval-shaped, glandlike organ, dark red in color. It is located in the upper left side of the abdominal cavity, just below the diaphragm, and behind the fundus of the stomach. It is soft and pliable and is the largest structure of the lymphoid system. Its size varies in different people and at different times in the same person. The spleen enlarges during infectious diseases and decreases in size in old age. The spleen, although an extremely useful and functional organ, can be removed if necessary with no harmful effect.

The chief functions of the spleen are:

hemopoiesis—the formation of lymphocytes, monocytes, and plasma cells.
phagocytosis—the removal and destruction of microorganisms, faulty platelets, and old erythrocytes; and the salvaging of globin and heme contents of the erythrocytes to be returned to the bone marrow and liver for later use.
storage area for blood in the splenic pulp.

The Tonsils

The tonsils are three pairs of small, round masses of lymphoid tissue, that filter out bacteria and other foreign matter, and play a part in the formation of lymphocytes. Their names and locations are:

palatine—located at the back of the throat
lingual—located at the root of the tongue
pharyngeal (also called *adenoids*)—located at the back of the roof of the pharynx

The Thymus

The thymus is a bilobate, grayish-pink structure of lymph tissue, located in the mediastinum, extending into the neck, to the lower border of the thyroid gland, behind the sternum. The thymus plays an important part in the immune system as a source of lymphocyte formation (T-cells) that destroy foreign substances. Its maximum development, relative to body size, is during early childhood. It is largest at puberty, after which it begins to atrophy, so that it has almost disappeared by extreme old age.

REVIEW 17.A

Complete the following:

1. The lymphatic system plays roles in the __Cardiovascular__ and __immune__ systems.
2. The lymphatic system includes __lymph nodes__, __spleen__, __tonsils__, and __thymus__.
3. The lymphatic structure resembles that of __veins__, including __valves__ to prevent backflow.
4. Five areas where lymph glands are located are __Lower Jaw__, __neck__, __axilla__, __groin__, and __knee__.
5. The lymph nodes have two major functions, __remove bacteria__, and the manufacture of __white blood cells__
6. The largest structure of the lymphoid system is the __spleen__.
7. One major function of this structure (in 6 above) is __Storage__.
8. There are __3__ pairs of tonsils.
9. The tonsils are the __palatine__, __lingual__, and __pharyngeal__.
10. The thymus plays an important part in the __immune__ system.

THE IMMUNE SYSTEM

The immune system consists of cells and chemicals that protect the body against invasion of foreign substances and maintain its general health. Weak immune system responses can result in failure to combat infections or malignancies, whereas excessively strong responses can result in *hypersensitivities* or *autoimmune disease* reactions.

Nonspecific Immune Mechanisms

There are many mechanisms in the various systems of the body that are involved in the prevention of infection and disease. The integumentary system (Chapter 8) provides both a physical and a chemical barrier (cerumen, sebum, and sweat) thereby blocking or killing invading organisms. The cardiovascular system (Chapter 9) produces granulocytes that function in phagocytosis and detoxification of foreign proteins. The respiratory system (Chapter 10) provides chemical and mechanical barriers through the action of the mucous membranes, which trap and kill disease organisms, and coughing and sneezing mechanisms which expel them. Other mechanisms include the actions of saliva and hydrochloric acid, products of the gastrointestinal system (Chapter 11), urine from the urinary system (Chapter 12), and tears from the eyes (Chapter 16), which wash foreign substances out of the body and can limit the growth of organisms or kill them outright. The more direct functions of the lymphatic system in the destruction of invading organisms have been described above.

There are also other substances involved in protection of the body against disease. There are natural body chemicals, such as *histamines* and *prostaglandins,* which produce vasodilation and inflammation, resulting in greater blood flow. This causes a rise in the number of leukocytes, leading to increased phagocytosis. Chemicals called *pyrogens* (*pyr* - means fire) are released by invading bacteria and by the defending leukocytes. These chemicals stimulate the nervous system, affecting the body temperature and producing fever, further increasing phagocytic action.

Complement refers to a group of approximately 12 proteins normally present in the globulin of blood serum. These proteins are given the name complement because they complement (complete or perfect) antibodies that activate the proteins to produce inflammation and destroy invading cells.

Interferon is a natural cell protein protecting the body against infection and possibly some types of cancer. Viral infection causes cells of the body to produce interferon, which attaches itself to noninfected cell surfaces. The interferon stimulates production of other antiviral proteins that directly interfere with and block further viral growth and infection.

Specific Immune Mechanisms

Specific immunity is the response of the defenses of the body to specific substances that are recognized as harmful and are attacked. Substances that are capable of producing such immune system reactions are called *antigens.* Antigens can be foreign to the body, such as bacteria, viruses, and pollen, or can be part of the body's own immune mechanisms.

There are two chief types of lymphocytes that are extremely important in the production of specific immunity, called *B-cells* and *T-cells.*

B-cells, which are formed as stem cells in the red bone marrow, migrate as immature B-cells, mainly to the lymph nodes. B-cells produce proteins called *antibodies* (*immunoglobulins*—also called *immune gamma globulins*). The immature B-cells are activated by contact with antigens. These activated B-cells quickly reproduce and develop into two types of cells, *plasma cells* and *memory cells.* The plasma cells produce an outpouring of antibodies that attack the sources of the antigens. Antibodies work by binding to antigens in the blood, preventing them from functioning. This produces inflammation; activates the globulin proteins (complements); and attracts eosinophils, macrophages, monocytes, and neutrophils, resulting in phagocytosis of the invading organisms. The memory cells are stored in the lymph nodes until some of them are exposed to the specific antigen that activated their production. Once activated, these then change into plasma cells, resulting in an outpouring of the specific antibodies that attack the source of the antigen. The remaining memory cells, with the ability to recognize the activating antigen, produce long-term immunity to that antigen (Figure 17.2).

The initial antibody response, before memory cell development, takes some time to produce sufficient antibodies to be effective, and usually some disease develops. Little or no disease occurs after the memory cells are available to produce antibodies.

T-cells are also produced as stem cells in the red bone marrow, maturing in the thymus, and stored in the lymph nodes. There are three types, *T-effector, T-helper,* and *T-suppressor.*

T-effector cells have several functions. They produce proteins, called *lymphokines,* which stimulate inflammation and phagocytosis. They are attracted to antigens produced by viruses, tumors, or transplanted foreign tissue on the surface of cells, and dissolve those "infected" cells. Like the B-cells, T-effector cells also can become *memory cells,* responding rapidly and vigorously to the presence of previously encountered antigens on cell surfaces, also producing long-term immunity to such antigens.

T-helper cells increase the immune response of both the T-effector and the B-cells.

T-suppressor cells suppress, or limit, the immune response of the T-effector and B-cells.

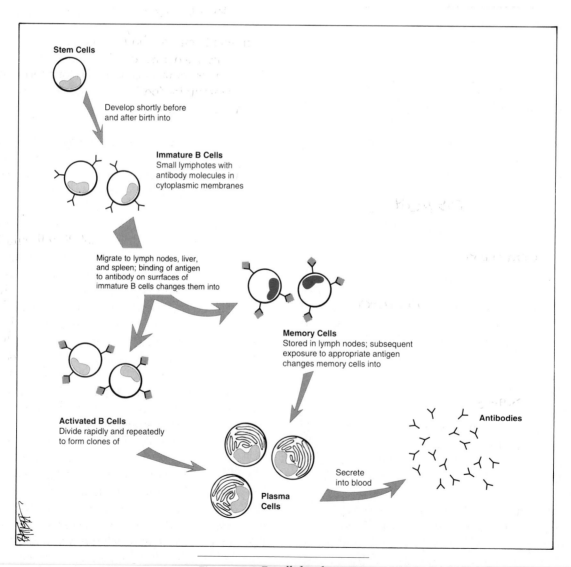

Figure 17.2 B-cell development.

The combined action of the T-helper and T-suppressor cells regulates the immune responses of the T-effector and B-cells.

A third type of lymphocyte, *null cells,* do not have the surface molecules that characterize B-cells and T-cells and are not able to develop into memory cells. This type includes *natural killer cells (NK cells)* and *killer cells (K cells)* and, like the T-effector cells, kills the target tumor cells and viral-infected cells by lysis. Their action may be enhanced by interferon or inhibited by prostaglandins.

The antibody-based part of the immune system, referred to as *antibody-mediated* or *humoral* immunity, primarily attacks invaders freely floating in the blood. The T-cell and null cell components, referred to as *cellular (cell-mediated)* immunity, primarily attack invaders infiltrating cells of the body.

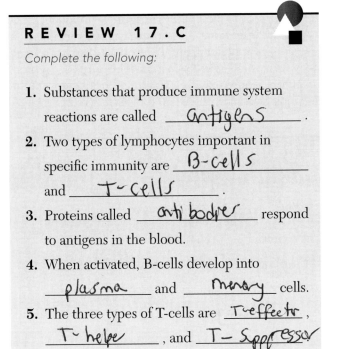

R E V I E W   1 7 . C

Complete the following:

1. Substances that produce immune system reactions are called ___Antigens___ .

2. Two types of lymphocytes important in specific immunity are ___B-cells___ and ___T-cells___ .

3. Proteins called ___antibodies___ respond to antigens in the blood.

4. When activated, B-cells develop into ___plasma___ and ___memory___ cells.

5. The three types of T-cells are ___T-effector___ , ___T-helper___ , and ___T-suppressor___ .

Acquired Immunity

Long-term specific immunity develops in response to the presence of antigens that arouse the various immune system responses. Immunity may be *natural* or *artificial, active* or *passive.* Natural immunity develops through the body's ordinary exposure to daily living. Artificial immunity is achieved by vaccination. Active immunity develops through the body's own immune response, whereas passive immunity is achieved through antibodies transferred from an external source.

Natural, active immunity is illustrated by exposure to measles (without benefit of previous vaccination). The immune system fights the infection until it has been brought under control, providing long-term immunity.

Natural, passive immunity is illustrated by the transfer of the antibodies of a pregnant woman to the fetus or from a mother to her breast-fed infant, which provides temporary, partial immunity.

Artificial, active immunity is illustrated by vaccination with weakened or dead infectious agents, or specific antigens, introduced into the body to arouse the immune system (as in vaccination for diphtheria, measles, whooping cough, etc.).

Artificial, passive immunity is illustrated by the introduction into the body of substances artificially produced outside of the body, such as antibiotics, gamma globulin, and interferon, providing immediate, temporary immunity.

Immunity may be short or long term, depending on the production of memory cells. Active immunity usually produces memory cells, and is long term, whereas passive immunity does not produce memory cells and is of much shorter duration.

Problems. There are two major types of immune system problems. There may be (1) a weakness or deficiency in the effectiveness of the system or (2) an excessively strong reaction by the system.

Immune weakness or deficiency. Problems producing deficiencies in the immune system can arise from congenital factors in which B-cells and T-cells may develop inadequately in number or effectiveness. An example of this is the condition known as *severe combined immunodeficiency disease* (see Related Terms list). In addition, inadequacies in availability of protein, stress problems that depress antibody formation, diseases that affect the effectiveness of lymphocytes, depletion of lymphocytes and granulocytes by previous infections, and suppression of the system by drugs to prevent tissue rejection in transplants or grafts all represent conditions in which the immune system is limited in effectiveness.

Excessively strong reaction. In some situations the immune system response to an antigen produces excessive inflammatory reactions and other *hypersensitivity* complications, for example, those in allergic conditions such as hay fever, hives, and asthma. Perhaps the greatest problem of overreaction is in *autoimmune* diseases, in which the system does not adequately distinguish between foreign antigens and those of its own cells and the body's tissues are attacked by its own antibodies. Diseases of this sort include *rheumatoid arthritis,* where joint tissue is attacked (Chapter 18); *myasthenia gravis,* in which the action of the neurotransmitter acetylcholine is affected (Chapter 7); *thrombocytopenic purpura,* in which platelets are destroyed (Chapter 9); *multiple sclerosis,* where the myelin sheath is attacked (Chapter 15); and *systemic lupus erythematosus,* in which skin, blood vessels, kidneys, and genetic material are attacked (Chapter 18).

REVIEW 17.D

Complete the following:

1. Immunity can be ___natural___ or ___artificial___ and ___active___ or ___passive___.

2. The transfer of antibodies by a mother to a fetus is an example of ___natural passive &___ immunity.

3. Two types of immune system problems are ___weakness___ and ___strong reaction___.

4. Immunity may be short or long term, depending on the production of ___memory___ cells.

5. Rheumatoid arthritis is an example of a(n) ___autoimmune___ disease.

Biotechnology and the Immune System

The immune system can be manipulated to develop vaccines and treat diseases. Most vaccines for viral or bacterial diseases use either a related *pathogen* (disease-producing organism), such as cowpox in the development of the smallpox vaccine, or a killed or severely weakened pathogen (polio and cholera). Recent developments, based on identifying the genetic character (DNA) of pathogens, are leading scientists toward the production of vaccines for previously resistant diseases such as tuberculosis, malaria, influenza, and AIDS.

DNA vaccines are produced by using safe genetic material from the particular pathogen and generating large quantities of this material by implanting it into relatively benign bacteria or viruses. When introduced into the body, these vaccines can trigger immune responses, especially cell-mediated responses, against the pathogenic agent. This is particularly useful against diseases in which the pathogen hides within the cells of the body, where the humoral (antibody-mediated) immune mechanism cannot reach it. DNA-based immune therapy can also be used to generate increased cellular immune response to cancer cells and is expected to have a significant place in cancer treatments.

Not only are DNA vaccines capable of producing strong cellular immunities, but they are safer than traditional vaccines, because unlike weakened or defective batches of killed pathogens, they cannot accidentally start infections. In addition, DNA vaccines can use common genes from a variety of disease-related organisms such as influenza or AIDS viruses. In time, a single vaccine may be capable of arousing immune responses to all of the related disease strains.

REVIEW 17.E

Complete the following:

1. A ___pathogen___ is a disease-producing organism.

2. Cowpox is related to ___smallpox___.

3. Safe genetic material is implanted into ___benign___ bacteria and viruses to produce DNA vaccines.

4. Another term for antibody-mediated immunity is ___humoral___ immunity.

5. DNA vaccines are ___safer___ than traditional vaccines.

ANATOMY

active immunity immunity developed by stimulating the body's own defenses.

adenoids see *pharyngeal tonsils.*

antibody a protein substance that interacts with a specific antigen to protect the body.

antigen substance that triggers the formation of specific antibodies, which react against the antigen.

artificial immunity immunity derived by vaccination, from a source outside the body .

B-cells lymphocytes that form and mature in the bone marrow, producing antibodies.

cellular immunity immunity produced by T-cell and null cell lymphocytes (also called *cell-mediated* immunity).

cisterna chyli (sis-ter'nah) saclike reservoir for collection of lymph, and origin of the thoracic duct.

complement a group of proteins normally present in blood serum that produces inflammation and destruction of invading cells.

hemopoiesis lymphocyte, monocyte, and plasma cell formation (also called *hemapoiesis* and *hematopoiesis*).

histamine natural body chemical that produces vasodilation and inflammation.

hilum depression where vessels and nerves enter the spleen.

humoral immunity immunity produced by antibodies.

hypersensitivity excessive immune system response to antigens.

immunoglobulins antibodies produced by B-cells (also called *immune gamma globulins*).

interferon a natural cell protein that protects against infection by stimulating production of other antiviral proteins.

killer cell (K cell) one type of null cell lymphocyte that kills tumor and viral-infected cells by lysis.

lienic (splenic) capsule membranous envelope enclosing the spleen.

lymph relatively colorless tissue fluid containing leukocytes, proteins, and water.

lymphatic duct channel conveying lymph, specifically the right and left (thoracic) lymphatic ducts.

lymphatic vessel channel conveying lymph.

lymph follicle (fol'i-k'l) saclike collector of lymphoid substances, chiefly beneath the mucous surfaces.

lymph nodes glandlike masses of lymphatic tissue varying in size from dots to bean-sized bodies, identified by their locations along the course of lymphatic vessels.

lymphocytes several types of leukocytes that either produce antibodies or carry out phagocytosis.

memory cells lymphocytes that can recognize previously encountered antigens, and react quickly.

memory response rapid lymphocyte response to previously encountered antigens.

monoclonal antibodies antibodies grown (cloned) in quantity from a single cell, for vaccine use.

natural immunity immunity produced by natural body defenses such as antibodies or killer cells.

natural killer cells (NK cells) one type of null cell lymphocyte that kills tumor and viral-infected cells by lysis.

null cells lymphocytes that do not become memory cells, and destroy target cells by lysis.

passive immunity immunity directly produced by sources external to the body.

pathogen disease-producing organism

phagocytosis removal and destruction of foreign bodies, platelets, and erythrocytes, and salvaging of globin and heme contents.

pharyngeal tonsils tonsils located at the back of the roof of the pharynx (also called *adenoids*).

plasma cells activated B-cells that produce antibodies for specific antigens.

prostaglandin natural body chemical that produces vasodilation and inflammation.

pyrogen chemical released by invading bacteria and defending leukocytes that stimulates the nervous system to increase body temperature.

right lymphatic duct lymphatic duct draining the lymph from the upper right quadrant of the body.

sinusoids sinuslike capillaries with specialized function.

spleen largest lymphoid system structure, a flattened, oval-shaped, glandlike organ located in the upper left side of the abdominal cavity.

red splenic pulp lymphatic tissue permeated with sinusoids filled with blood.

T-cells lymphocytes maturing in the thymus.

T-effector cells type of T-cell that produces lymphokines and can become memory cells.

T-helper cells type of T-cell that increases immune responses of T-effector cells and B-cells.

T-suppressor cells type of T-cell that suppresses the immune responses of T-effector cells and B-cells.

thoracic duct left lymphatic duct draining lymph from all but the upper right quadrant of the body.

thymus gland bilobate, grayish-pink structure of lymph tissue in the mediastinum that develops the T-cell lymphocytes from stem cells.

tonsils three pairs of small, round masses of lymphoid tissue.

white splenic pulp sheath of lymphatic tissue that surrounds the arteries of the spleen.

PATHOLOGIC CONDITIONS

Inflammations and Infections

acquired immune deficiency syndrome (AIDS) see Chapter 18.

actinomycosis see Chapter 18.

AIDS-related complex (ARC) see Chapter 18.

filariasis tropical parasitic disease, transmitted by a mosquito carrying *Filaria nematode* larvae, causing granulomatous inflammation and obstruction of lymph channels, with pain, blindness, swelling of extremities, and development of elephantiasis and pachyderma (Chapter 18).

infectious mononucleosis (mon"o-nu'kle-o'sis) acute, contagious, viral infection, caused by the Epstein-Barr virus (may be present in latent form in most human leukocytes and activated to pathogenicity by an immune suppression response), resulting in an abnormal increase in mononuclear leukocytes in the blood (Chapter 18).

lymphadenitis (lim-fad"e-ni'tis) inflammation of the lymph nodes.

lymphangitis (lim"fan-ji'tis) inflammation of one or more lymphatic vessels.

paratyphoid fever *Salmonella* bacterial infection similar to typhoid but not as severe, involving lymphoid mesenteric tissues and the intestines (Chapter 18).

splenitis painful inflammatory condition of the spleen.

sporotrichosis (spo"ro-tri'ko'sis) common, chronic, fungal infection caused by *Sporothrix schenckii*, characterized by skin ulcers and multiple subcutaneous granulomas along lymphatic channels, with rare involvement in muscles, joints, bones, and lungs.

Hereditary, Congenital, and Developmental Disorders

Gaucher's disease (go-shaz') hereditary splenic anemia (Chapter 18).

hypertrophy of thymus congenital enlargement of thymus.

leukocyte adhesion deficiency (LAD) a genetic defect resulting in inability of leukocytes to adhere to other cells, rendering a significant part of the immune system helpless.

severe combined immunodeficiency disease (SCID) congenital immune system deficiency disease in which the individual must be kept in a sterile environment ("bubble") to prevent illness or death from infections.

Other Lymphatic and Immune System Disorders

accessory spleen small mass of splenic tissue, sometimes found near the spleen in a peritoneal fold.

Banti's disease splenomegaly resulting from portal hypertension.

gammopathy disorder in which there are abnormal levels of gamma globulin in the blood.

lymphadenectasis (lim-fad"e-nek'tah-sis) dilation of a lymph gland.

lymphadenopathy disease of the lymph nodes.

lymphangiectasis (lim-fan"je-ek'tah-sis) swelling of lymphatic vessels.

lymphatic leukemia leukemia combined with hyperplasia and overactivity of the lymphoid tissue (also called *lymphocytic leukemia*, and *lymphoid leukemia*).

lymphedema (lim"fe-de'mah) swelling caused by blockage of the lymphatic vessels.

lymphorrhea discharge of lymph from a cut or torn lymph vessel.

lymphostasis (lim-fos'tah-sis) obstruction to the lymph flow.

myasthenia gravis muscular disease with suspected autoimmune involvement (Chapter 7).

multiple sclerosis neural demyelinating disorder of suspected autoimmune origin (Chapter 15).

rheumatoid arthritis destructive collagen disease of autoimmune origin (Chapter 18).

splenomegaly enlargement of the spleen.

systemic lupus erythematosus (SLE) chronic disease of suspected autoimmune origin involving many organ systems individually or in a variety of combinations (Chapter 18).

thrombocytopenic purpura systemic condition with suspected autoimmune origin (Chapter 9).

thymolysis destruction of the thymus.

thymopathy any disease of the thymus.

thymus hyperplasia enlarged thymus.

Oncology*

giant follicular lymphoma* (lim-fo'mah) malignant lymphoma marked by follicle-like nodules in the lymph nodes (also called *giant follicular lymphadenopathy* and *Brill-Symmers disease*).

Hodgkin's disease* malignant, progressive, painless condition marked by the enlargement of the spleen, lymph nodes, and lymphoid tissues (also called *granulomatous lymphoma, multiple lymphadenoma, lymphogranuloma,* and *lymphomatosis granulomatosa*).

Kaposi's sarcoma* (kap'a-sez) malignant neoplasm affecting the lymph nodes and other systems (Chapter 18).

lymphangioma (lim-fan"je-o'mah) tumor made up of newly formed lymph channels and spaces.

lymphangiosarcoma* malignant tumor of the lymph vessels.

lymphoma* lymphoid tissue tumors, usually malignant.

lymphomatosis* (lim"fo-mah-to'sis) development of multiple lymphomas in the body.

lymphosarcoma* (lim"fo-sar'ko'mah) general term for malignant neoplasm of lymphoid tissue.

SURGICAL PROCEDURES

angiotomy incision of a blood or lymph vessel.

lymphadenectomy (lim-fad"e-nek'to-me) excision of a lymph node.

lymphangiectomy (lim-fan"je-ek'to-me) excision of lymphatic vessels.

lymphangioplasty (lim-fan"je-o-plas"te) repair or replacement of a lymph vessel (also called *lymphoplasty*).

lymphangiotomy (lim-fan"je-ot'o-me) incision into a vessel of the lymphatic system.

lymphaticostomy (lim-fat"i-kos'to-me) making an opening into a lymphatic duct.

splenectomy removal of the spleen.

splenopexy fixation of the spleen.

splenorrhaphy repair of the spleen.

splenotomy incision of the spleen.

thymectomy removal of thymus.

LABORATORY TESTS

AIDS serology tests Blood tests to diagnose and screen for antigens or antibodies to the human immunodeficiency virus (HIV).

Enzyme-linked immunosorbent assay (ELISA) detects antibodies to the AIDS virus. False positives may occur and the Western blot test is used as a confirmation.

Western blot test detects the presence of HIV in blood serum.

angiotensin-converting enzyme (ACE) blood test used to assist in diagnosis of Gaucher's and Hodgkin's diseases.

complement assay blood test to measure serum complement levels, which increase or decrease according to type of disorder (e.g., increased levels in rheumatoid arthritis, decreased levels in systemic lupus erythematosus).

DNA analysis method of producing unique genetic profiles of individuals. The genetic material (DNA) is extracted from samples of blood, skin, semen, or hair, and separated into strands by enzymes that cut the strands into unequal pieces. These pieces are sorted by a process called electrophoresis, tagged by radioactive probes, and exposed to x-ray film, producing a series of black bands similar to the bar codes used in supermarket checkouts.

° Indicates a malignant condition.

EXERCISES THE LYMPHATIC AND IMMUNE SYSTEMS THE DEFENDERS OF THE BODY

Exercise 17.1   Complete the following:

1. The two ducts in the lymphatic system that receive the lymph and empty into the subclavian veins are called _thoracic duct_ and _right lymphatic duct_.

2. A _fibrous capsule_ encloses lymph nodes.

3. There are _3_ pairs of tonsils.

4. One function of the tonsils is _plays a part in leukocyte formation_.

5. Other than the lymphatic system, the thymus plays a part in the _immune_ system.

6. The largest structure of the lymphoid system is the _spleen_.

7. The thymus is the source of _T-cell_ formation.

8. Two natural body chemicals that produce vasodilation and inflammation are _histamines_ and _prostaglandins_.

9. A natural cell protein protecting against infection and possibly cancer is _interferon_.

10. _antigens_ are substances recognized as harmful and attacked by the immune system.

Exercise 17.2   Matching

_E_ 1. lymphatic vessels   A. filters
_G_ 2. cisterna chyli   B. natural killer
_J_ 3. spleen   C. firelike chemicals
_A_ 4. lymph nodes   D. protein group
_I_ 5. tonsils   E. beaded appearance
_H_ 6. thymus   F. hypersensitivity
_C_ 7. pyrogens   G. storage sac
_D_ 8. complement   H. T-cells
_B_ 9. null cells   I. palatine
_F_ 10. allergy   J. glandlike

Exercise 17.3   *Identify each listed part from Figure 17.3 in numbered blanks below.*

Axillary lymph nodes

Cervical lymph nodes

Inguinal lymph nodes

Popliteal lymph nodes

Submandibular lymph nodes

Cisterna chyli

Lymph vessels

Spleen

Thoracic duct

Thymus

1. _Submandibula lymph nodes_
2. _axillary lymph nodes_
3. _lymph ~~nodes~~ vessels_
4. _inguinal lymph nodes_
5. _popliteal lymph nodes_
6. _cisterna Chyli_
7. _Spleen_
8. _thoracic duct_
9. _thymus_
10. _cervical lymph nodes_

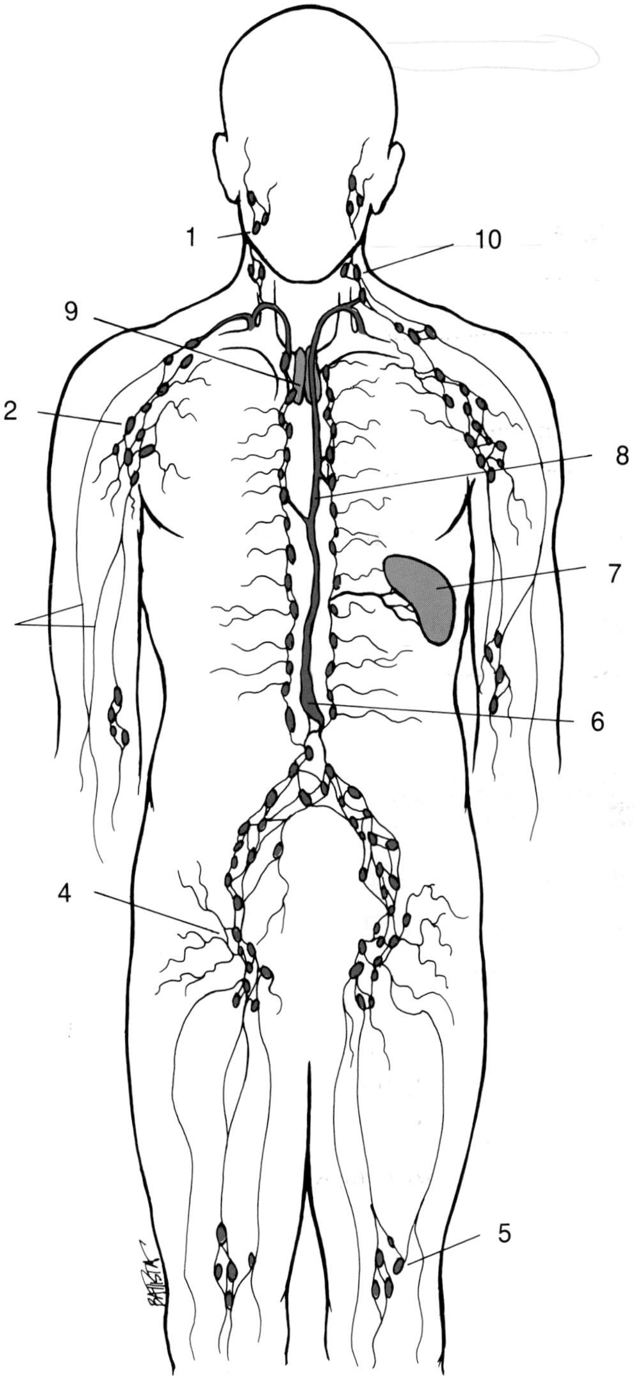

Figure 17.3 Principal organs of the lymphatic system.

Exercise 17.4   *Multiple choice*

1. Inflammation of lymphatic vessels is called:
   a. lymphadenitis
   b. lymphangitis
   c. lymphedema
2. Chemicals released by invading bacteria and defending leukocytes are:
   a. histamines
   b. prostaglandins
   c. pyrogens
3. B-cells produce:
   a. antibodies
   b. antigens
   c. complements
4. B-cells have the ability to become:
   a. memory cells
   b. T-helper cells
   c. stem cells
5. A type of leukocyte is:
   a. interferon
   b. lymphokines
   c. null cells

6. Which of the following cannot become memory cells?
   a. B-cells
   b. null cells
   c. T-cells
7. Which of the following kill target cells by lysis?
   a. null cells
   b. B-cells
   c. T-cells
8. Recovery from exposure to a disease such as measles is an example of:
   a. natural passive immunity
   b. artificial active immunity
   c. natural active immunity
9. Weakness of the immune system is illustrated by:
   a. autoimmune disease
   b. severe combined immunodeficiency disease
   c. hypersensitivities
10. Rheumatoid arthritis is a disease in which the immune system reaction is:
    a. excessively strong
    b. excessively weak
    c. natural passive

Exercise 17.5   *Give the meaning of the components of the following words and then define the word as a whole. Suffixes meaning* pertaining to or state or condition, *shown following a slash mark (/), are not to be defined separately. Before reaching for your medical dictionary, check the Related Terms list in this chapter.*

1. Lymphadenitis:
   lymph _lymph_
   aden _glands_
   itis _inflammation_

2. Splenectomy:
   splen _spleen_
   ectomy _surgical removal_

3. Thymoma:
   thym _thymus_
   oma _tumor_

4. Lymphocytopenia:
   lympho _lymph_
   cyto _cell_
   pen/ia _deficiency_

5. Immunodeficient:
   immuno _immune system_
   deficient _inadequate_

CROSSWORD PUZZLE

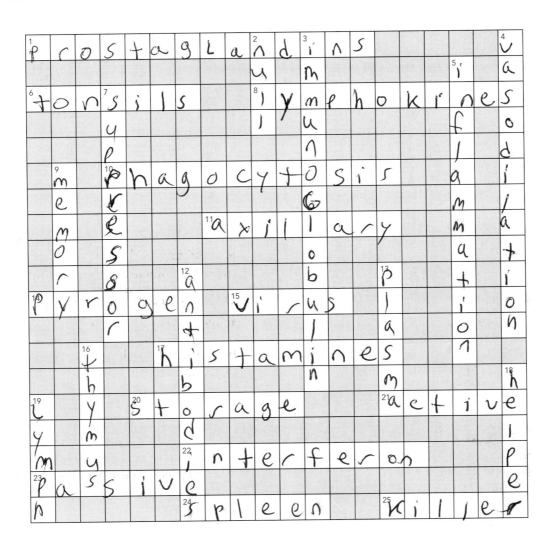

ACROSS

1. Body chemical producing vasodilation
6. Small mass of lymphoid tissue
8. Proteins produced by T-effector cells
10. One of the functions of the spleen
11. A group of lymph nodes
14. Fever-producing chemical
15. Type of invading organism
17. Body chemicals producing vasodilation
20. One function of the spleen
21. Type of immunity
22. Natural cell protein
23. Type of immunity conferred by vaccination
24. Largest structure of lymphoid system
25. Type of lymphocyte that uses lysis

DOWN

2. A third type of lymphocyte
3. Antibody produced by B-cells
4. Blood vessel enlargement caused by natural body chemicals
5. Results in greater blood flow
7. Type of T-cell
9. Type of B-cell or T-cell that recognizes a specific antigen
12. Proteins produced by B-cells
13. Cells producing antibodies against antigen sources
16. Source of lymphocyte formation
18. Type of T-cell that increases the immune response
19. Fluid carried by lymphatic vessels

HIDDEN WORDS PUZZLE

```
P U L T R Y V L H M P I W M L E M Q N O R G L Z Z P U A
A U T O I M M U N E Z T X X I R Q U D Z D G J T R L L P
C P C L L X C Z O S M R O F M Z F D F P C A U E O O F X
P W L Z F B F H D H V O G P M A J Z U F A U Y C Z R O T
T E F D C N Q M C F L U P J U U Q I O I B S L Q X D C I
L W X R W J J J Y K U H W C O N V G V Q B E S S C P S R Q
O W K G U M Y W S D Y A R T I F I C I A L M N I V D I K
G X Z I C Y J W L E W E J S T E B P J E K V J S V B F O
W Q L H Q U R J A V R H R E Y Q S Q Q F I B H T F E X R
P J E L M U W G L G S U B M A N D I B U L A R E X F J D
V I V P R W C F B R D Y M I D B R M S G L S S R L Q N Q
T E C W P D C K U T R K V T N C O M P L E M E N T P H W
Q C M B F P A Q R L V C Y S T P B U V L R H W A Y P E U
U C U U E I M N Q C H Y P E R S E N S I T I V E H U L R
S L Y B S F U O T S Q T L Y M P H O C Y T E I S B O B I
N X Y V D R H D K I B K C K J T G G M L X Z V Z O C O B
X U L P Y V V E V E G S Y O G A E L E T F U X P S L N K
S E J G G T M S L J R E F F E C T O R D L R Y V C W L N
V K K Y P V G Q N V L L N A N T I B O D Y Y C B B H V Y
K C G N F J K J E N E P X U A I W U D S W M W X W T G E
K C D I V C K F I R V C E S T V C L T M F T Q F G H I W
H H G O E X O Y Y Y O T N L U E U I J W F E Q J E M F D
L A U G X R U L Y X G S L P R X U N D E U X Y D N A C V
N Y Q H A E F L L L D R A B A L L T A X E Q T C O R V C
C C E C N Q D O B E K N K V L N V H T H H E X T H D H B
```

Can you find the 20 words hidden in this puzzle? All hidden word puzzles will have words running from top to bottom, left to right, and diagonally downward.

HYPERSENSITIVE

AUTOIMMUNE

EFFECTOR

NATURAL

HELPER

IMMUNOGLOBULIN

COMPLEMENT

ANTIBODY

ANTIGEN

ACTIVE

SUBMANDIBULAR

ARTIFICIAL

IMMUNITY

PASSIVE

SERUM

HEMOPOIESIS

LYMPHOCYTE

CISTERNA

KILLER

NODES

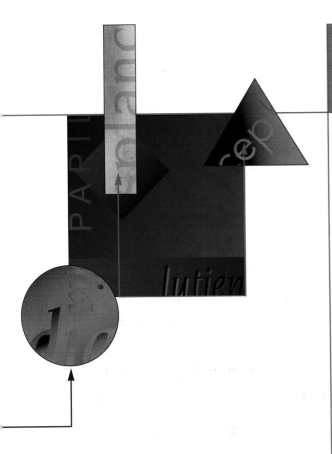

Multiple-System Diseases

a l i s t o f c o n d i t i o n s

a f f e c t i n g m u l t i p l e

s y s t e m s

In the preceding chapters, diseases and abnormal conditions have been listed under the appropriate anatomic systems. This method of classification, however, does not take into consideration all the diseases and congenital anomalies that affect more than one system. Multiple descriptions of each disease or anomaly would be required if they appeared under individual systems. To eliminate this duplication, we have chosen to list and describe many of these diseases in this chapter.

OVERVIEW

In multiple-system diseases, a "target" organ may be involved primarily, but as the disease advances and constitutional symptoms develop, other organs become progressively affected. This is particularly true of many infections, especially immunodeficiency diseases, which begin with a symptom in one body system and progressively spread to involve other systems.

It's a **FACT**

According to the World Health Organization, more than 25 million people worldwide have already been infected with HIV, and 30 to 40 million cases are predicted by the turn of the century.

355

Radiologic examinations often reveal characteristic findings in organs other than the primary system under investigation. The extent of spread of the disease process is evident in many body structures far removed from the primary focus, as in *acquired immune deficiency syndrome (AIDS)* and *lupus erythematosus (LE)*. It is also not unusual, in autopsies on stillborn neonates and those dying shortly after birth, to find a number of anomalies incompatible with life, including gross malformations of organs, atresia of passages, or heart defects that are not visually detected at birth.

The classification of diseases as "multiple-system" is now widespread since the advent of new and improved laboratory and radiologic procedures, as well as other diagnostic tests such as computer-assisted imaging techniques. These and other advances in medical knowledge make it possible to trace the extent of involvement of multiple systems in a disease.

No attempt is made here to list all the multiple-system diseases, since several medical writers have devoted separate texts to this subject.

The term *epidemiology* means the study of the frequency of occurrence, distribution, and causative factors of disease. There are specific terms that refer to the occurrence of disease.

> *Incidence*—how often a disease occurs in a population.
> *Prevalence*—the number of cases of a disease at a particular time.
> *Endemic*—a disease continuously present in a particular geographic area or population.
> *Epidemic*—a disease that affects large numbers of people at the same time in a particular geographic area.
> *Pandemic*—a disease that is epidemic throughout a country or the world.

■ RELATED **TERMS**   **MULTIPLE-SYSTEM DISEASES** A LIST OF CONDITIONS AFFECTING MULTIPLE SYSTEMS

PATHOLOGIC CONDITIONS

Inflammations and Infections

acquired immune deficiency syndrome (AIDS) infectious disease that produces a breakdown in the immune system and is transmitted by unprotected intercourse with an infected person; by contact with infected blood or blood products, contaminated needles, and infected donor organs; or across the placental barrier from mother to fetus. The disease process begins with infection by a retrovirus, *human immunodeficiency virus (HIV)*. This retrovirus destroys the ability of T-helper cells (a type of lymphocyte) to recognize invading pathogens, and also converts the T-cells into factories to reproduce the infecting virus, eventually leaving the body defenseless against even the most minor of infections. Eight to twelve weeks after initial infection, HIV antibodies begin to be produced, but there may be an extended incubation period that *can* last an average of ten years, during which time the virus may remain hidden in the lymph nodes. Although most cases take several months for HIV antibodies to be detected after initial infection, some may take as long as 24 months. *AIDS-related complex (ARC)* syndrome is an early condition in which symptoms of fatigue, weakness, fever, weight loss, diarrhea, and lymphadenopathy appear. The immune system's weakness allows many opportunistic infections to develop in one or more body systems, from sources that include protozoa, fungi, viruses, and bacteria. Life-threatening conditions common in full-blown AIDS include *Pneumocystis carinii pneumonia (PCP)* and *Kaposi's sarcoma (KS)*. Neurologic involvement is common, including such conditions as *AIDS dementia.* Some drugs, such as zidovudine (AZT) and lamivudine, are being used to inhibit progression of the disease. Newer drugs called protease inhibitors retard replication of the virus and, when combined with these drugs, offer hope of indefinite relief, if not actual cure.

actinomycosis (ak″ti-no-mi-ko′sis) fungal infection caused by the organism *Actinomyces*, characterized mainly by abscesses or granulomas of cervicofacial lymph nodes, abdominal organs, and pulmonary tissue.

AIDS-related complex (ARC) pre-AIDS syndrome, also known as *chronic lymphadenopathy syndrome* (see *acquired immune deficiency syndrome*).

alastrim mild form of smallpox (also called *variola minor*).

amebiasis (am″e-bi′ah-sis) protozoal infection with the microorganism *Entamoeba histolytica,* transmitted to humans by food and drink containing encysted forms of the microorganism, which affects the mucous membrane of the colon in the form of abscesses and ulcers and may also form abscesses in the liver, thoracic cavity, lungs, and skin.

anthrax bacterial infection of animals with the microorganism *Bacillus anthracis,* transmitted to humans by inhalation or handling of infected wool, hides, and carcasses, beginning with a lesion at the entry site of the infection, progressing to bloody, mucinous edema in many tissues and serous cavities, and may be fatal (also called *splenic fever, woolsorters'* or *ragsorters' disease,* and *malignant pustule*).

ascariasis (as″kah-ri′ah-sis) helminthic infection with the roundworm *Ascaris lumbricoides,* transmitted by ingestion of embryonated ova, which develop into adult worms in the intestines, but the worms may migrate to other organs.

botulism (bot′u-lizm) potent bacterial food poisoning with a high mortality rate, caused by the growth of *Clostridium botulinum* in food that has not been properly sterilized before canning or preserving. Symptoms include vomiting, abdominal pain, vision problems, central nervous system symptoms, motor disturbances, dyspepsia, coughing, dilation of the pupils, and muscle paralysis (*botulus* means sausage, and the disease derives its name from its first recognition in improperly cooked sausages).

brucellosis (broo″sel-lo′sis) bacterial infection caused by a species of *Brucella,* infecting humans through contact with infected animals or products such as meat, milk, and cheese, with lesions in many organs (also known as *undulant, Malta,* and *Mediterranean fevers*).

candidiasis (kan″di-di′ah-sis) *Candida albicans* fungal infection, involving superficial lesions of moist areas such as the respiratory tract, vagina, and mouth (*thrush*—common in HIV infections), with rare endocardial and systemic infections (also called *moniliasis, candidosis,* and *oidomycosis*).

cat scratch disease usually benign bacterial infection caused by the bite or scratch of a cat, which produces lymphadenitis but can also become more severe and manifest as osteomyelitis, arthritis, hepatitis, pleurisy, and other conditions (also called *cat scratch fever*).

chickenpox highly contagious childhood disease, caused by herpes zoster virus, with vesicular eruptions on face and trunk and possible complications, including pneumonia, myelitis, Guillain-Barré syndrome, encephalitis, meningitis, and Reye's syndrome (also called *varicella*).

cholera (kol′er-ah) acute bacterial infection caused by *Vibrio cholerae,* contracted from contaminated water, food, hands, and utensils; beginning with an acute diarrhea and progressing to vomiting, cramps, and severe dehydration, which may result in renal failure.

chronic fatigue syndrome (CFS) disabling fatigue following a viral-like condition, cause unknown, with symptoms that may include bone and muscle pain, low-grade fever, adenopathies, headaches, sore throat, memory problems, depression, and sleep difficulties. Remission of symptoms usually occurs spontaneously (also called *chronic fatigue and immune dysfunction syndrome—CFIDS*).

cryptococcosis (krip″to-kok-o′sis) a *Cryptococcus neoformans* fungal infection involving the lungs and spreading to any part or organ of the body, especially the central nervous system, fatal if untreated (also called *torulosis, Buschke's disease,* and *European blastomycosis*).

cytomegalovirus disease (CMV) herpes infection with large inclusion bodies in infected cells, most often found in salivary glands, ranging from asymptomatic to severe. Transmitted across the placental barrier, or, postnatally, through contact with body secretions, transfusions, renal and bone marrow transplants (postimmunosuppressive consequence), sexual relations, and kissing. It produces lesions throughout the body, particularly brain, liver, lungs, kidneys, and spleen (also called *salivary gland virus disease,* and, in infants, *cytomegalic inclusion disease*).

dengue (deng′e) eruptive febrile disease, caused by arbovirus infection transmitted by the Aedes mosquito, with rash and systemic symptoms. Although mild, it is so painful that it has been nicknamed "breakbone fever."

dengue hemorrhagic fever shock syndrome (DHFS) severe form of dengue fever, with all its symptoms plus hemorrhage, prostration, shock, and possible death. Common in tropical and subtropical regions, it is also transmitted by the Asian tiger mosquito, found in much of the United States.

Ebola hemorrhagic fever named for the river in Zaire (Congo), this lethal filovirus (threadlike virus) infects with symptoms of headache, fever, blood clots, and hemorrhages disseminated throughout the body, ultimately leading to death.

echinococcosis (e-ki"no-kok-ko′sis) a tapeworm, *Echinococcus granulosus*, infecting humans through drinking water, food, or hands contaminated by animal feces, produces hydatid cysts in liver and lungs (also called *hydatid disease*).

filariasis tropical parasitic disease, transmitted by a mosquito carrying *Filaria nematode* larvae, causing granulomatous inflammation and obstruction of lymph channels, with pain, blindness, swelling of extremities, and development of elephantiasis and pachyderma.

hantavirus diseases rodent-borne aerosol viruses producing a variety of diseases, including a severe hemorrhagic fever with chills, headache, respiratory, gastrointestinal, and renal involvement, found primarily in Asia. A pulmonary variety, found in the southwest United States, produces acute respiratory distress syndrome (ARDS). Another variety (Seoul) has been found in rats in many large U.S. cities and is suspected of causing acute and chronic renal disease and hypertension in humans.

infectious mononucleosis (mon"o-nu′kle-o′sis) acute, contagious, viral infection, caused by the Epstein-Barr virus (may be present in latent form in most human leukocytes and activated to pathogenicity by an immune suppression response), resulting in an abnormal increase in mononuclear leukocytes in the blood. Symptoms include fever, malaise, sore throat, lymphadenopathy, liver dysfunction, and enlarged spleen, with possible effect on the brain, meninges, and myocardium.

Kawasaki's disease childhood disease, etiology unknown, apparently noncontagious, usually appearing after a viral infection, with complete recovery in almost all cases. Symptoms include fever; reddening and inflammation of eyes, nose, mouth, and throat; red rash on the trunk; and swollen lymph glands and hands and feet, with desquamation of extremities. Complications include heart arrhythmias and coronary artery rupture (also called *mucocutaneous lymph node syndrome [MLNS]*).

leishmaniasis group of diseases, caused by one of a number of species of protozoa that belong to the genus *Leishmania*, transmitted to humans by the bite of insects. Varying symptoms include splenomegaly, cutaneous lesions, ulcers, granulomas, leukopenia, lymphatic involvement, and frequent involvement of the mucosal surfaces of the nose, mouth, and upper respiratory tract, which, if untreated, may be fatal to young children.

leprosy chronic communicable disease caused by the microorganism *Mycobacterium leprae*. Symptoms include granulomatous lesions in the skin, mucous membranes, and peripheral nervous system, which may result in progressive anesthesias, paralysis, ulceration, atrophies, gangrene, and mutilation (also called *Hansen's disease*).

Lyme disease tick-transmitted, spirochete-caused disease with symptoms of bull's-eye red rash, fever, headache, chills, nausea, vomiting, fatigue, muscle and joint pain, and swollen lymph glands, which, if not treated, progresses to a second stage that may affect joints (Lyme arthritis), the nervous system, or heart.

malaria protozoan parasitic (*Plasmodium* genus) infection transmitted through the bite of an infected female mosquito of the genus *Anopheles*. Involves the liver, spleen, and bone marrow and is characterized by recurrent attacks of chills, fever, and sweating.

mumps contagious viral infection affecting the salivary glands, usually the parotid, manifested by fever and inflammation, and if contracted after puberty, may affect the testes, ovaries, pancreas, and meninges (also called *parotitis*).

paratyphoid fever *Salmonella* bacterial infection similar to typhoid but not as severe, involving lymphoid mesenteric tissues and the intestines.

periarteritis nodosa inflammatory disease, etiology unknown, of the coats of the small- and medium-sized arteries of the body, with multiple-organ involvement, including nodular swellings, hypertension, jaundice, hepatomegaly, motor weakness, foot and wrist drop, and skin lesions (also called *polyarteritis* and *panarteritis*).

plague several types of bacterial infection caused by *Yersinia pestis*, with bubonic, the best known type, spread by fleas of infected rodents, and characterized by buboes (enlarged lymph nodes), occurring in femoral, inguinal, axillary, and cervical areas, with infection spread by the circulation. The pneumonic type is spread by person-to-person contact; both types are septicemic, involving lungs and other organs.

rat-bite fever two types, contracted from an infected rat or mouse bite: a Far Eastern type, *Spirillum minus* spirochetal infection characterized by relapsing fever, lymphadenopathy and rash, lasting 4 to 8 weeks, with relapses common (also called *sodoku*); a U.S. type, caused by *Streptobacillus moniliformis* bacterium, characterized by fever, headache, malaise, nausea, vomiting, and rash on soles and palms, lasting 2 weeks (also called *Haverhill fever*).

relapsing fever spirochetal infection caused by various species of *Borrelia* and transmitted to humans by the bite of a tick or louse, characterized by petechial rashes and febrile and afebrile periods, with enlargement of the liver and spleen accompanying the fever.

rheumatic fever delayed consequence of an upper respiratory tract infection in children, caused by group A hemolytic streptococci, producing multiple focal inflammatory lesions, which may develop into migratory arthritis, carditis, chorea, erythema marginatum, and subcutaneous nodules, with the acute phase limited, but involvement of the heart may lead to permanent valvular damage.

Rocky Mountain spotted fever tick-borne rickettsial infectious disease (*Rickettsia rickettsii*) transmitted to humans by bite, beginning with fever, myalgia, and weakness, and progressing to hemorrhagic lesions and a rash; may prove fatal without treatment (also called *mountain fever, mountain tick fever,* and *spotted fever*).

rubella viral infection transmitted by direct contact, with symptoms of macular rash, rhinorrhea, sore throat, and conjunctivitis, and with the ability to cross the placental barrier, possibly causing infection of the fetus, which, in the first trimester, may result in a high frequency of developmental abnormalities without interrupting the pregnancy (also called *German measles*).

rubeola highly contagious viral infection, spread by direct or indirect contact, affecting the respiratory tract and reticuloendothelial tissues, with skin eruptions in the form of red papules usually preceded by coryza, lymphadenitis, conjunctivitis, photophobia, myalgia, cough, and fever, and may be followed by complications of bacterial pneumonia, otitis media, and encephalitis (also called *measles*).

scarlet fever bacterial infection caused by a group A hemolytic *Streptococcus*, transmitted directly or indirectly, characterized by an erythematous rash, fever, enlarged cervical lymph nodes, and sore throat and may disseminate, involving many organs (also called *scarlatina*).

schistosomiasis (skis″to-so-mi′ah-sis) helminthic infection caused by a species of fluke of the genus *Schistosoma.* Transmitted by wading or bathing in water contaminated by human waste. Characterized by pain, obstruction, and anemia, involving the bladder, rectum, lungs, spleen, intestines, and liver and its portal venous system.

***Serratia* infection** a species of gram-negative bacteria, *Serratia* is responsible for nosocomial infections (acquired during hospitalization for other conditions) including respiratory and urinary system infections, as well as bacteremia.

smallpox acute contagious viral infection, transmitted by direct or indirect contact, characterized by an eruption of papules, vesicles and pustules, fever, and prostration, which may occur in hemorrhagic form in the kidneys and lungs, with possible complications of arthritis, osteomyelitis, and other conditions (also called *variola*).

sporotrichosis (spo″ro-tri′ko′sis) common chronic fungal infection caused by *Sporothrix schenckii,* characterized by skin ulcers and multiple subcutaneous granulomas along lymphatic channels, with rare involvement in muscles, joints, bones, and lungs.

syphilis contagious sexually transmitted disease caused by the spirochete *Treponema pallidum,* which can also be transmitted transplacentally to a fetus from an infected mother (congenital syphilis). It initially produces a primary lesion (a chancre), with multiple skin eruptions, especially on the trunk in the second stage, and progressing to a tertiary (third) stage involving multiple organs of the body, especially the heart, blood vessels, and the central nervous system.

TORCH syndrome acronym for fetal or neonatal infection by one of the following agents: *Toxoplasma gondii,* other (90% of infections), rubella virus, cytomegalovirus, and herpes simplex virus. TORCH complications may result in stillbirth, growth retardation, abortion, or premature delivery.

toxic shock syndrome (TSS) infectious condition involving a penicillin-resistant strain of *Staphylococcus aureus,* characterized by fever, diffuse macular erythroderma, desquamation of palms and soles, hypotension, and involvement of three or more systems, especially gastrointestinal (vomiting or diarrhea), muscular (myalgia), mucous membranes, kidneys, liver, circulatory, and central nervous system (disorientation and alterations of consciousness). Previously, there was a higher incidence among females, linked to the use of superabsorbent tampons, which were believed to provide a growth medium for the bacteria. A change in tampon construction has dropped the female incidence markedly, and the syndrome is now mainly associated with sequellae of various surgical procedures.

toxocariasis infection caused by ingestion of dirt containing larvae of roundworms found in fecal matter of dogs and cats. These larvae migrate throughout the body, lodging in various organs such as the lungs, liver, brain, and eyes.

toxoplasmosis *Toxoplasma gondii* protozoal infection, carried by cats and other hosts, of two types: lymphadenopathic—resembling mononucleosis, with a disseminated type widely distributed to brain, meninges, muscles, skin, heart, lungs, and liver, with lesions in any or all, and passed from infected mother to fetus; congenital type, with CNS involvement, including blindness, brain defect, and death.

trench fever *Rochalimaea quintana*, a *Rickettsia* infection transmitted by body lice, with weakness, fever, leg pains, and a macular rash.

trypanosomiasis (tri-pan″o-so-mi′ah-sis) protozoal infection of two types: a Central and South American type (Chagas' disease) caused by *Trypanosoma cruzi*, characterized by conjunctivitis and lesions caused by infected insect bites, with possible lymphatic, heart, and brain involvement; and an African trypanosomiasis, caused by *T. gambiense* or *T. rhodesiense*, transmitted by the tsetse fly, with the central nervous system as the main target (also called *sleeping sickness*).

tsutsugamushi fever (soot″soo-gah-moosh′e) *Rickettsia tsutsugamushi* infection, transmitted from infected rodents by the bite of lice, fleas, mites, or ticks, with headache, fever, chills, rash, and possible neurologic symptoms, vascular lesions, and lymphadenopathy (also called *scrub typhus*).

tularemia (too″lah-re′me-ah) bacterial infection caused by *Francisella tularensis*, which is transmitted by direct contact with infected animals, insect bite (especially tick, horsefly, or deerfly), handling contaminated animal products, or eating undercooked infected meat. It is characterized by suppurative or granulomatous lesions and septicemia and can also involve the skin, eyes, lungs, lymph glands, and more rarely, the meninges (also called *deerfly fever* and *rabbit fever*).

typhoid fever a bacterial infection caused by *Salmonella typhi*, transmitted directly or indirectly, with food and water as principal vehicles. Characterized by rash, fever, cough, headache, delirium, and diarrhea, followed by splenomegaly and leukopenia and possible gastrointestinal hemorrhage or perforation (also called *enteric fever*).

typhus group of infections caused by a species of *Rickettsia*, transmitted by infected lice, fleas, mites, and ticks, with the central nervous system as the main target, but it can involve other systems, with fatalities in 20% of untreated cases.

yaws tropical disease caused by a spirochete, *Treponema pertenue*, produced by direct contact with a lesion (yaw) of an infected person. It is characterized by a primary lesion, followed by a secondary stage skin eruption, and tertiary lesions (gummas and ulcers) of the bones.

yellow fever acute viral disease transmitted to humans in tropical regions by the bite of a mosquito, *Aedes aegypti*, involving the liver, gastrointestinal tract, and kidneys in a systemic spread, causing characteristic fever and jaundice.

Hereditary, Congenital, and Developmental Disorders

congenital hemihypertrophy one-sided overgrowth of part of the body.

cystic fibrosis genetic disorder causing dysfunction of sweat glands, affecting the pancreas and respiratory system, with decreased pancreatic enzymes in feces and excessive sodium and chloride loss in sweat, characterized by excessive fat in feces, malnutrition, viscid sputum, and bronchitis (also called *mucoviscidosis* and *fibrocystic disease of the pancreas*).

Danlos' syndrome hereditary symptom tetrad (having four parts), including excessive extensibility of joints, fragility of skin, hyperelasticity of skin, and pseudotumors following trauma (also called *Ehlers-Danlos syndrome*).

Down syndrome congenital condition characterized by some degree of mental retardation, with physical features including a broad short nose, protruding tongue, short broad neck, prominent abdomen, short phalanges, underdeveloped genitalia, rounded face, slanted eyes, and defects that may involve the eyes, ears, heart, and extremities. Results from chromosomal aberration, especially an extra chromosome 21, which is more likely to occur in infants born to older women, or from an extra chromosome translocated to the end of a larger chromosome and not related to maternal age (also called *mongolism* and *trisomy 21*).

Fanconi's syndrome rare, recessive, familial disease characterized by congenital hypoplasia of bone marrow with various congenital defects of the musculoskeletal and genitourinary systems; also a form of rickets beginning in early life, marked by hypophosphatemia, acidosis, and renal glycosuria.

fetal alcohol syndrome (FAS) developmental anomalies of the fetus, with growth deficiencies, limb and craniofacial defects, and mental retardation, caused by chronic alcoholism of the mother.

fragile X syndrome the second most common diagnosable cause of mental retardation after Down syndrome, with macroorchidism, craniofacial abnormalities, and neurologic problems, primarily affecting males, but carried by the mother.

gargoylism inherited type of dwarfism involving bone and other tissue, caused by a disturbance in carbohydrate metabolism, which appears to be the result of an absence of one or more of a group of enzymes that break down mucopolysaccharides. Noticeable physical characteristics appear early in life, including large head, coarse facial features, broad saddle nose, wide nostrils, thick lips and tongue, and an open-mouth expression, followed by dwarfism, skeletal deformities, mental retardation, hepatosplenomegaly, corneal opacities, deafness, and cardiovascular defects (also called *Hurler's syndrome* and *mucopolysaccharidosis*).

Gaucher's disease (go-shaz') hereditary splenic anemia, with Gaucher's cells found in the brain, pituitary gland, hypothalamus, kidneys, lungs, adrenals, thymus, and intestinal lymphatics, and lesions from tumorlike accumulations of these cells in the bones.

hepatolenticular degeneration (hep"ah-to-len-tik'u-lar) familial disorder of copper metabolism, with cirrhosis of liver, splenomegaly, and degenerative brain changes.

Klinefelter's syndrome (klin-fel'terz) gonadal abnormality caused by chromosomal aberrations of 47 chromosomes with an XXY sex chromosome, producing testicular dysgenesis and azoospermia, with possible gynecomastia and mental deficiency.

Laurence-Moon-Biedl syndrome autosomal recessive syndrome composed of a number of anomalies, consisting of obesity, hypogenitalism, retinitis pigmentosa, mental deficiency, skull defects, and sometimes, webbed fingers and toes.

Lindau-von Hippel disease hereditary condition involving angioma of the cerebellum, usually associated with hemangioma of the retina, polycystic pancreas and kidneys (also called *cerebroretinal angiomatosis* and *von Hippel-Lindau disease*).

Marfan's syndrome hereditary condition involving some skeletal, vascular and/or ophthalmic defects, such as long, thin extremities and fingers, loose joints, aortal aneurysm, and lens ectopia.

neurofibromatosis type 1 (NF-1) genetic disorder, with 50% probability of transmission by a gene-carrying parent. Half of all cases are not inherited, but arise from a spontaneous genetic mutation. The condition is characterized by café au lait spots, neurofibromas in many systems of the body, skeletal dysplasias, and optic gliomas, with no known cure or effective treatment (also known as *von Recklinghausen's disease*).

neurofibromatosis type 2 (NF-2) less common form of neurofibromatosis, characterized by bilateral acoustic neuromas, presenile cataracts, gliomas, and meningiomas, often leading to deafness (also called *central neurofibromatosis* and *bilateral acoustic neurofibromatosis*).

Niemann-Pick disease hereditary disturbance of infantile phosphatide metabolism, marked by anemia and a leukocytosis with an increase in lymphocytes, neural involvement, and an enlarged liver and spleen (also called *lipid histiocytosis* and *Neimann's disease*).

phenylketonuria (PKU) (fen"il-ke"to-nu're-ah) autosomal recessive congenital disorder of phenylalanine metabolism with phenylpyruvic acid present in the urine. It is characterized by central nervous system symptoms with resultant mental deficiency, treatable, when detected early, to minimize deterioration.

porphyria (por-fi're-ah) group of rare inherited disorders characterized by excessive production of porphyrins in the hematopoietic tissues of the bone marrow and liver, producing pigmentation of the face, facial deformation, hairiness in some cases, sensitivity to light (particularly sunlight), vomiting, and intestinal disturbances. Patients must avoid sunlight, and are treated by injections of heme, a blood product. The condition has been linked, in theory, to the development of the werewolf and vampire myths (deformed features, drinking of blood, hairiness, going out only at night), including the finding that garlic (which supposedly repels these creatures) contains a substance that exacerbates the condition.

Prader-Willi syndrome congenital metabolic condition caused by lack of normal secretion of gonadotropic pituitary hormone, producing hypotonia, short stature, obesity, hyperphagia, sexual infantilism, and mental retardation.

progeria, juvenile rare disorder, etiology not well established, in which growth ceases and premature aging signs appear. Includes symptoms such as graying of the hair, wrinkling of skin, generalized fibrosis and tissue atrophy, atherosclerosis, and connective tissue tumors, with death occurring early in life (also known as *Hutchinson-Gilford syndrome*).

proteus syndrome condition affecting multiple systems, especially characterized by lumps and tumors producing varying degrees of disfigurement (also known as *elephant man's disease*—previously confused with neurofibromatosis).

Turner's syndrome female gonadal abnormality, caused by chromosomal aberration of a total of 45 chromosomes with only one X chromosome, producing an XO female karyotype. Characterized by features of hypogonadism after puberty, such as amenorrhea, lack of breast development, delayed epiphyses closure, possible dwarfism, mental deficiency, cardiovascular anomalies, and deafness.

Werner's syndrome hereditary syndrome of adults producing premature senility, premature gray hair, spindly appearance of extremities, glossy skin, loss of subcutaneous fat tissue, hyperkeratosis with skin laceration, cataracts, arteriosclerosis, diabetes, and underdevelopment of the sexual organs.

Williams syndrome rare congenital disorder, characterized by slow growth, mental retardation, pixielike features, aortic stenosis, and abnormalities of other organs (also called *pixie disease*).

Other Multiple-System Disorders

amyloidosis accumulation of waxy, starchlike glycoprotein in body tissues, causing dysfunction; caused by heredity, a primary disturbance of endogenous protein metabolism, or following another disease.

beribeni (ber″e-ber′e) vitamin B_1 (thiamine) deficiency disease, occurring chiefly in the Far East, resulting from a diet of polished rice, with symptoms including edema, cardiac pathology, and neuritis.

Caisson disease condition producing nitrogen bubbles in body tissues, affecting aviators, deep-sea divers, and others who work at great depths; caused by rapid pressure changes, causing disorientation, pain, and syncope (also called *bends* or *decompression sickness*).

calcinosis condition of unknown etiology, with deposition of calcium salts in skin, muscles, tendons, nerves, and bones.

cheilosis (ki-lo′sis) disease of riboflavin deficiency, characterized by fissures and scaling of the lips.

collagen diseases group of conditions in which collagen tissue is involved, occurring in rheumatic fever, systemic lupus erythematosus, scleroderma, and dermatomyositis, and other connective tissue diseases.

Cushing's syndrome pituitary basophilism, with excessive secretion of adrenocortical hormone, characterized by obesity, moon-face, oligomenorrhea in women, and lowered testosterone levels in men, with additional involvement of osteoporosis, hypertension, kyphosis, polycythemia, and muscular weakness in both sexes (also called *hypercortisolism*).

Dercum's disease condition occurring mainly in females, accompanied by painful fatty swellings and nerve lesions, which may cause death from lung complications (also called *adiposis dolorosa*).

erythroblastosis fetalis (e-rith″ro-blas-to′sis) excessive destruction of red blood cells, with overdevelopment of the erythropoietic tissues and/or organs. It becomes evident late in fetal life, or soon after birth, as a result of transplacental passage of an anti-Rh antibody produced in an Rh-negative mother as a reaction to the Rh-positive red cells of the fetus or by a transfusion of Rh-positive blood, with a possibility of also having an ABO incompatibility (also called *hemolytic disease of the newborn*).

gout condition in which there are urate deposits in the cartilages of the joints and an excess of uric acid in the blood, manifested by acute arthritic attacks, with some forms of gout involving severe constitutional disturbances, including renal impairment.

hemochromatosis disorder of iron metabolism that may arise from exogenous, idiopathic, or hereditary causes. Characterized by bronze pigmentation of the skin, diabetes mellitus, and hepatomegaly, with deposition of iron in parenchymal cells throughout much of the body, with liver cells particularly affected, and cirrhosis usually present (also called *bronze diabetes*).

ochronosis inherited or exogenous metabolic condition involving lack of homogentisic acid oxidase activity in the kidney and liver. It is preceded by alkaptonuria, with a peculiar discoloration of body tissues, resulting from the deposit of alkapton bodies in the sweat glands, sclera, cornea, conjunctiva, eyelids, and ears, as well as in the cardiovascular and genitourinary systems.

plumbism (plum′bizm) form of poisoning caused by the absorption of lead or one of the salts of lead. Symptoms include loss of appetite, colic, insomnia, headache, dizziness, and more severe conditions extending to albuminuria, hypertension, anemia, and neuropathy with paralysis. It is commonly found in children who eat lead paint chips in poorly maintained lead-painted quarters, with resulting encephalopathy and secondary mental retardation (*plumbum* means lead).

polycythemia vera disease, etiology unknown, involving increase in red blood cell mass and total blood volume, producing splenomegaly, flushed face, and ecchymosis of the skin, with symptoms including headache, vertigo, and epistaxis (also called *Osler's disease*).

Reye's syndrome acute, noncontagious, childhood condition of unknown etiology (failure of the immune system is suspected, along with toxins that might unbalance metabolism and lead to liver damage). It is characterized by encephalopathy and fatty hepatomegaly, with brain swelling and central nervous system damage, generally following viral infections, especially influenza A and B strains, and chickenpox, and usually beginning with fever, vomiting, fatigue, apathy, and progressing, if untreated, to coma and death in a proportion of cases (with some studies linking aspirin medication for viral conditions to toxicity that produces liver and brain damage).

sarcoidosis chronic disorder, etiology unknown, characterized by multisystem granulomatous formations in mucous membranes, lacrimal and salivary glands, liver, spleen, lungs, skin, and lymph nodes.

scleroderma disease involving hardening and shrinking of connective tissues, manifested by dermal fibrosis and fixation of the skin to underlying organs or structures, characterized by weakness, joint pains, edema of hands, and Raynaud's phenomenon. This syndrome is characterized by paroxysmal ischemia of the digits, progressing to systemic organ changes affecting skin, heart, esophagus, kidneys, lungs, etc. It can appear in a diffuse form with progressive fibrosis of internal organs, as well as of the skin of the trunk, face, and extremities (also called *systemic sclerosis*).

sudden infant death syndrome (SIDS) a seemingly healthy infant placed in a crib is later found dead. The etiology is unknown and no single mechanism has been found responsible. SIDS babies may have defects of adaptation, with current views focusing on abnormal sleep patterns related to disturbed autonomic activity, on vagus nerve and cardiorespiratory reactions, and immunologic, metabolic, and endocrine factors. It is now recommended that babies be placed on their backs for sleep. Monitoring systems have been developed that set off alarms when the breathing pattern is interrupted for an excessive period (also called *crib death*).

systemic lupus erythematosus (SLE) chronic disease of suspected autoimmune origin involving many organ systems individually or in a variety of combinations, including a generalized connective tissue disease for which diagnosis is made by the lupus erythematosus test (LE cell prep) and antinuclear antibody test (ANA). Most patients have arthralgia, less than half have the classic butterfly rash, some have renal disease, some have pleural effusion, and, commonly, anorexia, nausea, vomiting, abdominal pain, and lymphadenopathy are present. Exposure to sunlight or ultraviolet radiation exacerbates the disease.

Oncology*

adenocarcinoma* malignant epithelial neoplasm appearing throughout the different systems of the body, such as salivary glands, bronchi, large intestine, connective tissue, kidneys, etc.

carcinomatosis* widespread dissemination of cancer throughout the body (also called *carcinosis*).

Kaposi's sarcoma* (kap'a-sez) malignant neoplasm occurring in the skin and metastasizing to the lymph nodes and viscera, beginning with purplish papules on the feet that slowly spread, occurring most often in men, and associated with malignant lymphoma, diabetes, and other disorders (also called *multiple idiopathic hemorrhagic sarcoma*; see also under *acquired immune deficiency syndrome*).

LABORATORY TESTS

antinuclear antibody test (ANA) blood test to measure levels of ANA. Increased levels are positive for systemic lupus erythematosus, rheumatoid arthritis, chronic hepatitis, periarteritis nodosa, dermatomyositis, scleroderma, infectious mononucleosis, Raynaud's disease, and other diseases.

lupus erythematosus test (LE cell prep) blood test to diagnosis and monitor treatment for systemic lupus erythematosus.

sweat electrolytes test detects elevations of sodium and chloride levels in sweat, for diagnosis of cystic fibrosis.

trypsin activity test test on fecal matter to detect trypsin, for diagnosis of fibrocystic disease of sweat glands and other organs.

*Indicates a malignant condition.

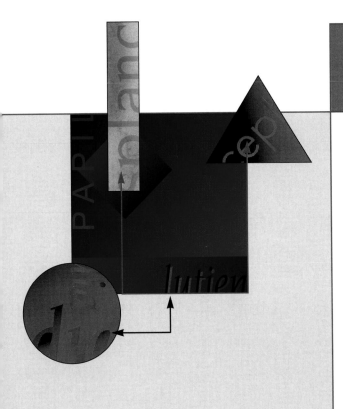

Adding to the Structure

This is the last of the five sections of *Learning Medical Terminology*. This section completes the building process by including the answers to all of the questions, exercises, and puzzles within the text, as well as additional enrichment material.

Appendix A lists commonly used abbreviations and symbols. Appendix B contains Latin and Greek combining forms that relate to numbers. The metric system and English equivalents for linear measures, weights, volumes, and temperatures make up Appendix C.

Samples of diverse types of hospital records and reports are presented in Appendix D. Appendix E covers medical insurance, managed care, and health maintenance programs. The various board-regulated medical specialties in the United States are listed in Appendix F. The answers to the chapter Review Questions, Exercises, and Puzzles appear in Appendix G.

Abbreviations and Symbols

A

A accommodation; acetum; angstrom unit; anode; anterior

a accommodation ampere; anterior; area

āā of each

A₂ aortic second sound (valve closure)

AB; ab abortion

Abd. abdomen

ABGs arterial blood gases

ABO three basic blood groups

AC alternating current; air conduction; axiocervical; adrenal cortex

a.c. before meals (*ante cibum*)

acc. accommodation

ACE adrenocortical extract

ACh acetylcholine

ACH adrenocortical hormone

ACTH adrenocorticotropic hormone

A.D. right ear (*auris dextra*)

ad lib. as much as desired (*ad libitum*)

add add to

ADH antidiuretic hormone

ADHD attention-deficit hyperactivity disorder

ADS antidiuretic substance

A/G; A-G ratio albumin-globulin ratio

Ag silver

ah hypermetropic astigmatism

AHF antihemophilic factor

AI aortic insufficiency

AIDS acquired immune deficiency syndrome

aj ankle jerk

Al aluminum

alb albumin

ALH combined sex hormone of anterior lobe of hypophysis

ALL acute lymphocytic leukemia

ALS amyotrophic lateral sclerosis

ALT alanine aminotransferase (formerly SGPT)

Alt. dieb. every other day (*alternis diebus*)

Alt. hor. alternate hours (*alternis horis*)

Alt. noct. alternate nights (*alternis noctes*)

Am mixed astigmatism

A.M.A.; a.m.a. against medical advice

AML acute myelocytic leukemia

amp ampule

ana so much of each

AO anodal opening; atrioventricular valve openings

AOP anodal opening picture

AOS anodal opening sound

A-P; AP; A/P anterior-posterior

A.P. anterior pituitary gland

A & P auscultation and percussion

APA antipernicious anemia factor

AQ achievement quotient

Aq water (*aqua*)

ARC AIDS-related complex; anomalous retinal correspondence

ARDS acute respiratory distress syndrome

ARF acute renal failure

arg silver

A.S. left ear (*auris sinistra*)

As arsenic

ASD atrial septal defect

ASH asymmetric septal hypertrophy

AsH hypermetropic astigmatism

ASHD arteriosclerotic heart disease

AsM myopic astigmatism

ASS anterior superior spine

AST aspartate aminotransferase (formerly SGOT)

Ast; As astigmatism

ATS anxiety tension state; antitetanic serum

AU both ears; Angstrom unit

Au gold

A-V; AV; A/V arteriovenous; atrioventricular

Av average; avoirdupois

AVR aortic valve replacement

ax axis; axillary

B

B boron; bacillus

Ba barium

BAC buccoaxiocervical

Bact bacterium

BBB blood-brain barrier; bundle branch block

BBT basal body temperature

BE barium enema

Be Beryllium

BFP biologically false positivity (in syphilis tests)

Bi bismuth

Bib drink

bid; b.i.d. twice a day (*bis in die*)

BM bowel movement

BMR basal metabolic rate

BMT bone marrow transplant

BP blood pressure; buccopulpal

bp boiling point

BPH benign prostatic hypertrophy

BRP bathroom privileges

BSA body surface area

BSP　bromsulphalein

BUN　blood urea nitrogen

BWS　battered woman syndrome

bx　biopsy

C

C　carbon; centigrade; Celsius

c̄　with

C_{alb}　albumin clearance

C_{cr}　creatinine clearance

C_{in}　inulin clearance

CA　chronologic age; cervicoaxial

Ca　cancer; calcium

CABG　coronary artery bypass graft

$CaCO_3$　calcium carbonate

CAD　coronary artery disease

Cal　large calorie

cal　small calorie

Cap.　let him take (*capiat*)

CBC; cbc　complete blood count

CC　chief complaint

cc　cubic centimeter

CCl_4　carbon tetrachloride

CCU　coronary care unit

CF　cystic fibrosis

cf　compare; bring together

CFT　complement-fixation test

Cg; Cgm　centigram

CH　crown-heel (length of fetus)

$CHCl_3$　chloroform

CH_3COOH　acetic acid

CHD　coronary heart disease

ChE　cholinesterase

CHF　congestive heart failure

$C_5H_4N_4O_3$　uric acid

C_2H_5OH　ethyl alcohol

CH_2O　formaldehyde

CH_3OH　methyl alcohol

Cl　chlorine

CLD　chronic liver disease

CLL　chronic lymphocytic leukemia

cm　centimeter

CMR　cerebral metabolic rate

cms　to be taken tomorrow morning (*cras mane sumendus*)

CMV　cytomegalovirus

c.n.　tomorrow night (*cras nocte*)

CNS　central nervous system

c.n.s.　to be taken tomorrow night (*cras nocte sumendus*)

CO　carbon monoxide

CO_2　carbon dioxide

Co　cobalt

COPD　chronic obstructive pulmonary disease

CPC　clinicopathologic conference

CPD　cephalopelvic disproportion

CPR　cardiopulmonary resuscitation

CR　crown-rump length (length of fetus)

CRF　chronic renal failure

C-section; CS　cesarean section

CSF　cerebrospinal fluid

CSM　cerebrospinal meningitis

CT; CAT　computerized (axial) tomography scan

CTS　carpal tunnel syndrome

Cu　copper

$CuSO_4$　copper sulfate

CVA　cerebrovascular accident; costovertebral angle

CVD　cardiovascular disease

cyl　cylinder

D

D　dose; vitamin D; right (*dexter*)

DAH　disordered action of the heart

D/C　discontinue

D & C　dilation (dilatation) and curettage

DC　direct current

DCA　deoxycorticosterone acetate

Deg　degeneration; degree

Det.　let it be given (*detur*)

dg　decigram

dieb. tert.　every third day (*diebus tertiis*)

diff　differential blood count

dil　dilute; dissolve

dim　one half

DCE　discoid lupus erythematosus

DNA　deoxyribonucleic acid

DOA　dead on arrival

DOB　date of birth

DPT　diphtheria, pertussis, tetanus (vaccine)

DRG　diagnosis-related group

dr　dram; ʒ

DSM　*Diagnostic and Statistical Manual of Mental Disorders*

DTR　deep tendon reflex

DTs　delerium tremens

Dx　diagnosis

E

E　eye

EAHF　eczema, asthma, and hayfever

EBV　Epstein-Barr virus

ECG; EKG　electrocardiogram; electrocardiograph

ECHO　echocardiogram; echocardiography

ECT　electroconvulsive therapy

ED　erythema dose; effective dose

ED_{50}　median effective dose

EDC　estimated date of confinement

EEG　electroencephalogram; electroencephalograph

EENT　eye, ear, nose, and throat

ELISA　enzyme-linked immunosorbent assay (AIDS test)

Em　emmetropia

EMB　endometrial biopsy; eosin-methylene blue

EMC　encephalomyocarditis

EMF　erythrocyte maturation factor

EMG　electromyogram

EMS　Emergency Medical Service

ENT　ear, nose, and throat

EOM　extraocular movement

EPR　electrophrenic respiration

ER　emergency room (hospital); external resistance

ERG　electroretinogram

ERPF　effective renal plasma flow

ERT　estrogen replacement therapy

ESR　erythrocyte sedimentation rate

EST　electroshock therapy

Et　ethyl

ext　extract

F

F　Fahrenheit; field of vision; formula

FA　fatty acid

FANA　fluorescent antinuclear antibody (test)

F & R　force and rhythm (pulse)

FBS　fasting blood sugar

FD　fatal dose; focal distance

FDA　Food and Drug Administration

Fe　iron

$FeCl_3$　ferric chloride

FH　family history

Fl; fld　fluid

fl dr; fl. dr.　fluid dram

fl oz; fl. oz. fluid ounce
FR flocculation reaction
FSH follicle-stimulating hormone
ft foot
FUO fever of undetermined origin

G

GA gingivoaxial
galv galvanic
GB gallbladder
GBS gallbladder series
GC gonococcus; gonorrhea
GFR glomerular filtration rate
GH growth hormone
GI gastrointestinal
GL greatest length (small flexed embryo)
GLA gingivolinguoaxial
Gm; gm; g gram
GP general practitioner; general paresis
gr grain(s)
Grad. by degrees (*gradatim*)
Grav I, II, III, etc.; Grav 1, 2, 3, etc. pregnancy one, two, three, etc. (*gravida*)
GSW gunshot wound
gt drop (*gutta*)
GTT glucose tolerance test
gtt drops (*guttae*)
GU genitourinary
Gyn gynecology

H

H hydrogen
Hb; Hgb hemoglobin
H₃BO₃ boric acid
HBV hepatitis B-virus vaccine
HCG human chorionic gonadotropin
HCl hydrochloric acid
HCN hydrocyanic acid
H₂CO₃ carbonic acid
HCT; Hct hematocrit
HCVD hypertensive cardiovascular disease
HD hearing distance; hemodialysis
h.d. at bedtime (*hora decubitus*)
HDL high-density lipoprotein
HDLW distance at which a watch is heard by the left ear
HDRW distance at which a watch is heard by the right ear

He helium
HEENT head, eye, ear, nose, and throat
Hg mercury
Hgb hemoglobin
HIV human immunodeficiency virus
HNO₃ nitric acid
H₂O water
H₂O₂ hydrogen peroxide
HOP high oxygen pressure
h.s. at bedtime (*hora somni*)
HSV herpes simplex virus
H₂SO₄ sulfuric acid
Ht; ht height; total hyperopia
Hy hyperopia

I

I iodine
¹³¹I radioactive isotope of iodine (atomic weight 131)
¹³²I radioactive isotope of iodine (atomic weight 132)
IBD inflammatory bowel disease
ICP intracranial pressure
ICS; IS intercostal space
ICSH interstitial cell–stimulating hormone
ICT inflammation of connective tissue
ICU intensive care unit
Id. the same (*idem*)
I & D incision and drainage
IH infectious hepatitis
IHD ischemic heart disease
IM intramuscular; infectious mononucleosis
IOP intraocular pressure
IQ intelligence quotient
IU immunizing unit
IUD intrauterine device
IV intravenous
IVP intravenous pyelogram
IVT intravenous transfusion
IVU intravenous urogram; intravenous urography

K

K potassium
k constant
Ka cathode; kathode
KBr potassium bromide
ke kilocycle

KCl potassium chloride
kev kilo electron volts
Kg kilogram
KI potassium iodide
kj knee jerk
km kilometer
KOH potassium hydroxide
KS Kaposi's sarcoma
KUB kidney, ureter, and bladder
kv kilovolt
kw kilowatt

L

L left; liter; length; lumbar; lethal; pound
L & A light and accommodation
lb pound (*libra*)
LB large bowel (x-ray film)
LBBB left bundle branch block
LCM left costal margin
LD lethal dose; perception of light difference
LDL low-density lipoprotein
LE lupus erythematosus
l.e.s. local excitatory state
LFD least fatal dose of a toxin
LFTs liver function tests
LH luteinizing hormone
Li lithium
LIF left iliac fossa
lig ligament
Liq liquor
LLL left lower lobe (of lung)
LLQ left lower quadrant
LMP last menstrual period
LP lumbar puncture
LPF leukocytosis-promoting factor
LTH luteotrophic hormone
LUL left upper lobe (of lung)
LUQ left upper quadrant
LV left ventricle
L & W living and well

M

M myopia; meter; muscle; thousand
m meter
MA mental age
Mag large (*magnus*)
MBD minimal brain dysfunction
μCi; μc microcurie

μμ micromicron

mcg; μg microgram

MCH mean corpuscular hemoglobin

MCHC mean corpuscular hemoglobin concentration

mCi; mc millicurie

MCV mean corpuscular volume

Me methyl

MED minimal erythema dose; minimal effective dose

mEq millequivalent

mEq/L milliequivalent per liter

ME ratio myeloid-erythroid ratio

MG myasthenia gravis

Mg magnesium

mg milligram

MHD minimal hemolytic dose

MI myocardial infarction

MID minimum infective dose

ML midline

ml milliliter

MLD median lethal dose; minimum lethal dose

MM mucous membrane

mm millimeter; muscles

mmHg millimeters of mercury

mμ millimicron

Mn manganese

mN millinormal

MRI magnetic resonance imaging

MS multiple sclerosis; mitral stenosis; morphine sulfate

MSL midsternal line

MT medical technologist; tympanic membrane (*membrane tympani*)

mu mouse unit

MVP mitral valve prolapse

My myopia

N

N nitrogen

n normal

Na sodium

NaBr sodium bromide

NaCl sodium chloride

Na₂C₂O₄ $Na_2C_2O_4$ sodium oxalate

Na₂CO₃ Na_2CO_3 sodium carbonate

NAD no appreciable disease

NaF sodium fluoride

NaHCO₃ $NaHCO_3$ sodium bicarbonate

Na₂HPO₄ Na_2HPO_4 sodium phosphate

NaI sodium iodide

NaNO₃ $NaNO_3$ sodium nitrate

Na₂O₂ Na_2O_2 sodium peroxide

NaOH sodium hydroxide

Na₂SO₄ Na_2SO_4 sodium sulfate

NCA neurocirculatory asthenia

Ne neon

NG tube; NGT nasogastric tube

NH₃ NH_3 ammonia

Ni nickel

NPN nonprotein nitrogen

NPO; n.p.o. nothing by mouth (*nil* [or *non*] *per os*)

NRC normal retinal correspondence

NSAID nonsteroidal antiinflammatory drug

NTP normal temperature and pressure

NYD not yet diagnosed

O

O oxygen; oculus; pint

O₂ O_2 oxygen; both eyes

O₃ O_3 ozone

OB obstetrics

OB/GYN obstetrics and gynecology

OBS organic brain syndrome

OD right eye (*oculus dexter*); optical density, overdose

o.d. once a day (*omni die*)

Ol oil (*oleum*)

o.m. every morning (*omni mane*)

o.n. every night (*omni nocte*)

OPD outpatient department

OR operating room

O.S. left eye (*oculus sinister*)

os opening; mouth; bone

OT occupational therapy

OTD organ tolerance dose

OU each eye (*oculus uterque*)

oz ounce; ℥

P

P phosphorus; pulse; pupil

P₂ pulmonic second sound

P-A; P/A; PA posterior-anterior

P & A percussion and auscultation

PAB; PABA paraaminobenzoic acid

Pap test Papanicolaou smear

Para I, II, III, etc.; Para 1,2,3, etc. live births: unipara, bipara, tripara, etc.

PAS; PASA paraaminosalicylic acid

Pb lead

PBI protein-bound iodine

PCP *Pneumocystis carinii* pneumonia; phencyclidine hydrochloride (angel dust hallucinogen)

PCV packed cell volume

PD pupillary distance; prism diopter

PDA patent ductus arteriosus

PDR *Physicians' Desk Reference*

PE physical examination; physical education

PEG pneumoencephalography, percutaneous endoscopic gastrostomy

PET positron emission tomography

PFF protein-free filtrate

PGA pteroylglutamic acid (folic acid)

PH past history

pH hydrogen ion concentration (alkalinity and acidity measure)

Pharm; Phar. pharmacy

PI previous illness

PID pelvic inflammatory disease

PK psychokinesis

PKU phenylketonuria

PL light perception

PM postmortem; evening

PMB polymorphonuclear basophil leukocytes

PME polymorphonuclear eosinophil leukocytes

PMI point of maximal impulse

PMN polymorphonuclear neutrophil leukocytes

PMS premenstrual syndrome

PN percussion note

PNH paroxysmal nocturnal hemoglobinuria

PO; p.o. orally (*per os*)

p/o postoperative

PPD purified protein derivative (test for tuberculosis)

Pr presbyopia; prism

PRN; p.r.n. as required (*pro re nata*)

pro time prothrombin time (blood clotting test)

PSA prostate-specific antigen

PSP phenolsulfonphthalein (intravenous dye to test renal function)

PT physical therapy

Pt platinum; patient

pt pint

PTA plasma thromboplastin antecedent

PTC plasma thromboplastin component

Pu plutonium

PUO pyrexia of unknown origin

PVC premature ventricular contraction; pulmonary venous congestion

PVD peripheral vascular disease

PZI protamine zinc insulin

Q

Q electric quantity

q. every, each

q.d. every day (*quaque die*)

q.h. every hour (*quaque hora*)

q.h.s. each bedtime (*quaque hora somni*)

qid; q.i.d. four times daily (*quater in die*)

q.l. as much as desired (*quantum libet*)

q.n. every night (*quaque nocte*)

qns quantity not sufficient

q.o.d. every other day (*quaque otro die*)

q.p. as much as desired (*quantum placeat*)

q.s. sufficient quantity

qt quart

Quat four (*quattuor*)

q.v. as much as you please (*quantum vis*)

R

R respiration; right; *Rickettsia;* roentgen

Ra radium

rad unit of measurement of the absorbed dose of ionizing radiation

RAI radioactive iodine

RAIU radioactive iodine uptake

RBC; rbc red blood cell; red blood count

RCD relative cardiac dullness

RCM right costal margin

RE right eye; reticuloendothelial tissue; reticuloendothelial cell

Re rhenium

rect rectified

Reg umb umbilical region

REM rapid eye movement

Rep. let it be repeated (*repetatur*)

RES reticuloendothelial system

RF rheumatoid factor

Rh symbol of rhesus factor; symbol for rhodium

RhA rheumatoid arthritis

RHD relative hepatic dullness

RIA radioimmunoassay

RLL right lower lobe (of lung)

RLQ right lower quadrant

RM respiratory movement

RML right middle lobe (of lung)

Rn radon

RNA ribonucleic acid

R/O rule out

ROM range of motion

RPF renal plasma flow

RPM; rpm revolutions per minute

RPS renal pressor substance

RQ respiratory quotient

RT radiation therapy

RUL right upper lobe (of lung)

RUQ right upper quadrant

Rx take; prescription, therapy

S

S sulfur

S. sacral

s̄ without (*sine*)

S-A; S/A; SA sinoatrial

SB small bowel (x-ray film)

SC closure of semilunar valves

Se selenium

SD skin dose

Sed rate; SR sedimentation rate

seq. luce the following day (*sequenti luce*)

SGOT serum glutamic oxaloacetic transaminase (see **AST**)

SGPT serum glutamic pyruvic transaminase (see **ALT**)

SH serum hepatitis

Si silicon

SIDS sudden infant death syndrome

SLE systemic lupus erythematosus

Sn tin

SOB shortness of breath

Sol solution

sp spirit

SPECT single-photon emission computed tomography

sp. gr.; sp. G. specific gravity

Sr strontium

s̄s̄ one half (*semis*)

Staph *Staphylococcus*

Stat immediately (*statim*)

STD sexually transmitted disease

STH somatotrophic hormone

Strep *Streptococcus*

STS serologic test for syphilis

Sym symmetrical

T

T temperature; thoracic

t temporal

T₃ triiodothyronine

T₄ thyroxine

TA therapeutic abortion

TAT tetanus antitoxin; toxin-antitoxin; thematic apperception test

T & A tonsillectomy and adenoidectomy

tab tablet

TAM toxoid-antitoxoid mixture

TB tuberculin; tuberculosis; tubercle bacillus

TE tetanus

TEM triethylene melamine

TENS transcutaneous electrical nerve stimulation

Th thorium

TIA transient ischemic attack

TIBC total iron-binding capacity

tid; t.i.d. three times daily (*ter in die*)

Tl thallium

TLC tender, loving care

Tm maximal tubular excretory capacity (kidneys)

TP tuberculin precipitation

TPI *Treponema pallidum* immobilization (test for syphilis)

TPR temperature, pulse, and respiration

tr tincture

TRU turbidity-reducing unit

TS test solution

TSH thyroid-stimulating hormone

TUR; TURP transurethral resection of prostate

T.V. tidal volume

Tx treatment

U

U uranium; unit

UA urinalysis

UBI ultraviolet blood irradiation
UIBC unsaturated iron-binding capacity
Umb; umb umbilicus
ung. ointment *(unguentum)*
URI upper respiratory infection
US; U/S ultrasonic
USP *U.S. Pharmacopeia*
Ut dict. as directed *(ut dictum)*
UTI urinary tract infection
UV ultraviolet

V

V vanadium; vision; visual acuity
v volt
VA visual acuity
VC vital capacity
VD venereal disease
VDA visual discriminatory acuity
VDG venereal disease–gonorrhea
VDM vasodepressor material

VDRL Venereal Disease Research Laboratories (test for syphilis)
VDS venereal disease–syphilis
VEM vasoexciter material
VF field of vision
VHD valvular heart disease
VIA virus inactivating agent
VLDL very-low-density lipoprotein
VMA vanillylmandelic acid
VR vocal resonance
VS vital signs; volumetric solution
Vs venisection
VsB bleeding in arm *(venaesectio brachii)*
VSD ventricular septal defect
VW vessel wall

W

w watt
WBC; wbc white blood cell; white blood count

WD well-developed
WL wavelength
WN well-nourished
WR Wassermann reaction
Wt; wt weight

X

x-ray roentgen ray

Z

z symbol for atomic number
Zn zinc

SYMBOLS

> greater than
< less than
♀ female
♂ male

Latin and Greek Combining Forms for English Numbers

Number	Latin term	Greek term
one	uni-	mon-, mono-
two	duo-	dy-, dyo-
three	tri-	tri-
four	quadri-, quadr-	tetr-, tetra-
five	quinqu-	pent-, penta-
six	sex-	hex-, hexa-
seven	sept-, septi-	hept-, hepta-
eight	octo-	oct-, octa-, octo-
nine	novem-, nonus-	ennea-
ten	deca-, decem-	dek-, deka-
one half	semi-	hemi-
one and one half	sesqui-	
one hundred	centi-	hect-, hecto-, hecato-
one thousand	milli-	kilo-
one-hundredth part	centi-	
one-thousandth part	milli-	
first	primi-	prot-, proto-
second	secundi-	deut-, deuto-, deutero
third	tert-	trit-, trito-
fourth	quart-	
fifth	quint-	
ninth	non-, nona-	
twice, duplication	di-, dis-	dys-

The Metric System and Equivalents

The basis of measurement in science is a standard one, the metric system, in which the chief units are the meter, the gram, and the liter, which are always multiplied and divided by 10. Although the English system is still used in the United States, the metric system is the preferred system in medicine because of its logic and accuracy.

UNITS OF LENGTH

Metric Linear Decimal Scale and English (U.S.) Equivalents

10 millimeters	= 1 centimeter	= 0.3937 inches
10 centimeters	= 1 decimeter	= 3.937 inches
10 decimeters	= 1 meter	= 39.37 inches (3.2808 feet)
10 meters	= 1 dekameter	= 10.936 yards
10 dekameters	= 1 hectometer	= 19.884 rods
10 hectometers	= 1 kilometer	= 0.62137 mile
10 kilometers	= 1 myriameter	= 6.2137 miles
1 inch		= 2.54 centimeters *or* 25.4 millimeters
1 foot		= 3.048 decimeters *or* 304.8 millimeters
1 yard		= 0.9144 meter *or* 914.40 millimeters
1 rod		= 0.5029 dekameter
1 mile		= 1.6093 kilometers

UNITS OF WEIGHT

Metric Weights and English (U.S.) Equivalents

1 milligram	= 0.001 gram	= 0.015 grain
1 centigram	= 0.01 gram	= 0.154 grain
1 decigram	= 0.10 gram	= 1.543 grains
1 gram	= (1 gram)	= 0.035 ounce
1 dekagram	= 10 grams	= 0.353 ounce
1 hectogram	= 100 grams	= 3.527 ounces
1 kilogram	= 1000 grams	= 2.205 pounds
1 grain	= 0.0648 gram	
1 ounce	= 28.349 grams	
1 pound	= 0.453 kilogram	

UNITS OF VOLUME

Metric Liquid Measure Capacity and English (U.S.) Equivalents

1 milliliter (cc)		= 16.23 minims *or* 0.2705 fluidram *or* 0.0338 fluidounce
1 liter		= 33.8148 fluidounces *or* 2.1134 pints *or* 1.0567 quarts *or* 0.2642 gallon
1 fluidram		= 3.697 milliliters
1 fluidounce		= 29.573 milliliters
1 pint	= 16 ounces	= 473.166 milliliters *or* 0.473 liter
1 quart	= 2 pints	= 946.332 milliliters *or* 0.946 liter
1 gallon	= 4 quarts	= 3.785 liters

TEMPERATURE EQUIVALENTS

Conversion Rules

To convert Fahrenheit to Centigrade (Celsius), subtract 32 from the Fahrenheit temperature and multiply that figure by 5/9.

To convert Centigrade (Celsius) to Fahrenheit, multiply the Centigrade temperature by 9/5 and add 32 to the total.

Hospital Records and Reports

There are many different medical reports that are part of a patient's hospital record, such as the diagnostic evaluation and pathologic and x-ray findings.

A notation of surgical instruments, techniques, and medications used is a part of hospital records, and the medical secretary must consult reference sources and medical dictionaries to spell these names correctly. Names of drugs, in particular, change from year to year, but each medical records department should have a copy of the *Physicians' Desk Reference (PDR)*, as well as a list of approved drugs published by the American Medical Association. The names of surgical instruments and techniques may also be found in various references available in the medical records department. Correct identification and spelling should present no problem when sources for reference are available.

Not all reports follow the same format. Each facility has specific forms for particular reports. The sampling in this appendix is to familiarize the reader with a variety of records and reports. Many of the medical terms in the reports have been italicized to further assist in learning medical language.

ADMISSION NOTE

Neurologic Hospital Report

This 5-year-old black male child was admitted to the emergency room shortly after being involved in a two-car accident. Apparently, the patient was thrown about 20 feet from the car into a ditch. He was unconscious when removed from the ditch by ambulance drivers shortly after the accident. He was then taken to a nearby hospital, where he was examined. It is reported that the patient appeared to be having intermittent convulsive activity and that his pupils were midposition and reactive, with the left pupil possibly larger than the right. He was transferred to the Neurologic Hospital for further evaluation.

On admission to the emergency room of the Neurologic Hospital, he is said to have been having seizure activity, or at least some activity of rigid contraction of muscles, more or less in extension but with no true *clonic* seizure activity, and vomiting.

When seen by a neurologist a short while later, the patient was not having any seizure activity but was actually making some semipurposive movements with his extremities. He moved his extremities reflexly in response to pain, the movement being generally somewhat extensor in type but not true *decerebrate rigidity. Babinski's signs* were easily elicited. The patient was *comatose* but not groaning. He had rapid breathing with a definite tendency toward periodicity, suggesting *Cheyne-Stokes respiration.*

The patient's pupils were midposition and promptly reactive to light. They were sometimes equal in size, and sometimes the left was slightly larger than the right. *Optic fundi* and *otoscopic* examinations were negative. There was a 4-cm *semilunar* laceration in the right *parietal* region.

The left side of the thorax was dull to percussion, but the breath sounds were equal on the two sides. Abdomen was lax. There was no evidence of *intracranial* bleeding. There was a *contusion* of the right elbow and a contusion of the posterior thorax bilaterally that appeared a short while later. From the beginning, a dark discoloration was noted in the midthorax posteriorly. There was no *crepitus* on palpation over the thorax.

There was a healed incision from a cutdown on the *left greater saphenous vein* in the past, and there was a *pilonidal* dimple.

Impression
1. Cerebral contusion
2. Scalp laceration
3. Skull fracture (by x-ray examination)

CASE HISTORY

Admission Note
This 65-year-old white female was admitted because of persistent *epigastric* and lower *substernal* pain off and on for the last 1 month. It is especially bad in the night, waking

her up with an indigestion type of discomfort in the lower sternal area. After she gets up and walks around, she feels better. She has had a *myocardial infarction* in the past. She had a posterior myocardial infarction and since that time has been relatively symptom-free except for occasional *angina*. She had been taking nitroglycerin with some relief for angina. However, the pain was relieved usually by sitting up or changing positions. Because it was felt this could be cardiac or gastrointestinal or *hiatus hernia,* she was admitted to the hospital for a complete workup. She has had no nausea, vomiting, diarrhea, black bowel movements, etc.

Past History
Essentially negative except for myocardial infarct.

Review of Systems
HEENT: Negative; no complaints.
PULMONARY: Negative; no cough, sputum, *hemoptysis.*
CARDIOVASCULAR: Angina pectoris with some nitroglycerin for relief.
GI: See admission note.
GU: Negative; no frequency, burning, *dysuria.*
NEUROMUSCULAR AND ARTHRITIC: Has had some generalized arthritic discomfort off and on. However, has had no specific gallop or *rheumatoid arthritis,* mostly *osteoarthritis* symptoms.

Social History
Does not drink or smoke.

Family History
Essentially negative.

Physical Examination
GENERAL: Well-developed, well-nourished. BP 128/80, pulse 84.
HEENT: Eyes, ears, nose, mouth, and pharynx are negative. Fundi reveals some arteriosclerotic changes.
NECK: Negative.
LUNGS: Clear to percussion and auscultation.
HEART: Normal sinus rhythm, no murmurs. Tones good.
ABDOMEN: Liver and spleen are not palpable. Some slight tenderness in the epigastrium. Lower abdominal examination is negative.
EXTREMITIES: Reveal good peripheral pulses. Reflexes are equal and active throughout.

Impression
Rule out gastrointestinal disease.
Rule out *hiatus hernia.*
Rule out *duodenal ulcer.*
Arteriosclerotic heart disease with myocardial infarction in the past.

DISCHARGE SUMMARY

Final Diagnosis: *Idiopathic* convulsive disorder.
Chief Complaint: This is a second College Hospital admission for this 40-year-old black male who enters with the chief complaint of blacking out.
History of Present Illness: The patient was in excellent health until the day of admission when, without any warning or *aura,* he developed *tonic* and *clonic* muscle activity with complete loss of consciousness and his eyes rolled back (this was observed by his wife). This lasted less than 5 minutes. There was no tongue biting or *incontinence* of urine or stool. He returned to consciousness but with severe headaches and was confused and disoriented for about 45 minutes. He was first taken to Metropolitan Hospital, then College Hospital Emergency Room where a variety of tests were done including EKGs, times 2, which apparently were nonrevealing. He was sent to Dr. A's office. While waiting to see Dr. A, he suddenly felt sick to his stomach and had loss of consciousness and had a similar but less violent episode, again followed by confusion. He was then returned to the College Hospital Emergency Room for admission. For the past few days prior to admission the patient had been eating very little and working very hard. He had no prior history of preceding hunger, sickness, weakness, or *diaphoresis.* There was no history of any seizures or head trauma, febrile or serious childhood illness. The only medicine he takes is a nerve pill 4 times a day and a sleeping pill. The patient drank heavily until 10 years ago, one half case of beer per day, but has not had any ethanol since. The patient was in an auto accident 5 days prior to admission but without any head trauma. Denies any history of diabetes.

Past History: The patient had a *varicose* vein stripping 1 year ago. Denies any allergies. Medications are as above. No blood transfusions.

Review of Systems: The patient has had a *pruritic erythematous* localized rash over the right arm for several weeks.

Family History: Father is 77 years old, has high blood pressure and congestive heart failure. Mother is 74 years old, has low blood pressure. Brother is 36 years old, alive and well. There is no family history of seizure disorders. The patient works for the Smith and Co., Manufacturers. He smoked 2 packs of cigarettes per day for 10 years; quit 19 years prior to admission.

Physical Examination: The patient is a well-nourished, well-developed male complaining of headache and diffuse myalgia. BP is 150/65; pulse is 96 and regular; respiration 12; he is *afebrile.*
HEENT: Reveals that there are no *bruits.* Pupils are equal and reactive. Fundi reveal sharp discs. Ears are normal.
NECK: Supple, carotids 2+ and equal, no jugular venous distention. Thyroid is not enlarged.
SKIN: Reveals times 2 times 2 crowded *erythematous papules* on the right arm anteriorly; no nodes palpable.
CHEST: Clear to *percussion* and *auscultation.*
HEART: Reveals PMI 8 cm left of midsternal line in fourth intercostal space. S_1 and S_2 are normal. Physiologic split of S_2. There is a loud apical S_4.
ABDOMEN: Soft and nontender without any *organomegaly* or masses. Bowel sounds are normal. Pulses are 2+.
EXTREMITIES: Reveal no *cyanosis,* clubbing, or edema. Pulses are full.
RECTAL: Is normal.

NEUROLOGIC: Reveals patient is alert, oriented, intelligent, good recent and remote memory but slight confusion (for example, he could not remember his age). Speech was slightly slurred. Cranial nerves were intact. Motor coordination was intact as was sensory exam. DTRs were 3+ uniformly. Toes were downgoing. Gait was normal.

Laboratory Tests and Results: Admitting CBC was normal as was profile. EKG was also within normal limits.

Hospital Course: The patient had a brain scan and echo; both were within normal limits. LP was attempted but was unsuccessful. However, after the LP the patient developed severe *orthostatic,* throbbing-type headache, which finally remitted prior to discharge. Cervical spine films were also normal. EEG reveals a large amount of low voltage symmetric alpha rhythm. There were also a few bursts of medium voltage beta delta waves on frontal and temporal area. EEGs were consistent with a seizure disorder. The patient was started on Dilantin 100 mg, p.o., t.i.d., without any further seizure activity in the hospital.

Discharge Program: The patient was discharged to be followed by his doctor with medicine including Dilantin 100 mg p.o., t.i.d, and Benadryl 50 mg p.o., q.i.d for rash.

PHYSICAL EXAMINATION

GENERAL: An elderly, somewhat overweight, white male who is not acutely ill.

HEENT & NECK: Ears are negative; pupils react well; fundi show about a 1+ *sclerosis* of *retinal vessels;* no *papilledema* is noted. *Pharynx* is negative. *Thyroid* seems to be normal, but there are several tumorlike masses in the *supraclavicular* region on both sides. These masses are fairly movable, nonpainful, and do not seem to be tied down to surrounding tissue.

CHEST: Respiration equal on both sides; lungs fairly clear, with only an occasional *rale* in the base.

HEART: By *percussion,* heart would seem to be enlarged slightly to the left; rate is 92/min and regular. The blood pressure is 130/70. There is a Grade IV *systolic murmur* at the *aortic* area, transmitted upward to the vessels of the neck and also transmitted downward toward the *apex. Apical* murmur does not follow the transmission around to the *axilla,* as seen with *mitral* lesions. I believe the aortic lesion is the main one here. The pulse is rather slow rising, consistent with *aortic stenosis.*

ABDOMEN: Right lower quadrant scar, inverted Y appearance from a *strangulated hernia* and *appendectomy.* Inguinal regions contain some slightly enlarged lymph glands on both sides. Abdomen shows a normal-sized liver. To the right of the scar, there seems to be an *incisional hernia* that protrudes slightly through the weakened abdominal wall. Spleen is definitely enlarged and comes down about two fingers on inspiration.

GENITALIA: Testicles normal.

RECTAL: Enlargement of the prostate gland (1+).

IMPRESSION: Congestive heart failure due to *arteriosclerotic* heart disease with *aortic stenosis,* calcific in type. Lymphatic pathology, type unknown.

SURGICAL PROCEDURES

Number 1

SURGICAL PROCEDURE: D & C, total abdominal *hysterectomy,* bilateral *salpingo-oophorectomy,* and *lysis* of adhesions.

PROCEDURE: The patient was placed in the *lithotomy* position on the operating table, and the *perineum* and *vagina* were prepared with Ioprep. Pelvic examination revealed the presence of a *marital introitus,* with normal external *genitalia.* There was good anterior and posterior support of the vaginal wall. The vagina was clean and well *epithelized,* as was the *cervix,* which was normal in appearance. *Bimanual* examination revealed an irregularly enlarged *uterus* the size of an 8-week *gestation.* The *adnexal* areas could not be identified as such. The operative site was draped with sterile towels and sheets, and the interior lip of the cervix was grasped with a sharp-tooth *tenaculum.* The *endometrial* cavity was sounded to a depth of 4½ inches, after which the *endocervical canal* was dilated with a No. 20 Hank dilator. *Endometrial curettage* was performed, revealing *submucous leiomyomata.* The dilation and curettage (D & C) was then dispensed with.

The anterior abdominal wall was prepared with Ioprep; the operative site was draped with sterile towels and sheets; and a Pfannenstiel incision was then made. The anterior *aponeurotic* flap was elected off the *rectus,* and the *peritoneal* cavity was entered in a longitudinal fashion. Examination of the pelvis revealed an irregularly enlarged uterus covered with *submural* and *subserous leiomyomata.* There were also a number of adhesions between the bowel and the anterior abdominal wall from a previous appendectomy site. *Lysis* of adhesions was carried out to free up the bowel, after which the *infundibulopelvic* ligaments were incised, the anterior leaves to the round ligaments, the posterior leaves to the *uterosacral* ligaments. The round ligaments were then ligated with No. 1 chromic catgut suture. An elliptic incision was carried out between the two round ligaments in such a way as to elevate the bladder flap away from the lower *uterine* sement of the uterus. The uterine vessels were visualized, bilaterally clamped with Dr. Long clamps, cut, and ligated with No. 1 chromic catgut suture. The lower portion of the broad ligaments was bilaterally clamped with Dr. Long clamps, cut and ligated with No. 1 chromic catgut suture. The *cardinal ligaments* were identified, bilaterally clamped with Dr. Long clamps, cut, and ligated with No. 1 chromic catgut suture. At this point it was noted that the *vagina* had been entered, and the *cervix* was then circumcised from the posterior vaginal vault. Aldridge sutures were placed at the angles, using No. 1 chromic catgut suture, after which the vagina was closed in a purse-string fashion with a running No. 1 chromic catgut suture.

Examination of the operative pedicles revealed good *hemostasis* to be present, although it was estimated that the total blood loss during the operative procedure was around 750 ml. A unit of blood was started at this point, and the *peritoneum* was closed, extraperitonealizing the entire operative site with chromic catgut suture. The *rectosigmoid* was then placed in the pelvis, and the peritoneum was picked up and closed in a running fashion. The *aponeuroses* of the *external-internal oblique* muscles were reapproximated, using interrupted No. 00 cotton suture. The subcutaneous and subcuticular tissues were reapproximated, using running No. 1 Dermalon suture. Telfa and dry-gauze dressings were placed over the incision, after which the patient was returned to the recovery room in excellent condition.

Number 2

PREOPERATIVE DIAGNOSIS: Anterior mediastinal mass; rule out malignancy.
POSTOPERATIVE DIAGNOSIS: Anterior mediastinal mass; malignant; probably carcinoma; rule out *lymphoma.*
OPERATION: Mediastinoscopy with biopsy of anterior mediastinal mass and frozen section.
ANESTHESIA: General.
INCISION: Low cervical transverse incision.
FINDINGS: Several enlarged lymph nodes in the anterior mediastinum just to the left of the trachea with a large, hard, necrotic appearing mass, just to the right and just over the trachea.
PROCEDURE: After an adequate level of anesthesia was reached, the patient was prepared and draped in the usual sterile fashion. The above-mentioned incision was then made and carried down through the subcutaneous tissue, down through the *platysma. Hemostasis* was made and verified using curved Kellys and *electrocautery.* This brought into view the strap muscles, which were divided in a vertical direction using blunt and sharp dissection. Hemostasis was again made and verified using curved Kellys. The *isthmus of the thyroid* was visualized and an inferior thyroid vessel was clamped, cut and ligated, and tied with a No. 000 suture ligature of catgut. We then viewed the trachea and, using blunt dissection, the mediastinum was opened, just anterior to the trachea, with the above-mentioned findings. A large $1 \times 1\frac{1}{2} \times \frac{1}{2}$ cm of soft lymph node was removed just from the right of the trachea and sent out for frozen section. Frozen section revealed a malignancy, probably carcinoma, but with no chance of it being a lymphoma. While waiting for the results of the lymph node dissection, two more biopsies were taken from a hard, necrotic mass, just to the right of the trachea. Hemostasis was verified at this point and the strap muscles were approximated using interrupted sutures of No. 000 Tab-Dek. The platysma was then approximated using interrupted sutures of No. 4/0 Tab-Dek and the skin was approximated using interrupted suture of No. 4/0 Tab-Dek. The dressing was placed on the wound, and the patient left the operating room in satisfactory condition.
PACKS: None.
DRAINS: None.
FLUIDS: 1000 cc of D5 and lactated Ringer's.
ESTIMATED BLOOD LOSS: 50 cc.

Number 3

PREOPERATIVE DIAGNOSIS: Hodgkin's disease.
POSTOPERATIVE DIAGNOSIS: Same.
OPERATION: Exploratory laparotomy for staging of Hodgkin's disease with *splenectomy,* liver biopsy, and *periaortic node biopsy.*
ANESTHESIA: General.
INCISION: Midline.
FINDINGS: Enlarged spleen and a slightly mottled liver and a large periaortic lymph node.
PROCEDURE: The patient was prepped and draped in the usual manner following successful general anesthesia. A midline incision was made down through the skin and subcutaneous tissue into the anterior fascia. The fascia was incised sharply and the abdomen was entered with hemostasis achieved by fine ligatures. Exploration of the abdomen revealed the above findings. At this time attention was turned toward the splenectomy. This was achieved by first dissecting on the gastrohepatic ligament for the splenic artery, which was difficult to find. Subsequently, the stomach was retracted superiority and the lesser sac was entered. Dissection on top of the pancreas at this time revealed the splenic artery, and it was ligated in continuity with a No. 00 Poly-Dek ligature. Following this the spleen was dissected from its position by both blunt and sharp dissection brought into the midline abdominal wound. The pedicle of the spleen was then divided between large hemo clips without difficulty and the spleen was removed. A pack was placed in the left upper quadrant in the splenic bed and attention was turned toward a liver biopsy. Two sutures of No. 0 chromic were then placed in a figure-of-eight horizontal fashion such that a **V** was created at the edge of the liver and the liver between these two sutures was excised sharply. Another hemostatic suture was taken in the liver to ensure there would be no bleeding. Attention was then turned to the dissection of the periaortic region and lymph node biopsy. By the use of sharp and blunt dissection a portion of a large node in this region of the celiac plexus was excised. Small bleeders were suture ligated and a pack was placed here. Prior to closure, all the packs were removed. There was no evidence of bleeding and the abdominal wall was then closed with interrupted figure-of-eight Tom Jones No. 0 Tycron suture and the skin approximated with No. 4/0 silks.
PACKS: None.
DRAINS: None.
TUBES: NG tube in place.

The patient tolerated the procedure well and received 600 cc of lactated Ringer's. Estimated blood loss was 600 cc. Sponge count was correct, times two.

REPORTS OF ELECTROCARDIOGRAMS WITH CASE HISTORIES

During a cardiac cycle, the electrical changes in the heart will cause five distinct movements of the galvanometer string in the normal electrocardiogram. Three are directed upward, and two are directed downward. These five movements are designated a P, Q, R, S, and T. P, R, and T are directed upward, and Q and S are directed downward. The P wave is produced by spread of excitation wave over the *auricle*. The Q, R, S, and T movements, or deflections, are produced by the *ventricles;* the Q, R, S waves during the spread, and the T wave during the retreat, of the excitation wave. The P-R interval is the beginning of P to the beginning of QRS. The S-T interval is the interval elapsing between the end of the S wave and beginning of T.

Number 1

HISTORY: This 35-year-old white male was admitted to the hospital with symptoms of 6 weeks' duration, consisting of *malaise,* fever, and aching of various joints. Prior to admission he became *dyspneic* and had to sit up to breathe. A *systolic* murmur was noted on the day of admission. Physical examination revealed a temperature of 102° F; pulse rate of 130; respirations, 24; blood pressure, 90/60 mm Hg. Lungs were clear to *auscultation* and *percussion.* The heart was not enlarged, but there was a harsh *systolic* murmur in the *mitral* area. No *diastolic* murmur or thrill was noted. Abdomen and extremities were negative. Repeated blood cultures were positive for a *Streptococcus* of the *viridans* group, and the patient was given penicillin. *Tachycardia* persisted, and he developed congestive heart failure and died after an illness of approximately 4½ months.

ELECTROCARDIOGRAM: The QRS was 0.11 sec, and the right axis deviation was marked. Two days later the electrocardiogram showed a sinus rhythm with a rate of 84 per min. The P waves were low and the P-R interval was 0.24 sec. The QRS occupied 0.15 sec. The initial R wave in leads I and II was followed by a deep, wide S wave. In lead III the R wave was wide and was followed by an inverted T wave. The T waves were upright in leads I and II. The V leads were not taken. The initial axis of the QRS was calculated to be plus 76 degrees, and the final axis was calculated to be minus 178 degrees. The mean QRTS axis was calculated to be plus 172 degrees. The tracing was classified as a Type II right *intraventricular conduction block.*

Following autopsy the final anatomic diagnosis was considered to be rheumatic heart disease with *mitral* and *aortic valvulitis;* and *subacute bacterial endocarditis (Streptococcus),* with cardiac enlargement and Type II right *intraventricular conduction block* and congestive heart failure resulting from *myocardial* degeneration.

Number 2

HISTORY: This 36-year-old white female was admitted to the hospital because of *tachycardia* and a slightly elevated blood pressure on routine examination, which led to an electrocardiogram revealing a left intraventricular conduction block. She gave a history of exertional *dyspnea* and *palpitation* and at times a tight feeling in the interior chest. An occasional skipped beat was noted, especially at night. There had been no *orthopnea, angina,* or *hemoptysis.* Past history revealed the usual childhood diseases, with no scarlet fever or known rheumatic fever. She did have a history of one episode of *gonorrhea* and had been treated for *arthritis.* She also gave a history of *asthmatic* attacks following colds. Further, she had had *lymphocytic choriomeningitis,* with no complications or *sequelae* noted.

Physical examination revealed blood pressure of 140/90 mm Hg on the left and 146/96 mm Hg on the right. Weight was 135 pounds, and height was 63 inches. Temperature was 99° F; pulse rate, 100; and respirations, 18. Fundoscopic examination was normal. Lungs were normal to auscultation and percussion. The heart was not enlarged to inspection, palpation, or percussion. Heart sounds were of good quality, with no murmurs. *Blood urea nitrogen* level was 11.4 mg/100 ml; *cholesterol* level was 167 mg/100 ml; *fasting blood* sugar level was 98 mg/100 ml; *hemoglobin* level was 97%; and total *leukocyte* count was 8,900, with 68% *neutrophils,* 24% *lymphocytes,* 6% *monocytes,* 1% *eosinophils,* and *basophils.*

ELECTROCARDIOGRAM: This revealed a sinus rhythm with a rate of 84 per min. The P waves were normal. The P-R interval was 0.14 sec, and the QRS occupied 0.13 sec, with a wide notched R_1, and R_2. The R_3 was wide, and S_3 constituted the final portion of the QRS. The T waves were upright in the limb leads. The chest leads revealed a delay in the intrinsicoid deflection of 0.08 sec in V_6. The initial axis of the QRS was calculated to be plus 50 degrees, and the final axis was calculated to be 0 degree. The mean axis of the QRS was calculated at plus 41 degrees. The tracing was classified as Type III left intraventricular conduction block.

INTERPRETATION: At the time of discharge, her diagnosis was considered by exclusion to be *arteriosclerotic* heart disease; *coronary artery sclerosis;* and a Type III left intraventricular conduction block.

REPORTS OF ELECTROENCEPHALOGRAMS WITH CASE HISTORIES

Changes in electrical potential of the brain can be recorded by applying electrodes to the scalp and obtaining tracings of brain wave activity, which is called an electroencephalogram. The patterns of these brain wave tracings can be related to neurologic conditions, alterations of consciousness, and mental states and are used for diagnosing seizure and brainstem disorders and brain lesions or tumors.

Number 1

HISTORY: This 32-year-old black female had a skull fracture 3 years ago with unconsciousness for about 3 days. She began to have blackouts late this year, which have persisted and are now increasing in frequency, with up to three per week (they formerly occurred every 3 months). Severe headache for 5 to 10 minutes occurred during the first attack. The impression was a *chronic brain syndrome* associated with *trauma*.

ENCEPHALOGRAM: *Monopolar* leads from right and left *frontal, parietal, occipital, temporal,* and *anterior temporal* areas, bilaterally. *Bipolar* leads were also run. It was necessary to give sedation for sleep record.

RECORD: The waking frequency is a well-defined 9 per sec. Sleep shows random slowing. There are no *paroxysmal dysrhythmias* or *asymmetries.* Overventilation produce no buildup.

INTERPRETATION: Normal EEG.

Number 2

HISTORY: This 38-year-old white male stated he had had two *grand mal seizures* recently, occurring 5 months apart. He stated he had incurred a head injury at the age of 6 when he was hit on the head by a baseball.

ENCEPHALOGRAM: Monopolar and bipolar leads were placed on frontal, parietal, occipital, temporal, and anterior temporal areas.

RECORD: The basic waking alpha is 10 per sec. Light sleep frequencies show rather low-voltage (flat) random slowing with variable frequencies and occasional (1 to 3 per sec) waves (14 per sec spindles are average). There are no asymmetries. On two isolated occasions, larval "slow" spikes appeared in the right temporal and anterior temporal leads. Overventilation produced marked buildup and 2 to 4 per sec slow waves.

INTERPRETATION: Borderline normal record. Two questionable isolated spikes seen in the right temporal and right anterior temporal areas.

RADIOLOGIC REPORTS

Number 1

SALPINGOGRAM: Examination of the female pelvis after the transvaginal injection of contrast material shows that the uterine outline shows an *"arcuate"* uterine configuration. Some dilation and filling of the *endocervical* portion of the uterus are consistent with a local *endocervicitis.* Both fallopian tubes fill but the fimbriated end of the right tube is closed and forms a *hydrosalpinx.* A large dilated hydrosalpinx is also observed on the left, but after the injection of a second volume of dye a small amount of free peritoneal spillage is demonstrated.

IMPRESSION:
1. Arcuate uterus.
2. Endocervicitis.
3. The presence of a small hydrosalpinx is seen on the right, which is completely blocked.
4. A large hydrosalpinx is present on the left, but a small quantity of dye spills into the peritoneal cavity.

Number 2

BARIUM ENEMA, LARGE BOWEL: There has been a history of surgical intervention in the large bowel. On the filled film there are *diverticula* present in the *distal descending* and *sigmoid* regions, as well as in the *ascending colon.* There is overlapping of bowel in the *transverse colon,* and whether this represents redundancy or a side-to-side *anastomosis* could not be determined either fluoroscopically or radiographically. On the evacuation film there is noted contrast medium extending outside the bowel wall in the region of the *sigmoid diverticula,* and the possibility that these represent abscesses resulting from diverticulitis must be considered. The *terminal ileum* is visualized. No filling defects are seen.

Number 3

GALLBLADDER: The gallbladder is faintly visualized. No obvious stone is identified. The *cystic* and *common ducts* are seen and are within normal limits. There is good contraction following the fatty stimulus. Opaque medium is seen in the region of the *cecum* and *ascending colon.* The findings suggest a poorly functioning gallbladder.

Number 4

RETROGRADE AORTOGRAM: The retrograde aortogram gives good visualization of the aorta and its arterial branches. There is noted persistent narrowing in the first portion of the left *renal* artery, with some *poststenotic* dilation. The right renal artery shows no gross abnormality.

PATHOLOGY REPORTS

Number 1

GROSS: The specimen consists of approximately 10 ml of yellowish-white, very mucoid material (sputum), which is submitted for *cytologic* examination.

MICROSCOPIC: The *Papanicolaou smear* of sputum reveals sheets and strands of *mucus,* as well as a few *exfoliated stratified squamous epithelial cells* and some *bronchial epithelial cells.* No cells resembling carcinoma are seen within this sputum.

DIAGNOSIS: Papanicolaou smear of sputum negative for malignancy.

Number 2

GROSS: This specimen consists of three irregular pieces of liver tissue measuring 1 to 2 cm in length and 1 cm in width. They have a yellowish-tan color and are rubbery in consistency. The *hepatic* lobules are fairly distinct.

There is also a *vermiform appendix* measuring 12 cm in length and 0.8 cm in diameter. The *serosal* surface is smooth and glistening. The vessels appear markedly dilated and congested. On cut section, the appendiceal wall is 2 mm in thickness. The lumen is filled with a greenish-brown *fecal* material. The mucosa is moderately congested. No ulcerations are seen. The attached *mesoappendix* is 1 cm in width.

MICROSCOPIC: Section of the liver reveals a normal *lobular* pattern. The liver cells are pale because of a moderate increase in *glycogen* content. The *portal* spaces have a light increase in *lymphocytes* the *biliary ducts* and *portal veins* have normal features.

Sections of the appendix reveal an intact normal *mucosa*. The *lumen* is *patent* and filled with fecal material. In the *submucosa* there is a moderate increase in the fibrous tissue. The *lymphatic* tissue shows several *germinal* centers. The *muscularis* and *serosal* layers are unremarkable.

DIAGNOSIS: Liver with mild *cholangitis; fibrosis* of appendix.

Number 3

SPECIMEN: Rectal biopsy.
PREOPERATIVE DIAGNOSIS: *Ulcerative colitis.*
POSTOPERATIVE DIAGNOSIS: parasitic infestation.
GROSS DESCRIPTION: The specimen is submitted as "rectal biopsy." It consists of two fragments of gray-tan tissue, which measures 4 × 3 × 1 mm each. The entire specimen is submitted in a single cassette.
MICROSCOPIC: Sections show *rectal mucosa* and small portion of underlying *submucosa* and *muscularis mucosa.* A focal area of chronic inflammation is seen in the submucosa. This inflammation is composed of *plasma cells, lymphocytes,* and *eosinophils.* In this area, mucosal gland architecture has been interrupted and many of the glands show regenerative epithelium. No crypt abscesses are seen. There is no evidence of granulomatous disease. These changes are compatible with but not diagnostic of *ulcerative colitis.*
DIAGNOSIS: Chronic inflammation of rectum.

AUTOPSY REPORTS

Number 1

Male 68 years
CLINICAL DIAGNOSIS: Abdominal aneurysm.
   Primary
   1. *Arteriosclerosis* or thoracic and abdominal aorta, coronary arteries (advanced), and renal and mesenteric arteries (moderate).

2. Old occlusion of circumflex branch of left coronary artery.
3. Replacement of lower abdominal aorta by aorta-iliac bypass graft, bilaterally patent.
4. Old *dissecting aneurysm* of ascending aorta with large (1 × 1.8 cm) orifice.
5. Dilation of aortic annulus, moderate (90 mm). (History of murmur of aortic insufficiency, significance unclear in light of dissecting aneurysm.)
6. Small *fenestration* of aortic valve and patent guarded *foramen ovale.*
7. Dilation and hypertrophy of left ventricle of heart (750 g).
8. *Subendocardial myocardial infarct, anteroseptal* and *posterolateral,* old, with questionable valve (clinical history of rheumatic heart and recent small *apical infarct*).
9. Pulmonary congestion and edema.
10. *Arteriolar nephrosclerosis,* moderate.
11. Splenomegaly (350 gm).
12. Chronic passive congestion of liver and spleen.
   Accessory
   1. *Diverticulosis* of sigmoid colon and rectum.
   2. Pulmonary *emphysema,* diffuse, moderate.
   3. *Cholelithiasis.*
   4. Calcification in pulmonary hilar lymph nodes.
   5. *Osteoporosis,* moderately advanced.
   6. Small *adenocarcinoma* of the prostate in left posterior lobe.
   7. Nodular *hyperplasia* of prostate with dilation and trabeculation of the bladder, advanced.

Number 2

Female 74 years
CLINICAL DIAGNOSIS: Congestive heart failure.
   Primary
   1. Rheumatic *valvulitis* (mitral disease) (T-32, F-9136).
   2. *Cardiomegaly,* moderate (450 gm) (T-32, M-7200).
   3. Pulmonary *thromboemboli,* multiple, with infarcts of lower lobes of both lungs (T-28, M-5470, T-28, M-3710).
   4. *Hydrothorax* (1800 cc right side, 300 cc left side).
   5. Fibrous pleural adhesions, upper lobes, bilateral.
   6. Acute passive congestion of the liver and spleen, severe.
BACTERIOLOGY CULTURE: Blood (heart): no growth.
SUMMARY: This 74-year-old female was admitted 2 weeks ago in terminal stage of congestive heart failure secondary to rheumatic valvular disease involving the mitral valve with moderate cardiomegaly (450 gm). The lung changes show multiple thromboemboli with segmental infarcts as well as fibrosis of lung parenchyma (popliteal veins do not show any thrombi). The changes in the *viscera* are secondary to passive congestion.

Medical Insurance, Managed Care, and Health Maintenance Programs

The importance of processing medical insurance claims has increased tremendously during the past few years because a large percentage of the population now is covered by either a service or an indemnity-type of insurance with commercial firms. Additionally, there is Medicare under the Social Security Administration, state-sponsored Medicaid, and military service or federal agency programs.

Because of the proliferation of computerized records, it is becoming more and more necessary for personnel in hospitals and medical offices to be computer literate.

GENERAL RULES

When a patient first applies for treatment or care, it is necessary to establish immediately whether the patient has medical insurance. If the patient does, the name and address of the insured must be recorded exactly as they appear on the insurance identification card. In addition, the patient's age, policy number, insuror, and, if applicable, the group number and name of the employer, organization, or association through which the person is insured also must be recorded.

An "authorization for release of information" appears on many insurance forms and must be signed by the patient or an accepted representative so that medical information may be shared with the insurance claims adjudicator. In policies written by commercial companies, where there are provisions for certain services by physicians and hospitals, the patient should sign the authorization to pay the hospital or physician directly. Be sure the form is dated. This authorization appears on many insurance forms, but if there is none on the form, have the patient sign and date one that you have for this purpose.

It is always necessary to ascertain whether the patient's illness or injury is related to employment, since it may be covered under workmen's compensation laws or other employer liability laws. The forms for claims under workmen's compensation or other employer liability laws are processed in much the same manner as all other medical claims.

After the type of coverage is determined and the necessary authorizations obtained, there is usually no further need to be concerned with the insurance until the time comes for processing the claim. Before completing a claim, thoroughly read the instructions and all questions and be sure you understand them. Do not ever leave any blank spaces. Keep two points in mind when filling out insurance forms: the patient's welfare and the payment expected from the insurance carrier. Insurance reimbursements are benefits for the patient and a source of income for the physician.

All questions that arise over a claim should be referred to the proper insurance carrier, and if additional information is needed, your office will be contacted by one of their representatives.

When filing a hospital claim, include records of all diagnostic procedures, room fees, drug charges, surgical and medical procedures, uses of respirators, kidney dialysis machines, or any other therapy. In a medical office, patient records should contain all information necessary to complete claims.

Accuracy is essential, including spelling names and copying numbers correctly. Some policies contain a clause stating that if a claim is not filed within a prescribed time period, benefits are disallowed, making timelines of the utmost importance. Almost all claims are now filed electronically, but copies of completed claims should be kept for the record and to settle any disputes that may arise.

MULTIPLE INSURANCE POLICIES

It is important to identify by name all companies that insure the patient. Many insurance policies allow only a small amount toward fees and charges, whereas others allow larger benefits. Some insurance policies carry a pro rata clause or rider, which distributes the charges among different companies, in instances of multiple coverage, with each paying a fair share of the expenses involved. The patient may also be eligible for collection from a number of policies for any one illness. Claim forms for each of these policies will have to be filled out. It is important to note which insurance is primary, and which is/are secondary; this is known as coordination of benefits (COB).

MEDICAL CODING AND TERMINOLOGY

A primary consideration in filling out insurance claims is the need to use standardized, approved medical coding or terminology for all diagnoses and procedures. Diseases and disorders are identified and coded by a numerical designation found in the *International Classification of Diseases* (ICD) code book. The medical, surgical, and diagnostic services are similarly identified and coded numerically in the *Current Procedural Terminology* coding system (CPT).

In addition to the ICD and CPT coding, there has been a more recent development led by Medicare to classify patients into groups based on principal diagnosis, presence and type of surgical procedures, presence or absence of significant comorbidities (associated disease conditions) and complications, and other relevant criteria. This classification, known as *Diagnosis Related Groups* (DRG), was intended to categorize patients into groups that are clinically meaningful and homogeneous with respect to resources used and provides another basis for reimbursement for services rendered.

FEDERAL AND STATE HEALTH INSURANCE PROGRAMS

There are several government-funded health insurance programs administered by either the federal government or the individual states.

Civilian Health and Medical Program of the Uniformed Services (CHAMPUS)

A comprehensive health benefits program administered by the Department of Defense, without premium payment but with cost-sharing provisions, that pays for care delivered by civilian health providers to dependents of uniformed services personnel and retired uniformed services personnel and their dependents.

Civilian Health and Medical Program of the Veterans Administration (CHAMPVA)

A comprehensive health benefits program administered by the Department of Defense for the Veterans Administration, without premium payment, but with cost-sharing provisions, that pays for care delivered by civilian health providers to dependents of veterans with a permanent service connected disability or dependents of veterans who died while on active duty or as a result of a service-connected disability.

Medicare

Medicare is the federally funded Health Care Financing Administration (HCFA) health insurance program that covers approved hospital and medical costs for persons 65 years of age and older, as well as certain disabled persons younger than age 65.

The hospital insurance (part A), with no premium payment but with limited cost-sharing, pays for hospital patient care, posthospital care in a skilled nursing facility, and posthospital home health care. The hospital and the extended-care facility must be approved by, and be a participating Provider of Medicare.

The medical insurance (part B), with premium deducted from monthly Social Security payments, and with limited cost-sharing, pays for physician services, outpatient hospital services, and various approved medical services and supplies not covered by part A Medicare insurance.

Medicare specifies charges for diagnosis related groups (DRGs) and pays 80% of approved charges, with the balance paid by the patient or other secondary insurance (Medigap).

Forms are subject to revision from time to time, but copies of the latest forms and information can be sent directly to your office. Preprinted forms with physician name and provider number are available for a fee. Increasingly, Medicare encourages claims to be filed electronically by computer using Medicare-developed software or software that asks for input for all fields on the paper form. This information is then transmitted to Medicare digitally, thus speeding the reimbursement process.

Medicaid

A federally funded and supervised program of the Health Care Financing Administration, in cooperation with each state, administers its own program and sets up its own eligibility guidelines. There is no cost to the recipient, and coverage is usually dependent upon low income and/or disability, with the states choosing the providers and the delivery sites.

MANAGED CARE

Managed care is a fundamental shift in the health care system from more expensive reactive care to care that is more proactive. It uses financial incentives and controls to direct patients to providers for appropriate, cost-effective care and is intended to control the cost of health care by emphasizing prevention, early intervention, and outpatient care. A managed care system may include health insurers, medical groups, hospitals, and health systems.

Health Maintenance Organization (HMO)

Members of HMO managed care plans prepay a premium to receive comprehensive, coordinated medical services with co-payments. The main focus is on preventive medicine and control of health care costs. There is a "gatekeeper," the primary care physician (PCP), selected by the member from the HMO's list of caregivers, who coordinates all services to the patient, including referrals to specialists.

Physician/Hospital Organization (PHO)

PHO is an organized arrangement between hospitals and physicians to pursue managed care contracts. This system furthers cooperative activity with a level of independence to both hospitals and physicians, and offers patients continuity of care.

Preferred Provider Organization (PPO)

PPO is an arrangement between those who pay for health care (employers or insurers) and the health providers. Employers or insurers encourage members to use the providers who have agreed to supply services at a specified, negotiated rate (discounted fee-for-service). This is designed to reduce cost to the payer and supply additional patients to providers. Members have freedom-of-choice among in-network providers, including specialists, and are given incentives (lower deductibles and co-payments) to use those providers. When using out-of-network providers, members are responsible for a larger portion of the costs.

Point of Service (POS)

POS is a newer form of managed care combining broader benefits and low costs of an HMO plan (in-network) with higher costs but greater freedom of a PPO plan (out-of-network). This type of plan is sometimes called an open-ended HMO or PPO, with members encouraged to choose a primary care physician and use the existing network providers, but they may choose other physicians and hospitals for service. When a participating provider is used, benefits are provided as in an HMO, with no deductibles and small co-payments. If the provider is not part of the network, members pay a higher co-payment and frequently a substantial deductible.

TRADITIONAL INSURANCE PLANS

Indemnity Plans

An indemnity is a benefit paid by an insurance policy for an insured loss. An insurance company or group agrees to assume health insurance risk for its subscribers at a predetermined rate (premium). The insured individuals are reimbursed after filed claims are reviewed and processed. An indemnity plan usually has a maximum benefit (cap) and an annual deductible payable by the insured, and all costs above a fixed percentage are the patient's responsibility. Depending on how the plan is written, providers may be paid directly by the insurers or by the subscribers.

HEALTH MAINTENANCE

Many managed care plans have provision for health maintenance programs to minimize risk factors of acute and chronic disease conditions. These programs provide guidelines for developing managed health or wellness, in which the individuals take personal control of their lifestyle to pursue optimal health, well-being, and personal fitness. Basically, each person is empowered to reduce his or her own risk of coronary artery disease, osteoporosis, chronic obstructive pulmonary disease, cancer, and other diseases.

Before entering into any program, especially one involving exercise, participants undergo screening to assess current risk factors. The purpose of this is to enable program instructors to determine the need for a physician's clearance before an individual participates in the program. As an example, for an exercise program designed to reduce the risks for cardiovascular disease, a Health Risk Appraisal (HRA), completed by a prospective participant, would include factors such as age, family history, smoking status, hypertension, hypercholesterolemia, diabetes, and activity level. Table E.1 shows the criteria defining each of these risk factors.

Typically, after the risk factors from Table E.1 have been assessed, an individual is identified in one of the following three categories:
1. apparently healthy—individual is asymptomatic, appears to be healthy and has no more than one major positive coronary risk factors.
2. increased risk—individual has signs and symptoms suggesting cardiopulmonary disease or metabolic disease, and/or has two or more major positive coronary risk factors.
3. known disease—individual has been diagnosed with known cardiac, pulmonary, or metabolic disease.

Individuals in category 1, the *apparently healthy*, can participate in moderate intensity exercise without a physician's approval. Those in category 2, with *increased risk*, and those in category 3, with *known disease*, should be evaluated by a physician before participating. It is always a good idea to consult a physician before undertaking vigorous physical activity or exercise.

TABLE E.1 RISK FACTORS FOR CORONARY ARTERY DISEASE

Positive risk factors	Individual is "at risk" if
age	individual is male >45 years, or female >55 years; or female with premature menopause not using hormone replacement therapy
family history	father or other first-degree male relative had a myocardial infarction or sudden death before age 55 or mother or other first-degree female relative had a myocardial infarction or sudden death before age 65
smoking habits	individual currently smokes cigarettes
hypertension	blood pressure has been confirmed, on two separate visits, to be ≥140/90 mm Hg; or individual is on antihypertensive medication
hypercholesterolemia	total serum cholesterol >200 mg/dL; or high-density lipoprotein (HDL) <35 mg/dl
diabetes	individual has insulin-dependent diabetes mellitus (IDDM) and is either >30 years; or has had IDDM for >15 years; or if individual has non-insulin-dependent diabetes mellitus (NIDDM) and is >35 years
physical activity	individual is physically inactive, being sedentary and sitting a large part of the day and participating in no regular exercise or active recreation (i.e., softball, volleyball, basketball, tennis, etc.)

Modified in part from American College of Sports Medicine (ACSM): *Guidelines for exercise testing and prescription*, ed 5, Baltimore, 1995, Williams & Wilkins.

Medical Specialties

The American Board of Medical Specialties (ABMS) is concerned with establishing and maintaining standards of medical specialty practice. There are 24 individual boards that certify those physicians choosing to practice in the specialty areas (Neurology and Psychiatry are separate specialties under one board).

AMERICAN BOARDS OF MEDICAL SPECIALTIES

American Board of Allergy and Immunology
American Board of Anesthesiology
American Board of Colon and Rectal Surgery
American Board of Dermatology
American Board of Emergency Medicine
American Board of Family Practice
American Board of Internal Medicine
American Board of Medical Genetics
American Board of Neurological Surgery
American Board of Nuclear Medicine
American Board of Obstetrics and Gynecology
American Board of Ophthalmology
American Board of Orthopaedic Surgery
American Board of Otolaryngology
American Board of Pathology
American Board of Pediatrics
American Board of Physical Medicine and Rehabilitation
American Board of Plastic Surgery
American Board of Preventive Medicine
American Board of Psychiatry and Neurology
American Board of Radiology
American Board of Surgery
American Board of Thoracic Surgery
American Board of Urology

MEDICAL SPECIALTIES

Allergy and Immunology (A & I) are those specialties concerned with the identification and treatment of allergies and the study of immunity to disease. The physicians are called *allergists* and *immunologists*.

Anesthesiology (Anes) is the branch of medicine devoted to the administration of a drug or gas to induce partial or complete loss of sensation with or without loss of consciousness. The physician is called an *anesthesiologist*.

Colon and Rectal Surgery (CRS) is the surgical specialty dealing with surgery of the colon (large intestine) and the rectum and anus. The physician is a *proctologist*.

Dermatology (D) is the branch of medicine devoted to the study of the skin and its diseases. The medical specialist is called a *dermatologist*.

Emergency Medicine (EM) is the branch of medicine devoted to diagnosing, treating, and stabilizing trauma or crisis conditions.

Family Practice (FP) is the branch of medicine dealing with the care of all members of the family regardless of age or sex. The practitioner is often compared to one in general practice.

Internal Medicine (IM) is the branch of medicine dealing with diseases not usually treated surgically. The practicing physician is an *internist*. Subspecialties of *internal medicine* are:

Cardiology is the study of diseases of the heart. The physician is a *cardiologist*.

Endocrinology is the study of the endocrine glands and their internal secretions. The physician is an *endocrinologist*.

Geriatrics or Gerontology is the study and treatment of diseases of the aged. The physician is a *geriatrician* or *gerontologist*.

Medical Genetics (MG) is a specialty concerned with the application of genetic information to the diagnosis and treatment of genetic based disorders. Ph.D.s as well as M.D.s are certified in this specialty, and the practitioner is a *geneticist*.

Neurological Surgery (NS) is the surgical specialty concerned with surgical procedures on the nervous system. The physician is a *neurosurgeon*.

Nuclear Medicine (NuM) is the branch of medicine concerned with the development and use of radioactive equipment and substances in diagnosis and treatment.

Obstetrics and Gynecology (ObG) is the branch of medicine concerned with the care of women. Obstetrics is devoted to the care of women during pregnancy, labor, delivery, and puerperium (the physician is an *obstetrician*). Gynecology is devoted to the treatment of diseases of women, especially those of the genital, urinary, or rectal areas (the physician is a *gynecologist*).

Ophthalmology (Oph) is the branch of medicine devoted to the treatment of disorders of the eye. The physician is an *ophthalmologist.*

Orthopaedic Surgery (OrS) is the surgical specialty concerned with prevention and correction of deformities by use of surgical procedures. The physician is an *orthopedist.*

Otolaryngology (Oto) is the medical specialty dealing with the study and treatment of diseases of the ear (otology), nose (rhinology), and throat (laryngology). The physician is an *otolaryngologist.*

Pathology (Path) is the branch of medicine that studies the causes and effects of disease and the resulting changes in structure and function. The physician is a *pathologist.*

Pediatrics (Ped) is the branch of medicine concerned with care and treatment of children. The physician is a *pediatrician.* A subspecialty of pediatrics is:

> **Neonatology,** the branch of medicine that deals with the diseases and abnormalities of the newborn infant. The physician is a *neonatologist.*

Physical Medicine and Rehabilitation (PMR) is the branch of medicine devoted to the study and treatment of disease by mechanical and physical means.

Plastic Surgery (PlS) is the surgical specialty concerned with restoration and repair of physical damage and defects.

Preventive Medicine (PrM) is the branch of medicine dealing with the prevention of both physical and mental illness.

Psychiatry (Psyc) and Neurology (N) is the branch of medicine concerned with the structure and functioning of the nervous system and its diseases. Subspecialties include:

> **Psychiatry** is devoted to diagnosis, treatment, and prevention of mental illness. The physician is a *psychiatrist.*

> **Neurology** is devoted to the study of the nervous system and its diseases. The physician is a *neurologist.*

Radiology (Rad) is the branch of medicine concerned with the use of roentgen rays (x-rays) for diagnostic and therapeutic purposes. The physician is a *radiologist.*

Surgery (S) is the branch of medicine that treats deformities, defects, injury, and disease by use of surgical procedures. The physician is a *surgeon.*

Thoracic Surgery (TS) is the surgical specialty concerned with surgical procedures of the thorax (chest).

Urology (U) is the branch of medicine dealing with the study of the urinary tract in both sexes, and the male genital tract. The physician is a *urologist.*

Answers to Review Questions, Exercises, and Puzzles

CHAPTER 1   AN INTRODUCTION TO MEDICAL TERMINOLOGY

CHAPTER 1 EXERCISES

Exercise 1.1   *In any order:*

1. prefix
2. suffix
3. root
4. combining form

Exercise 1.2   *In any order:*

1. prefix: beginning or first part of a word
2. suffix: ending or last part of a word
3. root: foundation of a word
4. combining form: root with combining vowel to attach to another root or a suffix

Exercise 1.3

1. H
2. F
3. A
4. G
5. B
6. I
7. E
8. C
9. D

Exercise 1.4

1. T
2. F
3. F
4. F
5. F

Bibliography

Ackerman D: *A natural history of the senses,* New York, 1990, Random House.

American Psychiatric Association: *Diagnostic and statistical manual of mental disorders,* ed 4, Washington, DC, 1994, The Association.

Anderson KN, Anderson LE, Glanze WD: *Mosby's medical, nursing and allied health dictionary,* ed 4, St Louis, 1994, Mosby.

Asimov I: *Isaac Asimov's book of facts,* New York, 1979, Grosset & Dunlap.

Austrin MG: *Sony medical transcription program,* New York, 1974, Sony Corporation of America.

Berne RM, Levy MN: *Cardiovascualr physiology,* ed 7, St Louis, 1997, Mosby.

Carson RC: *Abnormal psychology,* ed 11, Reading, Mass, 1997, Addison-Wesley.

Department of Health and Human Services, Health Care Financing Administration: *Guide to health insurance for people with Medicare,* Washington, DC, 1996, US Government Printing Office.

Department of Health and Human Services, Social Security Administration: *Your Medicare handbook,* Washington, DC, 1996, US Government Printing Office.

Dorland's illustrated medical dictionary, ed 28, Philadelphia, 1994, WB Saunders.

Fordney MT: *Insurance handbook for the medical office,* ed 5, Philadelphia, 1997, WB Saunders.

Ganong WF: *Review of medical physiology,* ed 18, Los Altos, Calif, 1997, Lange Medical Publications.

Gilroy J, Holliday PL: *Basic neurology,* ed 3, New York, 1990, Macmillan.

Gleitman H: *Psychology,* ed 4, New York, 1995, WW Norton.

Gould JA III, editor: *Orthopaedic and sports physical therapy,* ed 3, St Louis, 1997, Mosby.

Guyton AC: *Textbook of medical physiology,* ed 9, Philadelphia, 1995, WB Saunders.

Irwin S, Tecklin JS, editors: *Cardiopulmonary physical therapy,* ed 3, St Louis, 1995, Mosby.

Jensen D: *The principles of physiology,* ed 2, New York, 1982, Appleton-Century-Crofts.

Kuby J: *Immunology,* ed 3, Salt Lake City, 1997, WH Freeman.

McAleer N: *The body almanac,* Garden City, NY, 1985, Doubleday.

Miller FF, Keane CB: *Encyclopedia and dictionary of medicine, nursing, and allied health,* ed 6, Philadelphia, 1997, WB Saunders.

Nuland SB: *How we die,* New York, 1993, 1993. Alfred A Knopf.

Nurnberg M, Rosenblum M: *All about words: an adult approach to vocabulary building,* Englewood Cliffs, NJ, 1966, Prentice-Hall.

Pagana KD, Pagana TJ: *Mosby's diagnostic and laboratory test reference,* ed 3, St Louis, 1997, Mosby.

Perry AG, Potter PA: *Clinical nursing skills and techniques,* ed 4, St Louis, 1997, Mosby.

Seeley RR, Stephens TD, Tate P: *Anatomy and physiology,* ed 2, St Louis, 1992, Mosby.

Selye H: *The stress of life,* New York, 1956, McGraw-Hill.

Stedman's medical dictionary, ed 26, Baltimore, 1995, Williams & Wilkins.

Taber's cyclopedic medical dictionary, ed 18, Philadelphia, 1997, FA Davis.

Thibodeau GA, Patton KT: *Anatomy and physiology,* ed 3, St Louis, 1996, Mosby.

Thompson JM and others: *Mosby's manual of clinical nursing,* ed 4, St Louis, 1997, Mosby.

Tierney LM Jr, McPhee SJ, Papadakis MA: *Current medical diagnosis and treatment,* Norwalk, Conn, 1996, Appleton & Lange.

Tilkian SM, Conover MB, Tilkian AG: *Clinical implications of laboratory tests,* ed 5, St Louis, 1996, Mosby.

Umphred DA, editor: *Neurological rehabilitation,* ed 3, St Louis, 1995, Mosby.

Varmus HE, Weinberg RA: *Genes and the biology of cancer,* Holmes, Penn, 1992, Scientific American Library.

Wilson EO; *The diversity of life,* Cambridge, Mass, 1992, Harvard University Press.

PERIODICALS

The American Scientist
Discover
The Journal of the American Medical Association
The New England Journal of Medicine
The American Journal of Nursing
RN
Science
Scientific American

Index